Praise for *Heal Your Drained Brain*

"A smart, science-based way to heal anxiety and insomnia."

— **Daniel Amen, M.D.**, *New York Times* best-selling
author of *The Brain Warrior's Way*

"Wow, so many easy ways to heal our brains. What I love
about this book is that I can start with just a couple of these
tips and they will still make a big difference."

— **Amy Newmark**, Editor-in-Chief of *Chicken Soup for the Soul*

"Dr. Mike does a terrific job in helping people to understand
ways they can use tools like mindfulness and breath work to
feel better, eat better, sleep better, and live with a sense of peace."

— **Dr. Susan Albers**, *New York Times* best-selling author of *50 Ways
to Soothe Yourself Without Food, Eating Mindfully,* and *Eat Q*

"Mike does an incredible job in helping readers
understand how the foods we eat are linked to
conditions like excess stress, fatigue, and insomnia."

— **Tana Amen, B.S.N., R.N.**, *New York Times* best-selling
author of *The Omni Diet*

"Our brain is the conductor of the symphony of our body.
Unwanted weight gain, insomnia, IBS, and even premature
aging are profoundly influenced by our mental processes.
This book is a powerful guide for anyone who wants to balance,
heal, and optimize their life by using the power of the brain."

— **Anthony Youn, M.D.**, America's Holistic Plastic Surgeon
and best-selling author of *The Age Fix*

"Spiking your blood sugar with processed foods doesn't just affect your waistline. In *Heal Your Drained Brain*, Mike will help you understand how they lead to conditions like fatigue, insomnia, and anxiety."

— **JJ Virgin**, *New York Times* best-selling author of *The Virgin Diet* and *JJ Virgin's Sugar Impact Diet*

"Chronic stress and anxiety affect us in profound and complex ways. *Heal Your Drained Brain* illuminates how these conditions link to digestive woes, high blood pressure, and even cancer. If you feel frazzled and fatigued, you need Mike's solutions ASAP! He reveals the pathway to a balanced brain and body, so that you can reclaim the energetic, joyful life we all crave."

— **Kristi Funk, M.D.**, founder of Pink Lotus Breast Center

Heal Your Drained Brain

ALSO BY DR. MIKE DOW

The Brain Fog Fix: Reclaim Your Focus, Memory, and Joy in Just 3 Weeks*

Diet Rehab: 28 Days to Finally Stop Craving the Foods That Make You Fat

Healing the Broken Brain: Leading Experts Answer 100 Questions about Stroke Recovery,* with David Dow and Megan Sutton, CCC-SLP

*Available from Hay House
Please visit:

Hay House USA: www.hayhouse.com®
Hay House Australia: www.hayhouse.com.au
Hay House UK: www.hayhouse.co.uk
Hay House India: www.hayhouse.co.in

DR. MIKE DOW

Heal Your Drained Brain

**Naturally Relieve Anxiety,
Combat Insomnia, and Balance
Your Brain in Just 14 Days**

HAY HOUSE, INC.
Carlsbad, California • New York City
London • Sydney • Johannesburg
Vancouver • New Delhi

Published and distributed in the United States by: Hay House, Inc.: www.hayhouse.com® • *Published and distributed in Australia by:* Hay House Australia Pty. Ltd.: www.hayhouse.com.au • *Published and distributed in the United Kingdom by:* Hay House UK, Ltd.: www.hayhouse.co.uk • *Distributed in Canada by:* Raincoast Books: www.raincoast.com • *Published in India by:* Hay House Publishers India: www.hayhouse.co.in

Cover design: Jason Gabbert
Interior design: Riann Bender
Indexer: Joan D. Shapiro

Hypnosis on pages 177–179 adapted from S. W. Chiasson, *A syllabus on hypnosis.* American Society of Clinical Hypnosis, Education, and Research Foundation (1973).

Recipes on pages 264–309 used with permission by Liana Werner-Gray and Donna Schwenk.

Images courtesy of Dr. Mike Dow.

Library of Congress Cataloging-in-Publication Data

Names: Dow, Mike, author.
Title: Heal your drained brain : naturally relieve anxiety, combat insomnia, and balance your brain in just 14 days / Dr. Mike Dow.
Description: 1st edition. | Carlsbad, California : Hay House, Inc., 2018. | Includes bibliographical references and index.
Identifiers: LCCN 2017040960 | ISBN 9781401952105 (hardcover : alk. paper)
Subjects: LCSH: Brain--Psychology--Popular works. | Mental health--Popular works. | Self-care, Health--Popular works.
Classification: LCC QP376 .D6935 2018 | DDC 612.8/2--dc23 LC record available at

https://lccn.loc.gov/2017040960

Hardcover ISBN: 978-1-4019-5210-5

10 9 8 7 6 5 4 3 2 1
1st edition, February 2018

Printed in the United States of America

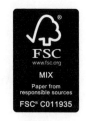
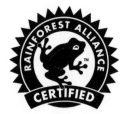

For Chris and our happy family.

Contents

PART III: The Brain Drain Super Fix

PART IV: Your Two-Week Plan

Introduction

It seems like everyone I know these days is way too stressed out. Whether they're patients, friends, or colleagues, I hear the same complaints from all of them: They're tired. They're anxious. They're working too much on not enough sleep. They have too many responsibilities but not enough energy. It's the same thing over and over and over again. Everyone is completely drained.

Adding insult to injury, the drain they're experiencing also manifests as symptoms in their bodies. There's weight gain. Irritable bowel syndrome. Ulcers. You name it. Stress leads to illness and disease.

The worst part is that the true solutions to these problems are both elusive and confusing. Turn to prescription antianxiety or sleeping pills, and there's a risk of dependence or making the problem worse in the long run. Many people are interested in natural remedies, but it's hard to know which ones actually work and which ones are just hype. That's why I've written this book—to separate the wheat from the chaff, so to speak. I created this comprehensive guide to healing drained brains because people need answers. All the depleted and downtrodden people out there are in desperate need of a solution.

The natural and clinically proven strategies in this book have helped me successfully treat even the most extreme and shocking cases of drained brains. I've had so many patients who have come to me as a last resort after going to countless doctors who haven't been able to help them.

Case in point: I recently treated two women with drained brains that included potentially life-threatening symptoms. Both were at the end of their proverbial ropes after no specialist could help. One had so much tension in her mind and body that she was unable to eat solid food. Her body would involuntarily regurgitate anything she ate, so she had been fed exclusively through a feeding tube for years. The other had a paralyzing phobia of needles, which was so intense she hadn't been to a doctor for years and had paid to be put under general anesthesia for simple blood work. I treated both women after they reached out for help to the show I was working on, and their journeys were shown on national television. As these women told me their stories, I realized that they—like so many people these days—were in dire need of hope. When none of the long line of doctors they'd visited provided treatment that worked, it compounded the problems and drained them even more. This led to a downward spiral that I knew could lead to serious illness or even death. My initial goal was to give both women a sense of hope. In my first session with the woman who couldn't eat solid food, I taught her a tool you'll learn in this book: diaphragmatic breathing. It worked so well that at the end of the session, she reported feeling hopeful for the first time in years. With the woman who had a paralyzing phobia of needles, I helped her reprocess the traumatic event that had led to her phobia while using cognitive behavioral therapy—a form of which you'll learn in this book as well. And so began their journeys to recovery. The moral of the story: If the antidotes in this book worked for their extremely drained brains, I know they will work for you.

I also know it's not just the people with extreme symptoms who need help. A few weeks after I worked with these young ladies, I was surprised to learn that all the producers who worked on this segment were also using diaphragmatic breathing. I was thrilled when one of them told me, "Wow! That really works! I can't tell you how much I needed that." Even the successful and "never-let-'em-see-you-sweat" types are secretly yearning for something to help them manage the stresses of everyday life.

The takeaway here is that there are indeed potent and clinically effective ways to heal a drained brain, and they're all here. I've combed through all the latest and greatest research and found the most effective, natural ways to heal stress, anxiety, exhaustion, and insomnia. In addition to learning about how your hormones affect your mood and your overall health, you'll learn practical tools such as energy-based cognitive therapy (EBCT), a protocol I created specifically for people who feel drained, which combines traditional and mind-body solutions. You'll also find a unique, three-level version of the clinically proven nondrug treatment for insomnia: cognitive behavioral therapy for insomnia (CBT-I). These solutions are incredibly multifaceted. You'll also get tools like autogenic training and progressive muscle relaxation to help you dissolve tension in your body. In addition to these techniques, I take you into your diet to show you what foods help you stress less and what foods help you sleep more soundly. I also jump into the hidden world of the gut bacteria that manufacture feel-good neurotransmitters and teach you easy ways to incorporate gut-healthy foods into your diet.

It's likely that doing just one of these things won't stop you from feeling drained, but by putting them all together, you harness the power of combination therapy. You know the old saying "The whole is greater than the sum of its parts." The two-week program in this book combines strategies that address mind, body, and spirit. The end result: less drain, more balance.

When you balance your brain, you experience countless rewards. You have more energy. You feel "normal" or "like yourself" again. You sleep more soundly and wake up looking forward to the day ahead. I know that when brains are balanced, people begin to create the lives they've always dreamed about. They become happier and healthier. They're more successful in their careers and their relationships. I can't wait for you to become the best version of yourself, and I look forward to the life you will create when you are no longer drained.

PART I

THE BIG DRAIN

CHAPTER 1

An Epidemic of Drained Brains

Sally felt like her life had been hijacked by stress, grief, and the unpredictability of our modern world. Five years ago, when she was 52, her youngest child was shot and killed in the line of duty as a police officer. Her mother had recently been diagnosed with dementia and was also recovering from hip surgery. Although Sally and her husband had been saving for their retirement, the recent ups and downs of the economy and general uncertainty of the world made them nervous about their future. Their health insurance premium and medication costs had doubled in the past few years. And since Sally's mother didn't have long-term care insurance, they worried about how they would afford the round-the-clock care they might need for her down the road. Sally worked a full-time job in addition to being her mom's primary caretaker.

After her son passed away, Sally became a chronic worrier. When something horrible and unpredictable happens to someone close to you, you feel as though something terrible could happen at any moment. In fact, you begin to look for anything that *could* go wrong—and headlines seemed to validate her fears and exacerbate her anxiety.

Ripples of anxiety affected Sally psychologically, physically, and spiritually. She felt jumpy and worn out during the day, and at night her sleep suffered. She had insomnia and periodic bouts of nightmares. Her anxiety also changed the way she perceived the world and life itself. She had visited various specialists to help her with an increasingly long list of complaints: insomnia, anxiety, indigestion, upset stomach, and a general lack of energy.

When Sally and I started to work together, she said, "I just wish I could feel peaceful again, and I wish I could shut off my worrying mind."

I wanted to hear more. What did she worry about?

"I worry that my mom isn't going to be okay or that we will run out of the money we need to give her the care she deserves," she said. "I worry that every time I feel sick I have some life-threatening illness. Every week, there's some new symptom I notice. I never used to be a hypochondriac, but I am now. I'm just so run-down all the time."

"Sally, it must feel like you're carrying the weight of the world on your shoulders. I can hear how heavy it is to walk around feeling like bad things are about to happen at any moment."

"It is," she exclaimed with tears in her eyes. "And I'm just tired of feeling this way. I tell myself to think positively, but it doesn't seem to work. I've tried so many meds. Some of them work okay, but they make me even more tired. I've gained thirty pounds in the past two years. I barely have the energy to get through most days—let alone exercise. I'm starting to believe I'll never feel like my old self again. I used to be a pretty happy and carefree person."

I felt tremendous compassion for Sally. She was being robbed of a vibrant, well-lived life by a drained brain. Treating her brain was essential to help her get back her life in the short term and preserve her health in the long term. While the short-term effects of being drained—anxiety, energy depletion, and insomnia—are uncomfortable, the long-term effects can be life threatening. Living in a perpetually drained state increases the risk of dying from a heart attack, stroke, or cancer. Treating a drained brain is as vital for your physical health as it is for a healthy state of mind.

A DRAINED WORLD

Sadly, Sally isn't alone in feeling like her brain has been drained. When you look at the statistics, it's clear that many people are experiencing the type of stress that leaves them feeling drained:

- As of 2017, the American Psychological Association found the first significant increase in the average level of stress in Americans since their nationwide survey was launched in 2007. On a scale from 1 to 10 with 1 being "little or no stress" and 10 being "a great deal of stress," the overall average reported stress is now 5.1.[1]

- Anxiety-related disorders are the most common mental illness in the U.S., affecting 40 million adults (National Institute of Mental Health) with 350 million people affected worldwide. They affect 18.1 percent of the population in a given year—twice as many people as mood disorders like depression. An even higher number experience anxiety but don't meet the criteria for a diagnosable anxiety disorder.[2]

- People with anxiety are *four times* more likely to develop high blood pressure, the leading cause of death worldwide.[3] Postmenopausal women who have panic attacks have *triple* the number of stroke or coronary events like heart attacks.[4] People with heart disease are twice as likely to have a heart attack if they also have anxiety.[5]

- Fifty to seventy million Americans currently suffer from sleep disorders.[6] According to the Centers for Disease Control and Prevention (CDC), 30 percent of Americans report symptoms of insomnia and 50 million Americans report an insufficient amount of sleep. Insomnia is responsible for an estimated $63.2 billion in lost workplace productivity.[7]

- Sales of both over-the-counter and prescription sleep aids are skyrocketing. In just five years, the number of prescriptions written for sleeping pills in the United States increased by over 10 million prescriptions: 47 million in 2006, 60 million in 2011 according to IMS Health. They're causing more problems than ever. From 2005 to 2010, there was a 220 percent increase in emergency room visits due to the sleeping pill Ambien.[8]

- New research shows that prescriptions for antianxiety benzodiazepines like Klonopin, Valium, and Xanax *tripled* between 1996 and 2013 in the U.S., while fatal overdoses from these drugs *quadrupled*.[9] According to the CDC, benzodiazepines account for 30 percent of prescription overdose deaths.[10]

DRAINED CITIZENS OF THE MODERN WORLD

It doesn't take something as tragic as a severe illness or the unexpected death of a loved one for you to experience the stress that results in becoming drained. It can be the loss of a job. Bankruptcy. A chronic illness. The end of a marriage. Child custody battles. Losing your shirt—as many people did—during the housing crisis or the recent ups and downs of the global economy.

Everything has changed, and it doesn't seem to be stopping. There seems to be no certainty about the future. A lack of predictability is evident in modern elections; polls have failed in accurately predicting the future. Mortgages are harder to qualify for. There are now more renters as fewer people own homes than in generations past. Millennials are less interested in owning homes than previous generations, which may buy freedom by sacrificing long-term stability. Rents have shot up in many cities. Commutes have gotten longer, and the average American who is employed full-time works an hour and a half more per week than they did a decade ago.

With so many baby boomers retiring and people living longer, Social Security, which many Americans depend on to cover basic living expenses, is in danger of running out of money. Brexit and a surprising U.S. presidential election outcome sent global markets on unpredictable roller-coaster rides, so even people who put money in a retirement account every year don't know how much they'll have left in their nest egg when they are ready to retire.

Pensions, the hope of Social Security for future generations, and "Cadillac" health insurance plans that cover nearly all your medications and doctor visits are disappearing. The cost of medications used to treat chronic illnesses have risen—by 100, 200, 500 percent, or more. Health-care laws are changing rapidly. We're more likely to live alone than in generations past, and so more people feel like they have to handle everything by themselves. There are more single parents trying to make ends meet. New businesses and tech start-ups go bust more often than they succeed, and the globalized economy also means a cutthroat world with razor-thin profit margins. Communities, countries, and political parties have become more polarized than at any time in recent history, and the disagreements have even led to anger and volatility.

It seems when one part of the world recovers economically, another region fails. The American stock market feels the ripples from Greece. A terrorist attack in Paris affects the Asian economies. When the UK votes to exit the EU, European markets nosedive—but so do the American and Asian markets.

While "big," clear-cut traumas and fears can certainly drain brains, more often in our modern world, the problem is also instigated by the subtle ways our world has changed. Invisible changes in our food supply; streaming video services that have made sitting on the couch the new international sport; rapid-fire dating apps, which some people use as a short-term substitute for lasting connections that help us deal with stress; and the way we interact with media all contribute to the global epidemic of drained brains. The blinking lights on our cell phones create a nonstop, false sense of emergency; and stress hormones spike as we check our e-mails, texts, and social media accounts before we even get out of bed.

The processed foods more and more people around the world are eating don't just contribute to weight gain, diabetes, and dementia; they can shrink the brain's hippocampus, a part of the brain that helps us remain resilient in the face of stress.

Our busy lives rarely include time for the activities that have been shown to help protect the brain, like exercise, meditation, or sautéing a healthy meal. Of course, stress and lack of sleep also create neurochemical states that make us more likely to overeat and zone out with social media and TV, which create downward spirals. Stress hormones run too high, and feel-good ones run low. Sleep problems result since stress can extinguish sleep-wake rhythms. And of course the more sleep deprived you become, the more stress, anxiety, and energy problems affect you the following day. Is it any wonder more and more people around the world turn to solutions like Xanax and Ambien regularly?

It seems everything we experience in our day-to-day lives—from our smartphones that wake us to the foods we eat all day long to the jobs we spend years of our life on—is set up to drain us.

BRAIN DRAIN PAIN

So what exactly does it feel like to be drained?

If you have a drained brain, you feel anxious, frazzled, and fatigued. You may say you're at the end of your rope. The proverbial gas tank of your brain that is usually filled with resilience, faith, patience, and perseverance is now running on empty. While your brain has a pretty amazing capacity to deal with challenges, it *can* become overloaded. When that happens, the world becomes overwhelming, both on the large and small scale. In the bigger picture, world events seem impossible to deal with, and in your personal life, every obligation or relationship or organized outing feels overpowering. Your body holds tension, and your brain generates worry. Sleep, concentration, and motivation become problematic. Psychological worry leads to physical consequences. Chronic conditions— everything from heart disease to cancer to digestive issues—are exacerbated, and new diseases are more likely to develop. This problematic response makes everyday tasks difficult, and you "just wish [you] had a break"—though it takes a bit more than a simple break to recover.

There is another condition that has similar symptoms: brain fog—and I think it's important to differentiate between these two so you make sure to treat the condition you actually have.

Both brain drain and brain fog cause problems with mood, energy, attention, and sleep. And both can lead to self-medication in the form of drinking or overeating.

While brain-drained individuals often experience anxiety, people with brain fog often become depressed. They have a muddy depression that leaves the world looking gray, as opposed to the bright-orange-hued world of someone with a drained brain.

Brain fog is also more closely associated with the accumulation of plaques in the brain that can cause "senior moments" or dementia.

While energy problems are common in both conditions, the fatigue that comes with brain fog is the result of a brain that's slowing down or becoming clouded with inactivity. For people with a drained brain, the lack of energy is caused by too much activity in the brain, which leads to an overactive sympathetic nervous system and the exhaustion phase of the stress response.

Even though brain drain and brain fog are different conditions, they do often go hand in hand. Brain fog can lead to brain drain, and vice versa. When you start to notice memory problems and brain fog, you may start to feel anxious and worry about your future. Now you're feeling drained in addition to experiencing fog. Or you're chronically drained, which means high levels of a stress hormone that reduces blood flow to the brain, which can eventually lead to brain fog in its worst form: Alzheimer's disease. Untreated brain drain results in brain fog.

As I noted before, even with the overlap, it's important to know which condition you're facing as you move forward. Each is caused by a unique imbalance in your symphony of hormones—and to tune up the orchestra, you need to know which ones to balance. If you're yearning for a sense of relief, peace, and a good night's sleep so you can take back what the stress of modern living has taken from you, then brain drain may be your problem.

Now let's delve a bit more deeply into the hormone changes that occur when you have a drained brain.

CHAPTER 2

A Symphony of Draining Chemicals

The week I began writing this book was the week of the horrific terror attacks in Paris at the Bataclan concert hall and other locations. That week, I was with two good friends who are both television producers in New York City.

If there's one thing to understand about television producers, it's that they're used to dealing with stress 24 hours a day. Their job is to put out fires—all the time. Because of this, producers tend to be the kind of people who are unfazed by crises and stress. In fact, they often move toward—not away from them.

As I was talking to one of them, I was completely taken aback when she stopped me in the middle of our conversation about a TV segment she was producing and said, "I just can't take it. I mean what is going on in our world?! Paris?! I think I may need to get a prescription for Xanax or something. I'm just so anxious all the time now, and you know me: I'm used to stress. It's my job, so why am I freaking out?"

That same week my other friend told me about a trip she and her fiancé had planned. Months earlier, they had booked their first trip to Paris. It was going to be her first time going to Europe. But after the attack, their plans were ruined. She didn't feel safe visiting this beautiful city, so they cancelled their trip of a lifetime—losing thousands of dollars and the chance to experience romantic moments they'd never forget in the process.

WHAT'S DRAINING YOUR BRAIN?

Many psychological phenomena in our brains evolved to keep us safe—but now they often backfire as they intersect with the unpredictability of our modern world, draining our brains and leaving us feeling anxious, frazzled, and fatigued. My friends had fallen prey to the first of these: *observational learning*. What does this mean? It means that people who simply see trauma and the pain of other people begin to feel the emotions of those actually experiencing it. And this has been borne out in research. Studies have shown that when people watch others who are displaying cues of pain and negative emotion, they begin to display their own negative response.[1] In fact, PTSD-like stress responses were present in people around the country who were nowhere near the Twin Towers on 9/11. While they were simply watching images, they experienced a stress response similar to the people who directly experienced the events of that day.[2] Research also shows more anxiety in people watching terrorism-related news compared with those watching other types of news.[3] Life can be a careful balancing act of staying informed about what happens in the world, which is generally a strength, and protecting our brains from too much negative information.

Just like the subjects in these studies, both of my smart, capable producer friends had high levels of anxiety because of something that happened thousands of miles away. Unlike a survivor of physical or sexual abuse, who experienced trauma firsthand, these women—like more and more people in the world these days—have higher levels of stress hormones as a result of observational learning.[4]

This phenomenon of observational learning paired with our modern world, which includes the 24/7 news cycle, news apps, and news channels that air footage of plane crashes, car chases, and shootings, fuels this type of learned anxiety. While observational learning helps people stay safe—they don't have to directly experience a traumatic event to know to avoid it—this phenomenon may now be doing some people more harm than good.

The next phenomenon draining our brains is called *negative bias*. Negative bias is the tendency for the brain to process and recall negative events more strongly than positive ones. If you touch a table and a hot stove for the first time, it's in your best interest for your brain to give priority to the memory of the hot stove over the table. Your brain is helping to keep you safe by remembering the negative event that resulted in a burned hand. By making the memory of this negative event stronger, you will likely avoid getting burned in the future. One prominent psychologist says the brain is like Velcro when it comes to negative experiences but like Teflon for positive ones.

You can see the power of negative bias even where people focus their attention. In various studies, researchers found subjects spend more time looking at negative photographs than they do looking at positive ones. They also blink more when studying negative words than positive words, which is an indicator of a stronger reaction to information that can lead to fear.[5] This helps explain the "if it bleeds, it leads" philosophy in news; your paying attention means you stay glued to that channel. And, of course, that means better ratings for that newscast.

Research also shows that people reason and think more about negative events than positive ones.[6] The peaceful confidence you once had is taken away as one defeat overshadows your plentiful successes. As your brain examines and stores these negative images, experiences, and words, it also drains itself by depleting your feel-good neurotransmitters and increasing stress hormones. And worse, as you dwell on these negative events throughout your day, your brain continues to drain.

The next phenomenon that drains brains is called *overgeneralization*, which was the subject of a famous study in the 1920s. In this experiment, a toddler was exposed to a white rat while the researchers made loud and scary noises every time the toddler touched the rat. The toddler then began to fear not just white rats but anything furry.[7] This infant's brain was overgeneralizing: expanding the coding of fear to include similar sensory experiences—no matter how strong or weak they were. A peripheral sighting of a small, white animal darting away would inspire fear just as much as an interaction with an actual white rat.

The same may be true for you. If you got rear-ended and remember the loud sound of screeching tires right before impact, *any* slight sound of screeching tires—or even any similar sound—can activate the "fight, flight, or freeze" response in your brain. If your brain reacts in this way, molehills become mountains.

How does this drain the brain? Overgeneralizing leads to more common activation of the stress chemicals that keep you fried and frazzled.

The final two psychological phenomena of the brain drain puzzle are *unpredictable danger* paired with *context conditioning*. In our modern world, we are less likely to be able to predict danger, and this wreaks havoc on our brains. Just a few decades ago, war zones were commonly encountered only by soldiers. Now every civilian is in danger of stepping into one. Horrific mass killings take place at bars, movie theaters, holiday parties, churches, and schools. Unlike people during the last world war who knew to head to the air-raid shelter after an alarm, many of our most horrific stressors have shifted from predictable to unpredictable danger.

Why is this unpredictable danger associated with higher rates of drain? In both animal and human studies, unpredictable shocks are worse than predictable ones. In classic Pavlovian conditioning, a neutral stimulus like a bell is paired with an unconditioned stimulus like food. The brain's unconditioned response, salivation, will then result after either stimulus. The same is true for negative events: pair a tone with a shock, and you fear the tone as well as the shock. With unpredictable shocks, there tends to be more context conditioning, which means that your brain doesn't merely pair the tone with the shock;

it pairs anything present in the environment at the time of the shock. What did the room look like when the shock occurred? What was the general feel or energy in the room like? These sense memories are stored, which can result in you fearing anything that was present when you had a negative experience—and this can operate at a conscious or unconscious level. This can turn you into an anxious person who is always on high alert, and you may go out of your way to avoid potentially fear-inducing situations.

When you do so, you are less likely to be able to take advantage of the healing side of conditioning: extinction. Extinction is essentially the brain taking an eraser to the fear it had previously sketched. The brain draws fear in pencil—not permanent marker. If you continue to hear tones you used to associate with a shock and don't receive one, extinction eventually occurs. This process happens more gradually than the initial stimulus-response pairing process. This is why I treat patients with phobias using gradual exposure therapy; it takes longer for the brain to unlearn fear than it did to learn it. Using the power of extinction is one of many ways you will begin to heal your drained brain.

When used in the right amounts at the right times, all of these phenomena can keep your brain in balance. When used too often or at the wrong times, they can do more harm than good. If you notice that you're feeling more and more drained, that's a signal that it's time to start rebalancing and replenishing your brain.

BRAIN DRAIN & YOUR NERVOUS SYSTEM

Feeling drained is the result of an autonomic nervous system that is unbalanced. The autonomic nervous system takes care of "automatics" like digestion, blood pressure, and healing. You don't have to consciously tell your body to digest your food after you eat or to release adrenaline to help you swerve out of the way of the car that slammed on its brakes. It takes care of these functions without conscious effort.

The autonomic nervous system has two parts that are like the two sides of a seesaw: the sympathetic and parasympathetic nervous system. The sympathetic nervous system triggers your fight, flight, or freeze response, which releases the stress hormones adrenaline, norepinephrine, and cortisol into the bloodstream.

The other side of that seesaw is the parasympathetic nervous system, which restores you with a calm state of rest and digest. It is what's responsible for bringing your three stress hormones into normal range after they've spiked due to stress.

In balanced brains, all three stress hormones go up together in times of stress and, thanks to the parasympathetic nervous system, gently come down like a wave falling because of hormones like acetylcholine and gamma-aminobutyric acid (GABA). When cortisol levels go down, other brain balancers work well. For example, the anxiety reliever serotonin is able to work more effectively in the brain. Without stress hormones disrupting digestion, more brain-balancing neurotransmitters are made in your gut. This parasympathetic shift boosts your immune system, keeps digestion regular, and promotes healthy blood pressure. It's the feel-good, "rest and digest" phase that's the hallmark of the parasympathetic nervous system. Your mood improves, and energy is steady and boundless. You know you will easily recover from stress, so you feel resilient and confident. You wake up each day ready to face what lies ahead of you with excitement instead of dread.

However, in drained brains, the sympathetic nervous system is dominant. This leads to perennially high levels of stress hormones and perennially low levels of feel-good ones.

The stress hormones of a dominant sympathetic nervous system and feeling drained don't just leave you feeling worried and anxious; they rob you of energy. In fact, the end result of untreated brain drain is called the exhaustion stage. Hans Selye, who originated this meaning of the word *stress* in 1936, described the three stages of bodily response in what's called "generalized adaptation syndrome."

The first stage is alarm. During the alarm stage, the sympathetic nervous system takes over to mobilize the body and protect you from threat. This is the fight, flight, or freeze stage. If you've ever experienced the sensations of butterflies in your stomach, that's the physical sensation of blood flow being diverted away from your stomach and redirected to the organ systems and extremities that would assist you in running from a predator. In this stage, adrenaline primarily heightens the response of the body; norepinephrine primarily heightens focus in the mind.

The second stage is resistance. In the resistance stage, the sympathetic nervous system remains dominant so you can remain focused and alert to defend against perceived or actual threat. After the initial spike of adrenaline and norepinephrine, cortisol spikes take over to keep the accelerator pedal pressed.

With a balanced brain, these spikes of stress hormones would be followed by the engaging of the parasympathetic nervous system, but when the seesaw remains tilted toward the sympathetic nervous system, the third and problematic stage of generalized adaptation syndrome is entered: exhaustion. In this stage, your resources are gone, you feel frazzled and fatigued, and you become vulnerable to disease.

Cortisol stays high, or in some cases, it plunges and stays low. Either of these states wreak havoc on the body. Like high levels of cortisol, low levels are also problematic since cortisol can act as an "off" switch for other stress hormones. Cortisol also helps your body cope with prolonged stress by enabling it to maintain steady supplies of blood sugar, which would help supply a steady source of energy for a long-term stressor.

People with low levels of cortisol experience extreme fatigue, sleeping problems, weakness, memory difficulties, impaired concentration, and electrolyte imbalances.

When cortisol levels are too high, blood-sugar levels rise, which can lead to diabetes. Inflammation, which can lead to disease, becomes more prevalent. Permanently high cortisol can also prevent serotonin, a brain-balancing, anxiety-relieving hormone, from binding to certain areas in the brain. It also restricts blood flow. As a result, anxiety, insomnia, and other symptoms become more pronounced. This leads to negative thought patterns that can trick your brain into thinking it's in danger all the time as it stews, worries, and looks for evidence that you're not safe or going to be okay. When the brain thinks there's danger, it produces more cortisol . . . and the draining downward spiral continues.

The goal is to restore balance.

AUTONOMIC NERVOUS SYTEM	
SYMPATHETIC NERVOUS SYSTEM	PARASYMPATHETIC NERVOUS SYSTEM
Fight, flight, or freeze	Rest and digest
Blood flow to organs needed for quick getaway	Blood flow back to normal and digestion
↑ Stress hormones	↓ Stress hormones
↑ Heart rate, respiration	↓ Heart rate, respiration
↑ Anxiety, dread, panic	↓ Anxiety, dread, panic
↑ Alertness, activation	↑ Sleep, ease
↑ Adrenaline, norepinephrine, cortisol	↓ Adrenaline, norepinephrine, cortisol
↓ Acetylcholine, GABA, serotonin, melatonin	↑ Acetylcholine, GABA, serotonin, melatonin
↑ Physical disease	↑ Healing
↑ Inflammation	↓ Inflammation
WHEN DOMINANT → DRAINED	WHEN DOMINANT → BALANCED

BRAIN CHEMICALS

Now that you understand how your nervous system is the culprit in draining your brain, let's look more closely at the chemical messengers associated with these two branches of your autonomic nervous system and how they can become unbalanced in a drained brain. First we'll look at the three stress chemicals that drain the brain, and then we'll move on to six healthy brain balancers.

Brain Drainers

Adrenaline, norepinephrine, and cortisol are the hormones associated with the sympathetic nervous system and its fight, flight, or freeze response. These hormones rev you into high gear, which can help save your life if you're in true danger, but they drain your brain and body when they stay high for too long. The levels should ideally look like the rise and fall of a wave. Your sympathetic nervous system takes these hormones up, and then the parasympathetic nervous system brings them back down.

- **Adrenaline** is responsible for the immediate, primarily *physical* reactions of the sympathetic nervous system. Your heart races, blood is diverted away from digestive function and toward the muscles, you breathe more rapidly, the small airways in the lungs open wide to take in more oxygen, and the body's reserves of blood sugar and fats are released into the bloodstream to supply energy. Too much adrenaline can damage blood vessels and lead to heart attacks and strokes. Adrenaline is secreted by the adrenal medulla, located in the center of your adrenal glands. The adrenal medulla actually secretes the majority of your stress hormones. When activated by the sympathetic nervous system, the adrenal medulla produces a release of stress hormones made up of 80 percent adrenaline.

- **Norepinephrine** is responsible for the immediate, primarily *mental* reactions of the sympathetic nervous system. Your mind becomes sharp, focused, and vigilant. Like adrenaline, it also increases blood pressure and diverts blood flow away from digestion and into muscles. Norepinephrine accounts for the other 20 percent of the hormonal release from the adrenal medulla.

- **Cortisol** is responsible for your long-term stress response after the initial surge adrenaline and norepinephrine subside. It keeps the sympathetic nervous system engaged by the hypothalamic-pituitary-adrenal (HPA) axis, which includes the hypothalamus, pituitary gland, and adrenal glands.

Cortisol is secreted by the cortex which is the outside layer of your adrenal glands. There is also a healthy and mild cortisol rise—called the cortisol awakening response—that should occur every morning to help you wake up and get you going even if a stressor isn't present. The cortisol awakening response can spike too high when you're experiencing excess stress. If it doesn't rise enough, you can experience fatigue.

Brain Balancers

Acetylcholine, GABA, serotonin, melatonin, oxytocin, and endorphins are hormones and neurotransmitters associated with feelings of well-being, restful sleep, steady energy, and connection. In different ways, they all can help balance a drained brain. For example, acetylcholine brings heart rate back down after the brain drainers speed it up. Melatonin, in its inverse relationship with the brain drainer cortisol, helps you get restful sleep. Restful sleep can then help you keep stress hormones in check the following day. Healthy levels of GABA and serotonin make you less prone to worry and reactivity, which can prevent brain drainers from spiking too high in the first place. Although some aren't directly associated with the parasympathetic nervous system, there tends to be an inverse relationship with these feel-good chemicals and brain drainers. When these chemicals are in steady supply, the parasympathetic nervous system tends to be peaceful, and the rest-and-digest state is dominant. Remember, this state is linked to general health and happiness.

- **Acetylcholine** is the chief neurotransmitter of the parasympathetic nervous system, helping to counteract the brain drainers. Adrenaline made your heart beat faster. Now acetylcholine helps slow it down. By learning to activate your parasympathetic nervous system, you can naturally boost acetylcholine.

- **GABA** is the primary inhibitory neurotransmitter in the cortex that counteracts glutamate, which is an abundant excitatory amino acid found in your nervous system. Thus, this is another brain balancer that can turn down the volume when it has been turned up. GABA helps you feel relaxed and peaceful. When GABA levels are healthy, you can easily recover from stress. Low levels of GABA are also associated with the activated manic states in bipolar disorder and difficulty controlling impulses. Without this neurotransmitter, there is too much "excitability" or activation in the brain. Drained individuals often turn to benzodiazepines like Xanax, Klonopin, and Ativan to address their lack of GABA.

- **Serotonin** is one of your primary feel-good hormones. It counteracts anxiety and is associated with feelings of calmness, serenity, optimism, and self-confidence. While serotonin is manufactured primarily in your gut, sufficient levels of this hormone moving freely in the brain help you feel happy and calm. It binds more effectively in the brain when cortisol levels are low. Brain-drained individuals commonly are prescribed selective serotonin reuptake inhibitors (SSRIs) like Prozac, Paxil, Lexapro, and Zoloft to address a deficiency of this hormone in the brain. By blocking the amount of serotonin that can be reabsorbed by one neuron, more of it stays in the space between neurons. Then more of the feel-good hormone travels to the next brain cell, leaving you feeling happy and calm.

- **Melatonin** helps you to maintain healthy sleep-wake rhythms and sleep well. It helps you to get a good night's sleep and is also a potent antioxidant. In balanced brains, melatonin goes high at night when cortisol goes low— and vice versa in the morning.

- **Oxytocin** is the connection and cuddling hormone that helps you to bond to those you love. It allows you to form long-term relationships that can buffer you from stress.

- **Endorphins** are pain- and anxiety-relieving chemicals. The word *endorphin* is short for "endogenous morphine" but luckily endorphins don't cause addiction or dependence like morphine does. When you feel peaceful, relaxed, and pain-free euphoria, your body may be pumping endorphins.

In general, brain-drained individuals will have high levels of one or more of the brain drainers and low levels of one or more of the brain balancers. These combinations can make you prone to unique brain-draining symptoms and also make you more prone to specific mental illnesses. People low in acetylcholine may feel constant dread. Those with low GABA are prone to alcoholism and bipolar disorder. Low serotonin may lead people to feel anxious or perfectionistic and be prone to anorexia. Brain-drained individuals with low melatonin will have sleep disorders. If you have low oxytocin, you may feel lonely or more prone to develop PTSD. And with low endorphins, you may be prone to pain, bulimia, or even self-mutilation. These levels may also predict what you use to self-medicate: People with low GABA may try to use alcohol to feel at ease. Those with low serotonin may use sugar or processed carbohydrates since they release this hormone in the brain. Of course, it's usually more complex than this since hormones operate in a symphony that's unique for each person.

THE CHEMICAL FOOTPRINTS OF DRAINED BRAINS

All right! Let's look at some of the variations on levels of those brain drainers that result in you feeling fatigued, frazzled, and fried. Remember: in a balanced brain, adrenaline and norepinephrine spike as the primary wave as the result of encountering a stressor. Then, cortisol spikes as the secondary wave. Both waves spike gradually and then fall gradually. Here's what it looks like:

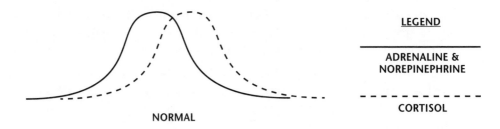

NORMAL

LEGEND

ADRENALINE &
NOREPINEPHRINE

CORTISOL

However, in drained brains, this doesn't happen. There are four distinct subtypes, which I refer to as the Light Drain, the Skyrocket Drain, the Drop Drain, and the X-treme Drain. You can see graphs of them below.

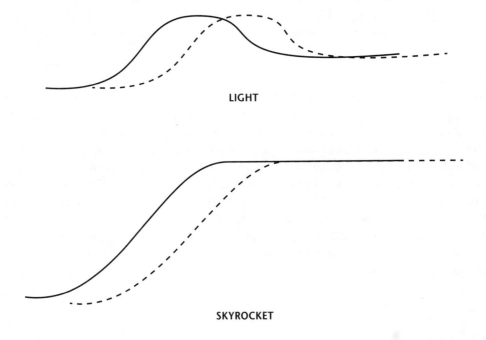

LIGHT

SKYROCKET

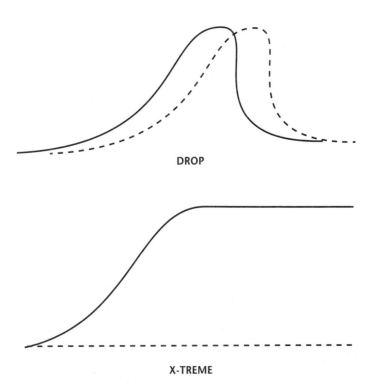

DROP

X-TREME

In the first two subtypes, adrenaline, norepinephrine, and cortisol go high and stay high. The difference between Light Drain and Skyrocket Drain is how fast and how high the chemical levels go. In Light Drain, which accounts for the majority of drained brains, all three hormones rise quickly and stay relatively high. This is the "garden variety" drained brain. In cases of Skyrocket Drain, all three stress hormones surge very high, very quickly and then stay there. With a brain that is Skyrocket Drained, panic attacks and extreme anxiety are often present.

In Drop Drain, the stress hormones have a blunted response: they begin to rise but then suddenly drop like a wave hitting a cliff. You feel stressed out initially but then lack the energy to get through the stressor.

In X-treme Drain, which is the worst case of brain drain, adrenaline and norepinephrine spike while cortisol remains low, leading to a state where you feel on edge but lack the energy that sufficient levels of cortisol provide. X-treme Drain is often the result of untreated milder forms of brain drain. It usually happens over time but can also happen quickly after one extreme trauma in the case of PTSD.

All these subtypes of drained brains are sympathetic nervous system dominant. This leads to perennially high levels of stress hormones and perennially low levels of feel-good ones.

The good news is that balancing the brain—no matter what combination of chemicals you have—tends to be fairly one-size-fits-all, because most brains balance themselves out when given the right tools. That's what this book is all about—giving you those tools. Be aware, however, that there are three low-cortisol conditions that this program does not address: a rare condition called Addison's disease, primary adrenal insufficiency caused by damage to the adrenal glands, and secondary adrenal insufficiency caused by changes in the pituitary gland or the discontinuation of corticosteroids. Adrenal insufficiency can cause chronic fatigue, weakness, and weight loss and can mimic some of the symptoms present in a high-cortisol, brain-drained state. These conditions can be serious. They should be screened for and treated. If you have risk factors for these conditions, like a family history of them or recent discontinuation of corticosteroids, report any symptoms to your primary care physician or treating specialist.

SHOULD I TEST MY CORTISOL LEVELS?

Most drained brain conditions like anxiety are diagnosed by self-reported symptoms, and part of the reason for this is that hormones and neurotransmitters (including the brain drainers and brain balancers you've learned about) are difficult and/or expensive to measure. However, cortisol levels can be easily measured by a fairly inexpensive saliva test that costs around $100.

A **diurnal cortisol test** takes saliva samples at four different points during the day: upon waking, before lunch, before dinner, and before bed. This accounts for the cortisol awakening response (cortisol should be higher in the morning and lower in the evening) and the 24-hour fluctuations of this stress hormone. Men and nonmenstruating women can use this test any day of the month. Menstruating women should use this test during days 19 to 21 of the menstrual cycle to get an accurate read. Your test results can help you determine which of the above chemical footprints of drained brain are affecting you. If your levels are too high, you may be experiencing one of the first three footprints of a drained brain. If they are too low but you are experiencing symptoms of a drained brain, this is an indication that cortisol has actually gone too low while adrenaline and/or norepinephrine are likely too high. Regardless of whether you have a drained-brain footprint that has cortisol that is mildly high, very high, blunted, or low (e.g., Light Drain, the Skyrocket Drain, the Drop Drain, or the X-treme Drain) this program can help you balance your levels (except for the Addison's disease, primary adrenal insufficiency, or secondary adrenal insufficiency).

The saliva-based diurnal cortisol test is available from ZRT Laboratory. Some states will allow you to buy a diurnal cortisol test from ZRT Laboratory directly, and this test is available online from Amazon and other vendors. Other states may not permit you to buy it directly but may allow you to buy it after you sign up for a free membership of CanaryClub.org.

Once you complete the Drained Brain program in Part IV, you may wish to do the diurnal cortisol test again to see how the levels have changed. (Menstruating women will need to wait until the next optimal testing window of their menstrual cycle.) That being said, most people will *feel* their brains balancing—and can simply retake the Drained Brain Quiz (which you'll take in a later chapter) to reassess their progress after completing the program.

POSITIVE STRESS

With all this talk of stress chemicals, I do want to point out that it isn't stress itself that's bad—it's an unbalanced brain that can't deal with stress. Even the brain drainers, while generally "bad," are sometimes "good" since they have a paradoxical effect when spikes are short-lived. Hans Selye didn't mean for the word *stress* to be negative. His definition is "the nonspecific response of the body to any demand or change." In fact, he later differentiated between eustress, or positive stress, and distress, or negative stress.

Positive stress can be helpful in our lives. For example, the stress of a reasonable deadline can sometimes be the best motivation to finish something. It spurs a short-lived adrenaline rush that can help us finish a task more quickly.

Paradoxically there are even times when intense stress can help balance the brain. There seems to be a depth and even spiritual appreciation in people who have recovered from trauma. You've probably heard at least one story of a near death experience that changed a person's whole perspective. In the '90s, the term *posttraumatic growth* was coined.[8] While there are, of course, negative aspects to experiencing trauma, there is also an upside. In fact, up to 90 percent of survivors report a positive aspect of posttraumatic growth; they pursue more fulfilling goals or have a renewed appreciation for life.[9] Life's stresses can make us more resilient when processed in a healthy way. One study showed older adults who got through significant stressful events like divorce were actually better able to deal with smaller, everyday stressors.[10]

We all have a point where eustress becomes distress. The way to best handle the stresses of life is to raise this point by balancing our brains.

CHAPTER 3

The Mind-Body Connection

Maria had a long medical history with some very complicated and difficult-to-treat illnesses, but the most troubling part of Maria's story was how anxious, sad, and scared she felt all the time. I'll never forget the first few minutes we spent together, because I immediately had a sense of how each day felt like a struggle for her. While I felt a tremendous amount of compassion, I also a felt a sense of inadequacy as I immediately knew she was looking to me as her "next great hope" in a long line of doctors she had turned to for relief.

Maria struggled with a variety of physical and psychological ailments, including irritable bowel syndrome, fibromyalgia, insomnia, and generalized anxiety disorder. She described herself as a hypochondriac and reported a list of other possible illnesses including chronic fatigue syndrome and possible parasitic infections. She'd tried both mainstream and alternative treatments, and nothing seemed to work. She felt hopeless and scared, and she was financially depleted from her health-care bills. Each new specialist she saw was supposed to be "the one," and with every new diet, regimen, or medication came a sense of disappointment when it didn't live up to her high expectations.

After hearing this history, one of the first things I did with Maria was to talk about the fact that I was not likely to be the answer to all her prayers. It was extremely unlikely her problems were purely psychological or purely physical. Psychological well-being affects physical health, and vice versa, in a very real and measurable way. For Maria, this had become a downward spiral. Worrying that originates in the mind can physically raise cortisol levels in the body, which leads to inflammation and lower levels of anxiety-relieving serotonin and GABA. This can negatively affect digestion and energy, and is associated with a variety of physical ailments. The more physical symptoms she felt, the more she worried. The more she worried, the more physical dysfunction was exacerbated. This cycle went on and on.

In more complex cases of brain drain like Maria's, a fix will usually be a combination of treatments that need to be put together in just the right amounts at the right time. It's like cooking a delicate soufflé. If you don't separate the eggs correctly or if you bake it for too long, you will ruin this delicately constructed work of art that seems to be effortlessly suspended in air when prepared just right.

Instead of cooking a complex dish with a variety of ingredients, Maria was trying to cook a soufflé with just one ingredient each time. One month, her problem was gluten, and she hoped a gluten-free diet would cure everything. The next, it was a brand-new prescription medication or supplement she would try. Then it was on to Chinese medicine and herbal remedies. The fact is most of Maria's treatments had some merit. But when used alone, none would be the silver-bullet cure she was hoping for.

As a psychotherapist, I began by asking Maria what she had learned about herself from her treatment thus far.

"Well, I learned that my body is just really messed up. I'm scared that nothing is going to work. I'm never going to feel normal."

She was in tears immediately.

"And lately, I'm scared that I have some rare, terrible illness, which only makes everything worse. I can feel my belly acting up right now because I'm getting upset. Of course, now I'm horrified and embarrassed because I'm afraid I'm going to have to run to the bathroom at any second—this is what happens. I already scoped it out before I came in here. It's so isolating. I don't want to attend social situations, and I certainly don't want to go on dates like this."

"I can see how hard this has been for you," I said, "and I appreciate the trust you've already placed in me by talking about your condition. When you just acknowledged your condition and fears right here and now with me, did it make your anxiety go up or down, or is it unchanged?"

"Well, I'm a little relieved that if I do run out of here, you'll know why," Maria said as her tears began to get softer, "and that helps a little bit I guess."

"And I'm sure that has actually decreased the likelihood that you'll have to run out since stress makes your stomach problems worse. And tell me about my response to you. Do I look horrified, judgmental, or grossed out right now?"

"Well . . . no," she said as she cracked a smile, "but you're a professional."

"I guess that's true," I replied, "but I'm also a human being who you just met. You had the courage to immediately share something with me that's embarrassing for you. I'm guessing you usually keep this a secret, so you're already doing something differently.

Do you think that maybe a piece of your anxiety comes from you overestimating people's responses? I wonder if that makes the anxiety and stomach pains worse."

"Yes," Maria said with tears in her eyes. "Probably. It does feels good to be able to talk about this with you and to feel like you understand me and that my condition makes sense to you. I feel like a crazy person most of the time, which is a big part of the problem."

I asked Maria if I could use hypnosis to help her retrieve old memories that could shed some light on her experience, because I had a feeling this was rooted in childhood trauma. We were going to look for times in her life where she had a similar feeling of "feeling crazy."

"Close your eyes for a second, and pay attention to that feeling in your body. I want you to just float back and look for the times in your life where you felt that same feeling."

Maria began to sob. "My mom!"

"What did your mom say to you?" I asked.

In our work together, Maria recovered the physical sensations of sickness that accompanied the first time she told her mother that she was being sexually abused by her neighbor. Her mother didn't believe her, and she kept the secret for months. Maria was aware of the abuse, but she had forgotten that feeling of being ill.

"Keeping that secret made me feel crazy. I kept that a secret for months until I finally told the school psychologist, and they arrested the guy," she said.

"When you talk about that, where do you feel that in your body?" I asked.

"My stomach," she replied.

"Tell me about it. If you were to give it a color, what color would that feeling be? Describe the texture to me."

"Well . . . I guess it feels heavy. Like dread," she replied, "Black. Churning. Like sludge I just can't escape. Oh my gosh. I can actually feel something moving in my belly as I'm talking about this."

Just like that. That was the how my treatment with Maria started. While this first interaction wasn't a cure, it was certainly a significant step in the right direction.

At the end of our session, I urged her to continue working with her primary care physician, gastroenterologist, acupuncturist, and other specialists, as each health-care professional has invaluable and appropriate expertise. I didn't want her to fall into her normal "all or nothing" approach to health care. While it is understandable to believe that something isn't working if it doesn't make you feel 100 percent better, it was important to understand that what she'd been doing was important. In fact, sometimes not responding to a treatment is helpful since it can help rule out a suspected cause, or it could help Maria and her providers figure out what wasn't working. Perhaps she would benefit from the wonders of combination therapy by putting effective treatments together. She might not feel a 100 percent improvement with one change, but when she started to put something that helped her 10 percent with five other strategies that also helped 10 percent, she'd get a 60 percent improvement. That's significant enough to improve one's quality of life.

Maria stuck with her other providers, and I became part of a team of health-care professionals she worked with. I continued to treat her on a regular basis for months, and we reprocessed the trauma that affected her brain and body in very real ways.

Together, we sorted out what part of her problems were related to untreated trauma, stress, and a drained brain. The beauty was that as our treatment progressed, she became the expert of her own experience and gained a sense of control over her health.

STRESS AND THE BODY

Maria's experiences are important because they show just how powerful our thoughts are in creating a drained brain—and how important healing a drained brain is in the long term. We need to learn to manage our thoughts to manage our stress to manage our health to manage our stress. It's all one big loop. The mind affects the body and the body affects the mind.

Just about every physical disease is affected by our brains and stress levels. Heart disease. High blood pressure. Cancer. Stroke. Obesity. Diabetes. Irritable bowel syndrome. Chronic fatigue syndrome. Crohn's disease. Ulcerative colitis. Fibromyalgia. Multiple sclerosis. Headaches. Migraines. Asthma. Chronic obstructive pulmonary disease. Herpes. HIV. HPV. The common cold. The flu. Shingles. Aging. Premature death. The list goes on and on.

No matter what specialists you have seen in your life for various conditions, they probably tell you that "managing stress" will help you with any ailment you may be facing. Stress can directly cause physical disease, contribute to it when mixed with other factors, or exacerbate symptoms and contribute to flares in existing ones. Unfortunately, the paradox is that "managing stress" is incredibly elusive when you're dealing with illness and the inherent fatigue, worry, pain, and malaise that come with it.

Physical disease and brain drain affect each other in multiple systems throughout your body. Pain creates negative thought patterns that can spike cortisol levels that then affect digestion and other bodily processes. Worry that begins in the brain activates the sympathetic nervous system, which affects the body as your muscles tense and your heart pumps more quickly. Stress can lead to the release of cholesterol and triglycerides into the bloodstream, which affects the heart and other parts of the body. Your immune system suffers as severe stress can reduce your natural killer (NK) cell activity that protects you against viruses and cancer cells by 50 percent.[1] Anticipation and stress can increase the numbers of bad bacteria like *E. coli* while decreasing good bacteria like *Bifidobacterium* and *Lactobacillus*, which can lead to digestion and mood problems.[2] The mind-body connection is indeed powerful. In fact, I think the term *mindbody*—spelled with no hyphen and referred to as a single entity—is a more accurate way to think about this relationship. They're far more connected than people think.

There are so many examples of how the mind and body are connected that there's no way I can give you an exhaustive list without boring the pants off you, but here are a few of my favorite examples, just to give you a taste.

First, let's look at irritable bowel syndrome (IBS) and upset stomach. These are the two most common digestive disorders, and they affect up to 20 percent of the American population. Worldwide, IBS itself affects 15 percent of the adult population, but it is still not well understood. While it is often treated with cognitive behavioral therapy and a variety of medications like antidepressants, the condition is often unresponsive.[3] This has a lot to do with the complex interplay of the mind and body. To most successfully treat illness, you have to use a whole-person-centered approach that requires far more effort and adherence to lifestyle changes than taking a pill. A 2007 study demonstrated the complex mind-body connection inherent in IBS. This study sought to see if psychological factors like personality traits, mood, and the way you perceive the illness increases the likelihood of being diagnosed with IBS. The answer was yes. This study used patients who were first diagnosed with gastroenteritis, a condition involving inflammation of the GI tract that usually only lasts for a few weeks. None of the patients had a history of IBS. Then researchers sought to see how the mind affected what happened next. Patients who had a tendency to interpret the initial physical illness in a pessimistic fashion were more likely to go on and develop IBS.[4] Thus, psychotherapy can help the minds of people prone to IBS by changing pessimism into optimism. This psychological tool can be combined with specific dietary restrictions (e.g., a low-FODMAP diet) that address the guts of people with this specific condition.

Another difficult to treat and debilitating condition related to mind-body brain drain is chronic fatigue syndrome (CFS), or myalgic encephalomyelitis, which affects up to 3 percent of adults.[5] In 2016, a breakthrough in research may have shed some light on the cause of this disease. Like other mind-body conditions, it is a real physical disease. After being exposed to a stressor, people with CFS get stuck in a metabolic state similar to hibernation in animals. Eighty percent of the metabolites, which help produce energy in cells, were decreased. This explains the extreme lack of energy; cells are in a nonaging, hypometabolic mode. Cells go into this hibernation-like state as a defense, but in people with CFS, they get stuck in it. While more research is needed, the lead researcher on this study hypothesized that the right diet and supplements could "wake" the body back up.[6] Even though more must be learned about the biological underpinnings of CFS, stress clearly plays a role in the potential development of the disease. Theoretically, extreme stress could trigger the cellular defense mechanism that leads to the development of CFS. Experiencing childhood trauma has been shown to increase the risk of developing the disease.[7] A study examining 30,000 veterans showed that the more stress and trauma the soldiers were exposed to, the greater the chance they had both PTSD and chronic fatigue syndrome–like illness.[8] In the largest study of chronic fatigue syndrome in children, published in 2016, researchers found the disease to be more common in teens than previously thought with 2 percent of 16-year-olds meeting diagnostic criteria. Stressed-out teens—those reporting financial difficulties in their family, housing problems, and a lack of maternal support— were more likely to have chronic fatigue syndrome.[9]

Another disease with strong mind-body ties is fibromyalgia, which affects somewhere between 2 and 8 percent of the population.[10] Fibromyalgia is characterized by chronic, widespread pain. Recently, there is more and more evidence that stress is one of many causes that also affects the progression of the disease. Research has shown that children with PTSD are more likely to be diagnosed with fibromyalgia.[11] This association has also been shown in adults. While I can't say the sexual abuse experienced by Maria, the woman I discussed at the beginning of this chapter, "caused" her fibromyalgia, research does show people with a history of sexual abuse are more likely to have the disease.[12] There are clearly complex biological and psychological risk factors at play. The disease has even been associated with the way people process serotonin, a neurotransmitter that many drained people are low in. An association was also shown between fibromyalgia and an anxious personality.[13]

Two other very common maladies that are the number one and number five leading causes of death are heart disease and stroke, respectively. Like digestive disorders, these diseases show very strong links to stress when you look at some of the shocking statistics. The American Heart Association says stress is one of the top precursors of cardiovascular disorders. Postmenopausal women who had panic attacks had *triple* the risk of experiencing a stroke or coronary event.[14] In another study, women with the most phobic anxiety were 59 percent more likely to have a heart attack and also more likely to die from one.[15] Other research shows that both men and women with an anxiety disorder and history of heart disease were *twice* as likely to have a heart attack compared with people with no anxiety disorder and a history of heart disease.[16] While hypertension, or high blood pressure, isn't directly caused by anxiety, there is a dangerous link. Triggering brain-draining cortisol spikes with too much stress or anxiety is associated with an increased risk of hypertension and thus heart disease. This association between anxiety and hypertension is present for all the different anxiety disorders a drained-brain person may be diagnosed with.[17]

Being drained in mind and body is also associated with diabetes and weight gain. Stress can indirectly cause diabetes. When you're stressed, levels of your main feel-good, stress-relieving neurotransmitter serotonin go down. When serotonin levels are low, you're more likely to crave and indulge in processed carbohydrates, flour, and sugar since carbohydrates release a surge of serotonin. Of course, doing this too often can cause diabetes.

Stress affects weight gain in complex ways. When the brain is drained and stress hormones spike, the body is more likely to store fat in the belly area. It's important to note that we all have to get through stressful situations; the difference is in *how* we get through these tasks. One study measured cortisol levels in women after they had to do the same stressful task: timed arithmetic. While all subjects felt taxed, it was the women who didn't have coping skills who were left feeling helpless. No surprise: these women had higher levels of cortisol in their body, and they were also more likely to have excess belly fat.[18] And although you're probably well aware of the dangers of obesity, it seems that this mind-body stress response could even be *more* hazardous to your health than you realize. Surprisingly, researchers found fit people who stored their fat in their midsection were more likely to die than those who were obese but who stored fat in other areas other than the midsection. The risk was quite pronounced—especially in men. Men with a normal body mass index (BMI) with excess belly fat were twice as likely to die as those with higher body mass indexes with fat stored in other places. Women with excess belly fat and a normal BMI showed a 32 percent spike in mortality risk compared with overweight women with fat stored in other areas.[19]

There is also a mind-body link to one of the scariest physical diseases: cancer. Your psychological stress response can increase the likelihood of the disease and speed its course. Personalities deemed "stress-prone" and that had poor coping skills were linked to both higher cancer incidence and poorer cancer survival.[20] While there is no direct cause-and-effect relationship, we know stress makes your body more hospitable to cancer cells and negatively affects your immune system. Stress hormones block anoikis, the programmed cell death that helps diseased cancer cells from spreading. When too many stress hormones are present, metastasis—the spread of cancerous cells from one organ or part of the body to another—is more likely to occur.[21] In 2016, a groundbreaking study demonstrated stress can create "cancer highways" through the lymphatic system. Scientists noted that cancer spread more quickly in mice who were stressed out. Previously, it was known that cancer can spread through the bloodstream since stress hormones increase blood vessel formation, which helps malignant cells spread. But this animal study also demonstrated that by activating the fight, flight, or freeze response and the resulting spike of adrenaline too often, lymph formation sped up. Stress hormones also changed the lymph vessels, which allowed the cells to escape faster. Thus, two disastrous changes were noted. First, new "cancer highways" out of the tumor were created for the cells to travel. Second, the speed limit went up so the tumor cells could flow more rapidly. Thus, the effect of stress on cancer is worse than previously thought since an entirely separate system has been shown to be affected by stress.[22]

It's important to note that just because these diseases have ties to stress and anxiety does not make them purely in people's heads or demonstrate a clear-cut cause-and-effect relationship between stress and contracting the disease. It's likely the interaction between something physical—like exposure to a virus—and one's genetically programmed and environmentally learned response to stressors then unleashes a cascade of responses in the body that may be difficult to undo. Remember: the word *psychosomatic* itself means mind (psycho) *and* body (somatic). You could say almost every disease or condition is technically psychosomatic, because which of them *doesn't* affect both mind and body?

STRESS AND THE BRAIN

Stress not only affects physical disease but also the very structure of our brains, making us even more likely to experience a drained brain. A number of studies have been done to shed light onto what happens in healthy people's brains when they go through something stressful. One study demonstrated a link between a smaller hippocampus in people who experienced long-lasting stress like childhood abuse.[23] Why does this matter? This part of the brain helps you remain resilient in the face of stress and is involved in mood regulation. It also helps you to monitor the safety of your environment and store dangerous images in your long-term memory so you can avoid them in the future. It does all these things as part of its duties of regulating your sympathetic and parasympathetic nervous systems. But chronic stress can confuse the hippocampus and lead to turning signals for cortisol "on" instead of "off," which can hardwire you into a constant state of fight, flight, or freeze. The hippocampus is also a very important part of the brain as we age, since it's one of only two areas of the adult brain where neurogenesis, the growth of new brain cells, is present. Neurogenesis in the hippocampus isn't just important for dementia prevention; it's also important to prevent anxiety, since the growth of brain cells in this part of the brain has been shown to reduce it.[24]

Another study utilizing brain scans was conducted at Yale in 2012. This groundbreaking study found that stress can shrink the brain fairly quickly if you're unable to handle it. It also showed shrinkage in another part of the brain: the prefrontal cortex. As it relates to mind-body brain drain, this part of the brain is responsible for physiological functions like blood pressure and glucose levels, which of course means havoc in the body when the system is faulty. The prefrontal cortex also acts as the brakes on stress, rumination, and impulsive behavior when other parts of your brain flood you with stress hormones.[25]

As I said before: The mind affects the body, and the body affects the mind. Stress and brain drain go hand in hand.

PITFALL THOUGHT PATTERNS

One form of stress that I see regularly when treating people with drained brains is what I refer to as *pitfall thought patterns*. These are simply negative ways of thinking that we can get trapped in—and when we do, they prevent us from reaching our highest potential, both psychologically and physically.

Here are the seven pitfall thought patterns that are linked to brain-draining conditions like anxiety and insomnia.

1. **Paralysis-analysis:** This type of thinking involves stewing and ruminating in anxious thoughts, preventing productive action from occurring. For example: "I wonder why Harmony got that account and not me. Does my boss like her better than me? I wonder if it's because of that mistake I made last month on that account. My boss said he wasn't mad, but maybe he was and just didn't want to tell me. He did give me a sort of funny look this morning. I'm so behind on this project, but I just can't stop thinking about this. I'm freaking out . . ."

2. **Permanence:** This type of thinking falsely assumes that just because something is a problem now, it will always be a problem. Mood-congruent recall in the brain lights up negative memories in the brain, creating the illusion that you've always been stressed and therefore will always be stressed in the future. For example: "Dealing with my dad's health problems is so hard, and it feels like it's never going to end. My life is hard, and it feels like it's always been this way. This dark cloud isn't going to pass."

3. **Personalization:** This type of thinking places the blame entirely on yourself for something not going your way. The error here is that there are multiple people as well as circumstances that are involved in unfavorable outcomes. Perhaps there were some things you'd like to change, but it's rarely *entirely* your fault just as it's rarely *entirely* the other person's fault. For example: "My divorce was my fault. It happened because I'm unlovable. I must not capable of being in a relationship. I'm weak."

4. **Pervasiveness:** This type of thinking allows something that is affecting one area of your life to spread to all areas of your life. For example: "What a stressful day! I can't deal with one more person. I'm going to skip yoga and get out of my dinner plans. I'd rather just sit alone by myself in front of the TV and eat pizza."

5. **Pessimistic:** This type of thinking considers the worst-case, catastrophic scenario. It dwells in the possible—not the probable. For example: "If I

don't get my anxiety under control, I'll probably start having panic attacks several times a day. How will I ever be able to work if I have uncontrollable panic attacks? If I started having one when I'm driving, I'd crash my car and kill someone. Maybe I'll get sent to prison. How would I ever live with that guilt?"

6. **Polarized:** This type of thinking has a binary, black-or-white pattern. The words *always* or *never* are frequently found in this type of thought pattern. For example: "I've always had sleeping problems. If my insomnia isn't 100 percent better, then I've failed. There are two types of people: good sleepers and insomniacs. I'm the latter."

7. **Psychic:** This type of thinking expects people around us to read our minds without us verbalizing what we need. It can also mean falsely assuming we know what someone else is thinking even when they haven't verbalized their opinion. For example: "My friends aren't helping me. Can't they see I'm struggling? They haven't even asked me how I'm doing tonight, and if you look at my face, you can see something's wrong. If they really knew me and cared about my well-being, they'd know this and would do something to help me feel better. I feel so alone."

When we don't address pitfall thought patterns, they can create self-fulfilling prophecies that turn irrational fears into realities. For example, worrying that you have a rare disease spikes cortisol levels. This depresses the immune system, and now you actually *are* more likely to develop diseases.

In traditional cognitive behavioral therapy (CBT), I help patients identify the pitfall thought patterns that are affecting them. When you're trapped in one of these patterns, life feels harder than it should, and you'll feel run-down. And it's not just your mood; you're actually changing your biology when you live in this state because you are stressed. Brain drainers like cortisol go up, while the brain-balancing neurotransmitters go down. As you now know, this can wreak havoc throughout the body. Muscles get tense. It becomes difficult to breathe deeply. Digestion suffers. This activates the feedback loop of stress, and it can be difficult to pull yourself out of the downward spiral of worry and fatigue. The autonomic nervous system gets caught in a sympathetic-dominant state. A negative thought creates negative action. A negative action creates tension. Tension creates negative mood states. Negative mood states lead to more negative thoughts, and so on. We do truly live in a mind-body state. Luckily, you'll learn a way to pull yourself out of these pitfall thought patterns through energy-based cognitive therapy, which you'll learn about in a later chapter.

CHAPTER 4

Wired for
Brain Drain

While we all experience pessimistic thoughts and pitfall thought patterns at one time or another, some of us are more prone to be affected by them. We are just genetically wired to experience the feelings that lead to a drained brain. That's exactly what the case was for Anthony, a young entertainment industry executive who was referred to me by his primary care physician. He experienced his first panic attack two years prior—a month after he was promoted to vice president at a television production company. The attack was frightening for him. He had always been an anxious person both as an adolescent and a young adult, but the panic attacks were especially troubling. Like many people with anxiety, there was also some mild depression present.

"Now I have about one predictable panic attack a month—usually before a big meeting," he said. "But others just come out of nowhere. The other day I was sitting at my desk and bam!"

I asked Anthony about what strategies were working for him.

"Well, Xanax works. But I don't want to be like the rest of my family. They all pop Xanax like candy. When I had to meet with our president the other day, I had taken two. I didn't have a panic attack, but I also didn't feel like I was on point either. And I felt groggy. My greatest fear is that I'm just cursed with bad genes that are going to make me anxious for the rest of my life."

I knew this wasn't the case—both as someone who has treated many people who seem to be wired for worry and as someone who comes from a family of worriers.

I remember being in the car with my grandparents as a kid. Any light tap on the brakes by my grandpa would elicit a response from my grandma. I can still picture it clearly: my grandma would gasp as she put her hand out and yelled, "*Ward!*"

My mom has the same startle response. Same gasp. Same hand. Same yell. It's why my stepdad jokingly calls her by my grandma's first name sometimes.

And then there's me. Always thinking about the future. Looking for evidence—usually financial or health-related—that I'm not going to be okay.

I know I have my mom's genes for worry. Pair that with some life experience—my parents' bankruptcy when I was 7 and my brother's stroke when I was 15—and you can see how nature and nurture collided to make me a worrier. Of course, there was evidence of my genetic tendency for anxiety before this; I was that inconsolable, wailing child at preschool who never wanted to be without his mom.

The two things I most frequently worry about today: money and health. My parents' financial ruin and losing everything taught me, "Even if you have it all, you can lose it all in a moment." Before the bankruptcy, we lived a charmed life. My father was a physician, and we had a home with ocean views. That was one day. The next, my parents filed for bankruptcy and divorced. We were left penniless after a big real estate deal went bad. I'm sure the stress of financial ruin weighed heavily on my father. In fact, his drained brain was a major cause of his first heart attack. The last one took his life a few years ago.

My brother's rare brain disease, which was diagnosed after he had a major stroke at the age of 10, stitched a similar message into my brain: "Even if there's no evidence of disease right now, you could be walking around with a life-threating condition." After all, that's what happened to my brother. It was what my personal experience told me was true with a capital *T*.

For people without a genetic tendency toward brain drain, these experiences may not have caused a significant amount of lasting stress. But for those people who are wired this way, it's important to understand that you need to be especially vigilant about caring for your brain.

It's also important to realize that you are not simply doomed to be anxious, overwhelmed, and drained. While you are more genetically prone to it, you have the power to overcome this through how you live your life.

This intersection between nature and nurture is an exciting part of science called epigenetics that looks at how your environment influences the expression of your genes. Studies in this area of research show that our genes just "load the gun." It's our life experiences that "pull the trigger" as genes are then "turned on" or expressed. This explains why only some people who have the mutated BRCA1 and BRCA2 genes actually develop breast cancer. People with these genes are more prone to breast cancer, but they aren't doomed to get it.

These genetic underpinnings help to explain why one soldier witnessing a horrific experience will be diagnosed with PTSD while the other witnessing the same event will show no symptoms. In fact, most soldiers don't develop PTSD. Of course the likelihood of a person—even those without a strong genetic tendency—being diagnosed with PTSD increases with multiple exposures to stress and trauma. Not surprisingly, soldiers who have been deployed to war zones multiple times are at a higher risk of developing PTSD than other soldiers.[1]

ARE YOU WIRED?

So how do you know if you're wired in a way that would make you more likely to experience a drained brain? Of course, having a panic attack is one way. Your startle response is another common way scientists predict people who may be wired for worry. Maybe you've seen evidence of your own startle response when you're in the passenger seat of a car or in a scary movie. And of course family history is another predictor since people with a family history of anxiety are more likely to be diagnosed with an anxiety disorder.[2]

The general way you approach life can show you if you are wired for brain drain. Just look at what you do when faced with big, scary, or unknown parts of life. Do you face them head on, or do you tend to shy away from them? If you are an "approacher," you may be classified as a sensation seeker. If you avoid, you may be classified as a sensation avoider. And your classification as a sensation seeker versus sensation avoider has been shown to correlate with worry and anxiety. If you are an "avoider," you are more likely to be wired to be easily drained.

Interestingly, the way you react to intense stimuli actually sheds light on what's going on in your brain. Sensation seekers process dopamine, the neurochemical of novel and thrilling experiences, differently. But since their brains tend to like and seek out dopamine, they are also more likely to engage in risky behaviors and struggle with addiction.[3] The upside of sensation seeking: they are less sensitive to stress and trauma and are less likely to be diagnosed with PTSD.[4] It's not just that they aren't bothered by intensely positive or negative stimuli; research shows they prefer it.[5] This personality trait has been shown to have strong genetic underpinnings, which is one reason addiction can run in families.[6] But it also means they're less susceptible to becoming drained; stressful events are less likely to cause lasting or problematic responses. This doesn't mean sensation seekers can't get brain drained, but it does likely provide them with an extra layer of protection against it when facing a stressor.

On the other hand, sensation avoiders shy away from novel or intense stimuli. Instead of craving the "upper" dopamine in the brain, they find too much of it overwhelming. Pair these genetics with a negative experience (nurture activating nature), and you will see a problematic stress response. In an animal study, sensation avoiders (e.g., nature) who were separated from mothers when they were young (e.g., nurture) later showed a heightened stress response as adults.[7]

If you're a sensation avoider, you are less likely to be diagnosed with addiction since alcohol, cocaine, and other drugs release dopamine—a neurochemical that sensation avoiders tend to find too activating. However, you may be more likely to experience brain drain as you release more stress hormones like cortisol and deplete your brain balancers like serotonin and GABA; this neurochemical response is more easily activated and longer lasting in sensation avoiders.

Your stress response is evident at a very young age. In an experiment with four- and five-year-old children, the kids had to meet the researchers and participate in 45 minutes of testing. They measured the children's cortisol levels before, during, and after the experiment. Healthy children had stress hormone levels that rose in response to meeting strangers and performing tasks and then went back to normal; these children also tended to be well behaved and displayed higher levels of self-regulation. In other children, the stress hormone either rose and stayed high or rose quickly and then dropped. These children were rated by their teachers as aggressive and lacking self-control.[8] In slightly older children, high levels of cortisol were linked to academic difficulties. The researchers' analysis demonstrated that this wasn't the result of low mental ability but rather the stress hormone affecting children's ability to learn.[9] Now, the high cortisol levels could be a result of either nature *and/or* nurture. But this research shows how early a drained brain can affect people and the potential course of their lives. Consider the stressed out 4-year-old labeled "aggressive" by teachers and how he or she may struggle academically as a result of that stress. He or she would likely receive very little positive feedback from parents and be shunned by peers, negatively affecting self-worth. The child would become an adult more likely to be in stressful situations like financial, relationship, and legal difficulties. The importance of learning healthy and natural stress management skills is vital, and the need begins at a very young age.

Another surprising way to know if you are wired for drain: you have high levels of verbal intelligence. A 2014 study found a correlation between verbal intelligence and anxiety. Specifically, high levels of verbal intelligence predicted worry and rumination. Subjects were likely to agree with the statement: "I am always worrying about something." The researchers believe that with verbal intelligence comes the ability to consider past and future events in more detail—leading to the pitfall thought pattern called paralysis-analysis as the person worries, stews, and ruminates, which doesn't do anything to create action that would solve the problem. In fact, this kind of thinking *prevents* action.[10]

Other research has shown an association between anxiety and general intelligence. In one study, subjects with generalized anxiety disorder tended to have higher IQs.[11] Perhaps a bit of ignorance is indeed bliss.

THE POWER OF YOUR GENES

Most people who are wired for brain drain know it. I suspect that if you didn't already know, you have a much better idea after reading the previous section. But *why* did this happen and *how* does it work?

One explanation for why some people are more wired for worry-induced drain is that this condition may have developed over time as a means of survival. For example, the researchers who found the correlation between higher IQs and generalized anxiety disorder suggest this may be a function of evolution. Whereas a nonanxious and intelligent person will detect some danger, the anxious and intelligent person will always be considering the possibility of danger. This would mean the anxiety and worry helped the person stay alive as he or she was perennially on the lookout for anything that could harm him or her.[12]

People wired in this way are not only more likely to see the danger but also apt to take quick physical action in response. People wired for worry and brain drain process threats in a different area of the brain: the motor-specific parts that help you to quickly move out of the way of danger. People who do not suffer from anxiety, on the other hand, process these threats in the temporal region of the brain, which leads to a more passive and less physical response to threats.[13]

Another possible evolutionary theory explains why women are more likely to be wired for worry and twice as likely to be diagnosed with anxiety, which is partially due to sex hormones. Levels of estrogen, progesterone, and testosterone affect corticotropin-releasing factor (CRF), which affects the nervous system and stress response. In animal studies, both males and females engaged in anxiety-related grooming when exposed to CRF, but this reaction was especially pronounced in females with higher levels of estrogen and progesterone. So what does this have to do with evolution? An enhanced stress response may help females be more responsive when protecting their young in the face of danger.[14]

The *how* of being wired for brain drain—how does it work—is still unclear, but there is definitely a genetic component.

Research with twins shows anxiety has a simple "genetic architecture." Genetic influences may be separated into two distinct categories. One study found generalized anxiety disorder, panic disorder, and agoraphobia were affected by one genetic factor. Specific phobias, on the other hand, were associated with a different one. Social phobia was influenced by both of these distinct genetic factors.[15] Despite these separate genes that affect different anxiety disorders, people with anxiety often don't stay neatly in one lane of their particular diagnosable condition. In fact, people with one anxiety disorder are more likely to be affected by other types of anxiety.[16] So, yes—your genes play a role.

Other research that's been done to determine how genetics affect anxiety found that 20 percent of adults are lucky enough to have a gene variation that results in less anxiety because it leads to lower levels of fatty acid amide hydrolase (FAAH).[17] FAAH is a chemical that prevents the breakdown of anandamide, a feel-good chemical known as the "bliss molecule," which is a naturally occurring marijuana-like substance. People with this genetic variation who use marijuana have been shown to experience less cravings for the drug when they stop using it. Unlike 80 percent of adults who don't have this mutation, this subset of people experience a similar, "natural" high all the time.[18]

When scientists tested mice, the mice with this variation spent more time in the open parts of a maze. This indicates that these mice felt fearless, free, and less stressed in general. In studies with both humans and animals, people and animals with this gene variation were also able to recover more quickly from stressful and fear-provoking situations.[19]

Genes also play a role in your mood in general. If you've ever wondered how much of your general feeling of happiness is genetic, one scientist has actually put a hard number on it. Using research from identical and fraternal twin studies, she determined that 50 percent of your mood is genetically determined. A minuscule 10 percent is based on life circumstances, and a whopping 40 percent is based on *your outlook*.[20] These numbers are actually good news for anyone who is *not* hardwired to be a happy-go-lucky person since they suggest there are many ways to change your overall mood. This scientific understanding also helps to turn off the kind of thinking that begins with "I'll be happy and stress-free when ____." Since just 10 percent of your mood is based on life circumstances, changing these circumstances will make some—but not much—of a difference. That small difference—like the joy of a nicer car or a small raise at work—tends to be fleeting. It reminds me of the quote: "There is no way to happiness; happiness is the way." You're better off targeting your outlook and the way you perceive the world since it results in more significant and lasting change.

THE UPSIDES OF ANXIETY

Most anxious people—myself included—know there are many good things about anxiety, worry, or stress. Anxiety is an easy thing to turn to in any situation because it feels protective. It may even be protective in some instances. Maybe your quick reflexes have saved you when the driver in the car in front of you unexpectedly stepped on the brakes. Or maybe it helped you prepare for a storm so you were living in comfort when other people were suffering.

Your worry may have led you to be an "overachiever" or a "planner." You may have gotten an advanced degree and found a high-level job that makes you not have to worry about your finances. And yes, your anxiety may have helped take you to this level. But if you let those traits go to the nth degree, you are sure to experience brain drain.

It's also been shown that anxious people may be kinder in general because they have more empathy and relate to others facing a difficult period. One recent animal study found that rats given an antianxiety medication were less likely to free a trapped companion since the drug—like the ones more and more people around the world have turned to—lessened their empathy.[21] Even rats will help other rats in need, unless of course they were too medicated to feel others' pain. Imagine how much empathy human beings may be stifling thanks to too much Xanax, Klonopin, and other benzodiazepines.

So yes, anxiety does have its upsides, but don't let that deter you from mitigating its effects. Just like most other aspects of life, it's fine in moderation.

CHAPTER 5

How Drained
Is Your Brain?

Hopefully by now you understand the biological and genetic underpinnings of becoming brain drained. Maybe you have begun to understand the "how" and "why" of anxiety, fear, and stress. In doing so, perhaps you have also started to "befriend" some of your anxiety as you see the ways it has kept you safe.

So now let's move on to seeing just how brain drained you are and how you might benefit from the information found in the rest of this book.

There are four main ways brain drain shows up. First, it can be related to *an external stressor*, something that has happened to you recently. Anyone who goes through a major life change like a loss or a divorce is going to experience a significant amount of stress. This is a very normal response. Just because it's an isolated event doesn't make the process any less difficult to get through.

Second, brain drain can be *psychological*. In these cases, brain drain is more inside job than external stressor. These people feel anxious most of the time because it's the way they experience life. Of course these people tend to feel even worse when an external stressor is present but will even persist in the absence of them. This state can be genetic, due to trauma, or even the result of seemingly benign choices like eating too many processed foods.

Third, brain drain can be *physical*. Many people experience physical symptoms when they are brain drained. Tension, digestive problems, and a racing heart are common manifestations of anxiety and stress. For some, brain drain presents itself physically with no awareness that the cause is stress-related. It can sometimes manifest as a physical condition like indigestion or irritable bowel syndrome when the true root is a drained brain. This can be especially true in certain cultures where it's more acceptable to have a physical health problem than a mental one.

Fourth, brain drain can be about *sleep*. Whether you have difficulty falling asleep or staying asleep, brain drain and sleep go hand in hand. Anyone who is tired will feel brain drained and have difficulty. Patience, calm, and ease are difficult for anyone to feel when they're not sleeping well. There is a chicken-or-the-egg relationship to anxiety and insomnia; anxiety can lead to insomnia, but insomnia can also lead to anxiety.

The following quiz will help you discover how drained your brain is and hopefully shed some light on the root of your drained brain. As you take the quiz, notice if you see your answers cluster in one or more of these four areas. External stressors are addressed in questions 1 to 4, psychological underpinnings in questions 5 to 12, bodily based drain in questions 13 to 17, and sleep in questions 18 to 20.

Add up your score to see just how brain drained you are.

THE BRAIN DRAINED QUIZ

I've lost someone close to me or have just had a significant relationship end recently.

    a.   yes: 4

    b.   no: 0

I have experienced a major trauma in my life like abuse, violent crime, war, or major accident.

    a.   yes: 4

    b.   no: 0

I have financial or legal problems.

    a.   yes: 4

    b.   no: 0

I have or someone close to me has significant health problems.

    a.   yes: 4

    b.   no: 0

I get stuck in negative thoughts.

    a.   never: 0

    b.   occasionally: 1

    c.   sometimes: 2

    d.   often: 3

    e.   all the time: 4

I feel nervous.

    a.   never: 0

    b.   occasionally: 1

    c.   sometimes: 2

    d.   often: 3

    e.   all the time: 4

It's hard to relax.

    a.   never: 0

    b.   occasionally: 1

    c.   sometimes: 2

    d.   often: 3

    e.   all the time: 4

I worry about how things could go wrong.

    a.   never: 0

    b.   occasionally: 1

    c.   sometimes: 2

    d.   often: 3

    e.   all the time: 4

It's hard to make decisions.

    a.   never: 0

    b.   occasionally: 1

    c.   sometimes: 2

    d.   often: 3

    e.   all the time: 4

I feel out of control of important things in my life.

    a.   never: 0

    b.   occasionally: 1

    c.   sometimes: 2

    d.   often: 3

    e.   all the time: 4

I feel stressed out.

    a.   never: 0

    b.   occasionally: 1

    c.   sometimes: 2

    d.   often: 3

    e.   all the time: 4

It's difficult to cope with all the things I have to do.

    a.   never: 0

    b.   occasionally: 1

    c.   sometimes: 2

    d.   often: 3

    e.   all the time: 4

My body feels tense.

    a.   never: 0

    b.   occasionally: 1

    c.   sometimes: 2

    d.   often: 3

    e.   all the time: 4

I am jittery.

    a. never: 0

    b. occasionally: 1

    c. sometimes: 2

    d. often: 3

    e. all the time: 4

I have digestive problems.

    a. never: 0

    b. occasionally: 1

    c. sometimes: 2

    d. often: 3

    e. all the time: 4

My heart races.

    a. never: 0

    b. occasionally: 1

    c. sometimes: 2

    d. often: 3

    e. all the time: 4

I have difficulty breathing.

    a. never: 0

    b. occasionally: 1

    c. sometimes: 2

    d. often: 3

    e. all the time: 4

I'm exhausted.

    a. never: 0

    b. occasionally: 1

    c. sometimes: 2

    d. often: 3

    e. all the time: 4

I have trouble falling asleep.

    a. never: 0

    b. occasionally: 1

    c. sometimes: 2

    d. often: 3

    e. all the time: 4

I have difficulty staying asleep.

    a. never: 0

    b. occasionally: 1

    c. sometimes: 2

    d. often: 3

    e. all the time: 4

SCORING:

9 or below: balanced brain
parasympathetic nervous system dominance

You move through the world with ease. You're able to move quickly through difficult and stressful events without getting bogged down by them. There aren't too many large stressors present in your life right now, and if there is one, you're good at dealing with the stress. Your brain is balanced with high levels of feel-good neurotransmitters and low levels of stress hormones. Your cortisol/melatonin levels also follow a healthy 24-hour cycle; one dips as the other rises. Also, your brain shows mild parasympathetic nervous system (rest and digest) dominance. When the sympathetic nervous system (fight, flight, or freeze) is activated, the pattern looks like a rolling wave: up briefly and then back down easily.

10–14: mild brain drain
mild sympathetic nervous system dominance

Your brain is somewhat drained. If sleep is a problem, your cortisol/melatonin levels are likely out of balance or are not following a 24-hour cycle. If it has more to do with stress, anxiety, or physical problems, it may be the result of mild sympathetic nervous system dominance. In this case, brain drainers like cortisol and adrenaline may be moderately high and one or two feel-good chemicals may run somewhat low. You are most likely experiencing the most common neurochemical footprint associated with this state: Light Drain. This quiz may offer some clues to which of the brain drainers and balancers are out of whack in mild cases. Questions 5–12 may indicate low serotonin and/or GABA since anxiety runs high, questions 13–17 may indicate high adrenaline and norepinephrine since they indicate physical problems, and questions 18–20 may indicate low melatonin and high cortisol.

15 or above: moderate to major brain drain
major sympathetic nervous system dominance

You're drained, and—chances are—you know it. You feel frazzled, stressed, fatigued, and exhausted quite often. If your stress response tends to go high and stay high, you may be experiencing the Skyrocket Drain form of sympathetic nervous system dominance. If you begin to feel frazzled but soon lack the energy to get through a crisis, your neurochemical footprint may be Drop Drain. Either way, you may consider yourself a worrier and have difficulty moving on after stressful events. Difficultly sleeping soundly is likely. There is probably one or more physical problems present, including problems with digestion or immunity. Additionally, your 24-hour cortisol/melatonin levels aren't peaking and dipping at the right time. If you've survived a severe and untreated trauma, your sympathetic nervous system dominance may be manifesting itself as X-treme Drain. This neurochemical footprint can also develop over time if Skyrocket Drain is left untreated. In X-treme Drain, adrenaline and norepinephrine are high, but cortisol remains low. Major sympathetic nervous system dominance also means you are likely low in most or all of the brain-balancing neurotransmitters: acetylcholine, GABA, serotonin, melatonin, oxytocin, and endorphins. Your sympathetic nervous system displays major dominance, and your parasympathetic nervous system is weak or nonexistent.

No matter how drained your brain is right now, don't worry about how bad it seems. The strategies I present in the rest of this book will help you balance your brain and bring you back to your regular self.

HOW TO USE THIS BOOK

Now that you understand what brain drain is and know where you stand on the spectrum, here's how you'll move forward with this book.

1. Part II will teach you about all the bigger-picture lifestyle changes that are important for creating and maintaining balance.

2. Part III will give you simple in-the-moment tools.

3. Part IV is a two-week program that puts the lifestyle changes and tools together in a simple, easy-to-use daily regimen.

You can use the quiz in this chapter as a baseline to track your progress. Retake the quiz after you finish the program or after you implement some of the other advice to see how much you've improved. Feelings are information. Your anxiety, stress, exhaustion, or insomnia are present in your life to say that you could be doing something differently to feel better and less drained. And that's exactly what we're going to do.

PART II

THE BRAIN DRAIN FIX

CHAPTER 6

Balance Your Blood Sugar

Janet was a 48-year-old woman who struggled with her weight and anxiety her entire life. Recently she was diagnosed with prediabetes, which only added to her worry. Although the diagnosis didn't surprise her, it was becoming more and more difficult for Janet to stop overeating and lose weight. Recently divorced, she felt insecure about her age and body. For Janet, a big bowl of pasta followed by ice cream comforted her on nights alone in front of the TV. Of course increasing anxiety means serotonin levels go down, creating more carb cravings since processed carbs, sugar, and flour release a surge of serotonin. In the moment, Janet felt better as she used carbs as self-medication. But the constant blood-sugar spikes would eventually turn her prediabetes into diabetes and lead to more weight gain, which would increase her insecurities and shrink her hippocampus, making her less able to deal with stress. This would, of course, lead to even more brain drain. This vicious cycle is what brought Janet to me. She needed help climbing out of this hole so she could feel better and create the life she wanted.

"It's just so hard," she said. "I look around at other people eating anything they want, and it makes me so angry. I gain five pounds if I have even a few pieces of bread. My metabolism makes it so much harder for me than other people, and it's only getting harder as I get older. Now that I'm prediabetic, I feel like I'm not allowed to eat anything good at all, and lately food has been the only thing that makes me feel better. Now I can't even do that. Honestly, I reach this point where sometimes I just give up and eat everything I'm not supposed to: fries, pasta, pizza, bread . . . I mean, what's the point of life if you can't enjoy bread?"

As I spoke more with Janet, I quickly came to realize that her brain imbalance was likely due in part to low serotonin levels, which meant we needed to work on raising those to counteract the dependence she felt on food. With a bit of digging into her past, we were able to figure out that Janet often found herself in a spiral of pessimistic thinking, believing that she wouldn't be able to handle life. By shifting the focus to her past successes and her strengths, we came up with a plan.

"So what does the powerful, confident Janet do differently in her life? Paint a picture for me. What does a typical day look like?"

"Well, I'd be eating healthy again. I used to love gardening and making caprese salad with the tomatoes and herbs in my garden," she said with a smile. "And I have so many friends I've been neglecting lately because I just haven't felt very social."

"Sounds like a great place to start," I replied, "so now you have your homework. And it also sounds like you're identifying other activities—like gardening and talking to friends—that will be your 'replacement therapy.' Those activities release the same serotonin that you now get through binging on carbs, and they'll help to mitigate the withdrawal symptoms and temporary cortisol spikes food addicts feel when they switch to healthier ways of eating. Think of gardening and talking to friends like a nicotine patch for a smoker—only better and more fun. Find other ways to boost feel-good serotonin through healthier activities."

THE ABUSER: SUGAR. THE VICTIM: YOUR BRAIN.

Part of Janet's story is probably relatable to most of us. Using food as self-medication is, after all, the most socially acceptable way to drug yourself. We all know that pints of ice cream put Band-Aids on worries and broken hearts. But sugar can be a disaster for your brain. It's vital for all of us to reduce the blood-sugar spikes lurking in all the tempting food most Americans are presented with 24/7.

Remember: these processed foods are extremely profitable to food companies and restaurants. The profit margin on soda and processed foods is sky high; the margin on healthy proteins and organic vegetables is pretty low. This means the processed foods and soda are marketed to you more heavily to keep the shareholders happy. While they tempt you to improve their bottom line, your waistline ends up paying the price. And as your waistline grows with blood sugar–spiking foods, your hippocampus shrinks. Remember, this is the part of the brain that helps you remain resilient in the faces of stress and helps mood regulation by controlling your sympathetic and parasympathetic nervous systems. It's also the part of the brain where the most neurogenesis, the growth of new brain cells, occurs.

As we discussed in Chapter 3, research has established the way extreme stress from childhood trauma can damage the hippocampus. But now we also know that sugar and other blood sugar–spiking food can wreak the same havoc as trauma or extreme stress. The result: high levels of brain drainers like cortisol which, in turn, can also lower levels of feel-good hormones like serotonin.

In a groundbreaking experiment published in 2016, baby rats were divided into four groups. Early childhood trauma was mimicked in one group by only giving these baby rats limited nesting material, which alters maternal behavior and spikes cortisol. This was meant to re-create the high-cortisol state of a child suffering extreme stress and neglect. These stressed rats were then subdivided into two groups: one that got food and water and one that got food and sugar water. Another group of baby rats who weren't subjected to the stressful early life experience also were divided into the same two groups: food and water or food and sugar water. Thus, there were four groups: stressed without sugar, stressed with sugar, unstressed without sugar, and unstressed with sugar.

The surprising results: the unstressed with sugar group had similar negative changes in the hippocampus as the two stressed groups subjected to trauma and neglect. The changes also affected the way cortisol was processed by altering its receptors in the unstressed with sugar group. The takeaway: we now know that spiking your blood sugar damages your brain in the same way as extreme childhood stress or trauma.[1]

This relationship has recently been demonstrated in studies with humans as well. In 2015, the first human study demonstrating associations between diet and hippocampus volume was published. This study looked at people who followed a "prudent" diet versus the blood sugar–spiking "Western" diet. The prudent diet was associated with a larger hippocampus, and the Western one was associated with a smaller hippocampus; and these relationships held true even when accounting for other variables like education or physical activity levels.[2]

Other studies have shown other parts of the brain and systems associated with stress are affected as well. In research published in 2015, we see what happens when people withdraw from an unhealthy, blood sugar–spiking Western diet: genes that affect stress are altered. When rats went from an unhealthy diet to a healthier one, cortisol spikes resulted. This highlights the fact that we can truly be addicted to unhealthy food, and withdrawal symptoms result when you try to cut back.

This study also showed changes in the amygdala, one of the parts of the brain affected by emotionally traumatic events and brain drain, when changes in diet occur. When rats went from the healthy diet to the unhealthy one, the receptor in the amygdala to which cortisol binds was negatively affected as well. This demonstrates that we truly can "numb" and self-medicate ourselves temporarily with unhealthy food.[3] Blood sugar–spiking foods have the power to neurochemically lure us with short-term pleasure and sedation while setting us up for long-term stress, anxiety, and a drained brain.

All of this really changes how we think about the relationship between drained brains and blood sugar–spiking foods. The link between blood sugar spikes with diabetes, obesity, and dementia had previously been established; now we can also put a decreased resiliency to stress and a drained, shrunken brain on that list. With all of the processed foods we eat, is it any wonder so many people struggle with stress and anxiety?

Another way that sugar affects your brain is by negatively affecting your sleep. In a study from Columbia University, people who ate the most sugar throughout the day had more arousals during sleep. These intrusions can pull you out of deep sleep without consciously waking you, so you may not even be aware your carbs are preventing you from sleeping well at night—except that you may notice fatigue and increased hunger the next day. Like too much alcohol, a big plate of pasta can create a sedated "food coma" that may help you fall asleep but then prevent deep sleep. Processed carbs like foods high in flour were also correlated with these sleep arousals, and unhealthy carbs can delay your body's release of sleep-inducing melatonin.

Of course, lack of sleep creates a vicious cycle since being sleep deprived makes it harder to deal with stresses you face during the day. And it also releases hormones that make you crave unhealthy foods that will spike your blood sugar, which of course will prevent the next night of good sleep. One study found men who slept for a shorter amount of time for just one night reported almost 50 percent higher hunger ratings compared with those who slept for 7 hours.[4] Lack of sleep also spikes your risk for a wide range of other disorders like heart disease and high blood pressure. And so the vicious cycle continues. The result: becoming drained.

The solution: Cut foods with a high glycemic index or load and replace them with lower glycemic index or load foods.

GLYCEMIC INDEX AND GLYCEMIC LOAD

What do I mean by "cut foods with a high glycemic index or load"? Basically, replace the foods that spike your blood sugar with foods that keep it steady. To determine which foods are draining and which are balancing, you can use their glycemic index (GI) and glycemic load (GL) measurements.

The glycemic index gives an approximate measure of how much a carbohydrate in a food raises your body's blood-glucose level. A high-GI food will raise your glucose level a great deal; a low-GI food will not. Beans, small seeds, and strawberries are examples of low-GI foods, with a ranking below 55. Medium-GI foods like basmati rice and bananas have a ranking between 56 and 69. High-GI foods, the ones so pervasive in our diet, have a GI of more than 70. White bread, white rice, pasta, cookies, candy, cake, and even most whole-wheat breads are all examples of high-GI foods.

The glycemic load (GL) measurement, which was created by researchers at Harvard, is based on the glycemic index but also takes into account the serving size of a food to more accurately calculate blood-sugar spikes. The numerical values are different since the GL is calculated by multiplying the GI by the number of carbohydrate grams in one serving of that food and then dividing by 100. Thus, a low-GL food has a ranking under 10; medium-GL foods have rankings between 10 and 20; high-GL foods have rankings 20 or above.

While many unhealthy foods are both high GI and high GL, like soda, candy bars, and donuts, the GL measurement does help to adjust for healthy foods like carrots that may have a high GI but a low GL since the average serving of carrots does not spike blood glucose levels. The takeaway: GI matters, but the *amount* of food you eat should be considered as well. Instead of getting caught up on the exact numerical ranking of a food's GI or GL or measuring serving sizes, we will focus on reducing the worst culprits of brain-draining blood sugar spikes—sugar, flour, and processed foods that also commonly have emulsifiers that cause inflammation of the gut and thus stress—while increasing the amount of whole foods like vegetables, fruits, natural sources of fiber, and healthy proteins and fats that protect the brain. High-GI and high-GL foods aren't just bad for your waistline; they profoundly negatively affect the brain and the body and even create growth factors that help cancer cells grow and divide.

For a list of GI and GL rankings for more than 100 common foods, check out this website: http://www.health.harvard.edu/diseases-and-conditions/glycemic_index_and_glycemic _load_for_100_foods.

REPLACING YOUR SWEETNESS

Since we're talking about sweets and sugar, I want to specifically address some of the swaps that people make to "eat healthier" while still having sweetness in their diet.

The first of these is replacing soda with fruit juice. While fruit juice is the lesser of two evils in this case, it's not a great choice for a couple of reasons. First, juicing fruit leaves the sugar while reducing the blood sugar–stabilizing fiber provided by the pulp and skin of the whole fruit. The result: apple juice can spike your blood sugar like chips or pasta.

While some people might argue that this sugar is okay because it's natural, this is unfortunately not the case. Fructose, the natural sugar in fruit, has actually been linked to anxiety. In an experiment looking at this relationship, rats were divided into two groups— one that ate a healthy diet and one that ate a diet high in fructose. These rats were then exposed to a stressor. Teenage rats displayed anxious behavior when facing the stressor, in addition to higher levels of cortisol. This affected genes that potentially lead to a dysfunctional stress response and decreased resiliency in the face of stress.[5]

So what's the solution here? If you're thirsty and want sweetness, aim for water and whole fruit. When you eat an apple whole, including its skin, you've got fiber to balance your blood sugar, protect your brain, and promote restful sleep. And bonus: when eaten more slowly as people tend to do when they chew, it also allows the fiber time to register in your brain as the feeling of fullness—something that is bypassed when downing a glass of fruit juice.

You can also feel free to drink vegetable juice since it doesn't have the sugar content of most fruit juices. Or if you just can't let go of fruit juice, dilute it with sparkling water or mix a little fruit juice with veggie juice to cut the blood sugar spike that can drain the brain. You can also drink unsweetened iced tea and zero-calorie stevia-sweetened beverages like Vitaminwater Zero as you ditch soda.

The other swap I want to address here is added sweeteners. Over the years, we've been told that agave is a healthy alternative to sugar. Unfortunately, this isn't true. The "goodness" of agave came as a reaction to the public's understanding that the high-fructose corn syrup, which began to replace cane sugar as a sweetener in the 1970s, was harmful. We were looking to natural sweeteners rather than the processed versions of white sugar and corn syrup. But agave—and natural sweeteners such as honey, molasses, and maple syrup—are all high in fructose.

Artificial sweeteners, like aspartame (Equal, NutraSweet), saccharin (Sweet'N Low), and sucralose (Splenda), have also been used to replace the sweetness of sugar while avoiding the calories that other sweeteners provide. However, these have been linked to obesity, possibly by recalibrating your taste buds to prefer sweet and blood sugar–spiking foods. They also reduce levels of good bacteria in the gut. That's important because when levels of good gut bacteria go down, anxiety rises.

The best option for adding sweetness is stevia, which has a GI of 0. Very limited amounts of real maple syrup and honey (especially manuka honey) are also acceptable since they both have relatively low GI values. Recent science has also shown both may contain valuable health benefits, including minerals that can combat stress. Manuka honey from New Zealand is the best form of honey since it may have health benefits like reducing reflux and digestive problems that many brain-drained individuals face. But use these two sweeteners in very small amounts as an occasional treat since they do contain fructose which, in large amounts, can lead to health problems and anxiety.

You can also look to other spices to take the place of sugar. For example, you can sprinkle cinnamon in your oatmeal or tea instead of sugar. By making this change, you'll prevent a brain-draining blood sugar spike. Cinnamon also has anti-inflammatory and antioxidant effects, whereas sugar creates inflammation.

BLOOD SUGAR–SAFE SWAPS

Replacing soda with another sweet beverage is one kind of swap, but we also have to take into account swaps for foods that may not seem sweet but actually rank high on the GI scale—things like rice, bread, and pasta that break down into sugar and spike your blood-sugar level.

These swaps are easier than you might think. Try sprouted, flourless bread instead of your favorite white or even whole-wheat bread. Instead of white rice or pasta, try mixing your veggies with quinoa or sprouted barley—or try cauliflower rice, which is now available in bags in the freezer or refrigerated section of most grocery stores. Instead of regular white pasta, try zucchini noodles or shirataki noodles. Instead of macaroni salad, try an organic egg or chickpea salad.

The general rule is to swap out your blood sugar–spiking simple carbs with vegetables or other more complex carbs, including brown rice, quinoa, barley, oatmeal, bulgur wheat, millet, couscous, and spelt. While complex carbs are still made of sugar, they break down more slowly, so they don't spike your blood sugar as much as bread.

Here are some other ideas that can help keep blood sugar in check:

- Cut the pasta in half and sub zucchini or spaghetti squash noodles for half. You can use a vegetable peeler or an inexpensive spiralizer to make the zucchini noodles.

- When choosing pasta, spaghetti spikes blood sugar less than shapes like macaroni. Thicker spaghetti spikes blood sugar less than thin spaghetti.

- When you do cook pasta, prepare it al dente style. Overcooking pasta increases its glycemic index, so set the timer for a minute or two below the suggested cooking time.

- When you're making pasta, use half as much pasta and add broccoli or cauliflower. When I make my favorite childhood treat, macaroni and cheese, I throw out half the pasta and add bulk with broccoli and cauliflower. (Of course, I also use organic milk and butter or olive oil.)

- At Subway, ask for your bread to be "shelled out" to cut your carbs in half. While you're at it, ask for low-glycemic veggies like spinach, tomatoes, olives, and green peppers. Load up on low-GI dressings like vinegar and mustard. Or when you get your sandwich, just eat half of the bread.

- When ordering pizza, ditch the deep dish or traditional for thin crust. Instead of eating four slices for dinner, eat a big salad with vinegar and olive oil first and then just one or two slices of pizza.

- Generally favor the recommended sources of healthier carbs in the program section of this book which include whole grains like quinoa and barley. In general, eat carbs in the presence of healthy fats and fiber, which can help reduce brain-draining blood sugar spikes.

These swaps are better for two reasons. First, they significantly bring down the glycemic load of your food: white and even most whole-wheat breads have a glycemic index in the 70s, whereas sprouted bread has a glycemic index in the 30s. And substituting spaghetti squash for half of your pasta cuts down your blood-sugar spikes significantly for that meal. With just one simple substitution, you'll have reduced your blood sugar spikes by at least half, which can help keep your hippocampus in tip-top shape. This will help you feel less drained and more balanced.

BLOOD SUGAR–SMART TIPS

In addition to the swaps above, there are some simple additions you can make to your diet that can minimize draining blood sugar spikes.

1. Eat raw or slightly cooked vegetables. The more you cook a vegetable, the more you may compromise the blood sugar–blocking capabilities of the fiber it contains. This fiber can minimize some of the blood sugar spikes created by carbs, especially when you eat the vegetable before the carb.

2. Use vinegar. Vinegar has been shown to keep blood-sugar levels in check by preventing some of the starch in bread or pasta from turning into sugar. You'll effortlessly lower your blood sugar by switching from store-bought salad dressings that often contain sugar to a simple blend of vinegar and olive oil.

3. Drink Tea. Tea may reduce the amount of glucose absorbed by the intestine, which reduces blood sugar spikes. So drink a glass of unsweetened, black iced tea at lunch. One study showed black tea did this better than other types of tea. White tea was second best at preventing blood sugar spikes and also contains very little caffeine, which makes it a great choice to accompany dinner at night.[6] This blood sugar spike protection is an added bonus to the stress-fighting compounds theanine and EGCG found in tea.

4. Enjoy some red wine. For those without a history of alcoholism or problem drinking, a glass of red wine with dinner may lessen blood sugar spikes by preventing intestinal glucose absorption and reducing your liver's production of glucose. One study found that red wine may be more effective at blocking glucose absorption than white wine.[7] One glass of wine can balance the brain, but more can drain it since excess alcohol increases cortisol levels.

Now that you know that blood sugar spikes can shrink your brain and make you more vulnerable to stress, I am going to tell you about foods that will not only keep your blood sugar balanced but also heal your body. By making these healthier alternatives a normal part of your everyday diet, you'll feel much better.

CHAPTER 7

Calm Your Brain

So you've eliminated the foods that are spiking your blood sugar. Now let's look at some of the foods that can help heal your brain—namely vegetables and whole fruit. But first let's pick up with Janet, who we met at the beginning of the last chapter.

I can happily report that Janet is now back to the vibrant, social, and happy version of herself she was once afraid was gone forever. She combined two of her favorite replacement activities—gardening and socializing—to help her get the serotonin she used to get from eating bread and pasta.

While it took her a few weeks to become an integral part of the group of friends she had been neglecting, Janet now sees her friends regularly. Hosting dinner parties as a self-proclaimed "healthy, organic foodie" with fresh rosemary, oregano, and thyme from her garden served over fresh, ripe tomatoes with olive oil has helped her lose weight without feeling deprived. Her blood-sugar levels have improved, which has helped her feel less anxious about her health.

Janet now reports the act of caring for these herbs and tomatoes helps her appreciate and savor every bite, so there is an inherent mindfulness to her healthy eating. The days of her turning to food as a substitute for what was missing in her life are over. Now she uses food as a way to bring people together, and by doing so uses it to celebrate how full her life is.

As Janet has begun to feel better about herself, she says improving other areas of her life is easier. With her newfound self-confidence, she travels more, loves hiking, and has begun dating again. Janet has created a brain-balancing snowball effect in her brain where every healthy choice she makes leads to another activity that promotes a sense of peace and well-being.

YOUR BRAIN'S FRIENDS: FRUITS AND VEGETABLES

As you know, sugar, flour, and other processed carbs can shrink the hippocampus, making you less able to deal with stress and draining the brain. But the antioxidants that are found in vegetables and whole fruits help protect the hippocampus from losing volume by combating oxidation—another process that can shrink this part of the brain. Fruits and vegetables are also full of fiber, which has been linked to more deep, slow-wave sleep. This is possibly due to the fact that fiber can slow digestion, preventing the sleep-disrupting blood sugar spikes.[1]

But eating more vegetables and whole fruits isn't *just* about preventing brain-shrinking blood sugar spikes. They also work in other, more complex ways to help protect your brain from stress and anxiety. They are rich in cofactors—the specific vitamins and minerals your brain needs to make your two primary stress-relieving brain boosters: serotonin and GABA. This is important because, as you'll recall, healthy levels of serotonin and GABA help you feel more optimistic and peaceful. You're less likely to engage in self-medicating behaviors like eating carbs in front of the TV by yourself and more likely to want to engage in healthy behaviors like exercise and connection with loved ones. Over time, this helps to keep cortisol levels down as you move through life with more peace and ease. This is vital since there is an inverse relationship between cortisol and brain balancers like GABA and serotonin. High levels of cortisol can block your body's production of both these brain balancers.

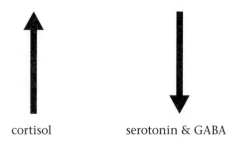

cortisol   serotonin & GABA

To heal brain drain, we need more healthy and natural ways to support serotonin and GABA as we reduce high cortisol. These two brain balancers can be made from the foods you eat. Let's look at a very simplified diagram of serotonin and GABA and how they are made from the amino acids with the help of cofactor vitamins and minerals that are found abundantly in healthy, low-GI foods like vegetables, whole fruits, healthy proteins, fats, and grains.

tryptophan (an amino acid found in foods like quinoa) → 5-HTP (the precursor to serotonin) → serotonin (an anxiety- and stress-relieving neurotransmitter)

Eating enough tryptophan-rich foods is vital in relieving stress and anxiety since this amino acid helps your body to produce soothing serotonin. For people who have been diagnosed with anxiety, a lack of tryptophan can lead to a relapse and panic.[2] But it's not *just* about getting enough tryptophan in your diet, because your body has trouble with this conversion if it's lacking in cofactors. What happens when your body doesn't have enough folate, vitamin B6, vitamin C, zinc, and magnesium from other healthy foods? Less soothing serotonin is made. Of course, the problems don't stop there. Since serotonin metabolizes into melatonin, you may also have trouble sleeping. This is especially true as people get older and melatonin production slows down. So if you really want to pacify and relieve your brain, eating a variety of healthy foods, including a diet rich in vegetables, whole fruits, and healthy proteins and fats, helps your body to get everything it needs to manufacture serotonin. After all, most of your serotonin is found in your gut—not your brain. Here's just one example of how to maximize serotonin production:

tryptophan (from quinoa) → folate (from spinach) → 5-HTP → vitamin B6 (from bananas), vitamin C (from raspberries), zinc (from chickpeas), and magnesium (from Swiss chard) → serotonin (stress less) → melatonin (sleep soundly)

Now let's look at the way your body makes your other soothing, brain-balancing neurotransmitter: GABA.

glutamine (an amino acid found in spinach) → GABA (an anxiety- and stress-relieving neurotransmitter)

This same principle also applies to GABA: your body has trouble making enough of this soothing neurotransmitter when your diet lacks the amino acid glutamine with vitamin and mineral cofactors found in healthy foods. Increasing levels of glutamine has been shown to increase anxiety- and stress-relieving GABA in the body by 30 percent.[3] So to help your body to make this stress-relieving chemical, it's vital to get enough glutamine through a wide variety of healthy foods to help provide cofactors needed for the conversion. Here's an example of a way to optimize GABA production with healthy foods:

glutamine (from spinach) → vitamin B6 (from carrots), magnesium (from broccoli), zinc (from pumpkin seeds) → GABA (brain-balancing neurotransmitter)

While GABA has fewer cofactors than serotonin, other vitamins and minerals, including potassium, magnesium, and zinc, help boost GABA release in other ways. Theanine, an amino acid found in tea, enhances GABA. Serotonin also enhances GABA production, so the vitamin C from raspberries that helped your body make serotonin can also then go on to synergistically support GABA levels.

Instead of obsessing over every vitamin cofactor or taking heaps of supplements with every vitamin and mineral known to man, here's a simple way to ensure you'll be getting the cofactors you'll need: eat seven servings of vegetables and whole fruits every day. (The only one that won't count in the program you'll follow: blood sugar–spiking white potatoes.) The proof this works? In 2013, a study of over 80,000 people found that people who ate that magic number of seven servings per day were less nervous and happier, and had higher levels of life satisfaction and well-being.[4] The average American only eats about three per day.

The link between seven servings and less stress makes sense for a variety of reasons. First, vegetables and fruit have antioxidants that combat the oxidation that shrinks the hippocampus. Second, you're less likely to crave unhealthy foods when you fill up on low-calorie, high-fiber veggies and whole fruits. Less overeating means fewer blood sugar spikes, which prevents potential volume loss in the hippocampus. Third, the fiber in vegetables and whole fruits promotes restful, restorative sleep. Better sleep means fewer unhealthy food cravings and more patience during stressful days. Fourth, vegetables and fruits are disease-preventing powerhouses that can help you avoid illness that would, of course, lead to stress. And finally, this large number of servings ensures you're getting the cofactors you need to naturally produce healthy levels of serotonin and GABA—keeping you happy, healthy, and calm.

ORGANIC VERSUS CONVENTIONAL

While eating organic is a good general rule of thumb, it can also be both hard to find organic foods and expensive to purchase them. Solution? Favor organic in general, but especially for fruits and vegetables that have been shown to be very high in pesticides when conventionally farmed. Strawberries and apples are notoriously "dirty" unless they're organic. Those that have a protective, nonedible shell like bananas and oranges tend to be "cleaner" in general. But if you only eat fruits and veggies with nonedible shells, you miss out on some of the wonderful sleep-promoting fiber found in edible fruit skins and vegetables with no protective shell.

The Environmental Working Group (www.ewg.org) does amazing work prioritizing which fruits and vegetables you should buy organic. Below is the complete list of the Environmental Working Group's results of pesticide tests of the most popular produce items in order from dirtiest to cleanest when conventionally raised. Anything near the beginning of the list is essential to buy organic. The closer it is to the end, the safer it is to buy conventionally raised:

1. Strawberries
2. Apples
3. Nectarines
4. Peaches
5. Celery
6. Grapes
7. Cherries
8. Spinach
9. Tomatoes
10. Sweet bell peppers
11. Cherry tomatoes
12. Cucumbers
13. Snap peas (imported)
14. Blueberries (domestic)
15. Potatoes
16. Hot peppers
17. Lettuce
18. Kale and collards
19. Blueberries (imported)
20. Green beans
21. Plums
22. Pears
23. Raspberries
24. Carrots
25. Winter squash
26. Tangerines
27. Summer squash
28. Snap peas (domestic)
29. Green onions
30. Bananas
31. Oranges
32. Watermelon
33. Broccoli
34. Sweet potatoes
35. Mushrooms
36. Cauliflower
37. Cantaloupe
38. Grapefruit
39. Honeydew melon
40. Eggplant
41. Kiwi
42. Papaya
43. Mangoes
44. Asparagus
45. Onions
46. Sweet peas (frozen)
47. Cabbage
48. Pineapples
49. Sweet corn
50. Avocados

CALMING COFACTORS

Let's look at dietary sources of these aforementioned amino acids along with their vitamin and mineral cofactors that help manufacture feel-good serotonin and GABA while keeping blood sugar in check. We'll also take a look at the specific ways they each can balance drained brains. Many of the natural, nutritional stress relievers on this list are found in vegetables and fruits, and others are also found in protein, including meat, fish, and dairy.

1. What to get: Tryptophan: Tryptophan is the amino acid that your body converts into 5-HTP and then soothing serotonin with the help of the cofactors folate, vitamin B6, vitamin C, zinc, and magnesium. Since serotonin is later converted into melatonin, it can also help you sleep better at night.

> **Where to get it:** chia seeds, sunflower seeds, flaxseeds, pistachios, cashews, almonds, hazelnuts, peanuts, soybeans, tofu, tempeh, cheese, buckwheat, wheat bran, wheat germ, quinoa, beans, salmon, cod, perch, meat, eggs, granola, milk, yogurt, chocolate, avocado, bananas, tamarind

2. What to get: Glutamine: Glutamine is the amino acid precursor to one of your body's main brain-soothing chemicals: GABA. Like other amino acids, it is involved in protein synthesis. By eating whole foods containing amino acids as part of a healthy, well-rounded diet, including the cofactors magnesium and vitamin B6, you will bring your body and nervous system back into blissful balance.

> **Where to get it:** beef, chicken, pork, fish, eggs, beans, cabbage, kale, parsley, beets, Brussels sprouts, dairy, milk, quinoa, almonds, pistachios, walnuts, seeds, peanut butter

3. What to get: Vitamin B6: Stress can lower vitamin B6 levels, so getting enough of it is vital when you're feeling drained. B vitamins are stress-relieving powerhouses, and vitamin B6 is essential since it acts as a cofactor for two brain-balancing neurotransmitters: serotonin and GABA. It helps your body to convert 5-HTP, which is manufactured from tryptophan, into serotonin and the amino acid glutamine into GABA. It's also involved in the production of melatonin, which helps promote sleep, which is why some melatonin supplements also contain B vitamins. Vitamin B6 is essential to your nervous system and supports healthy function of your adrenal glands, which can drain or balance your brain. It also helps your body turn the foods you eat into usable energy. It has even proven helpful in treating the symptoms of PMS and ADHD. Vitamin B6 deficiencies are common, and extreme deficiency can produce irritability, nervousness, and insomnia.

Where to get it: carrots, spinach, peas, bananas, sunflower seeds, pistachios, lentils, chickpeas, salmon, shrimp, turkey, beef, pork, milk

4. What to get: Folate (also known as vitamin B9): Stress also lowers levels of folate. Folate is a B vitamin that helps your brain convert the tryptophan in your diet into 5-HTP, which is then converted into calming, feel-good serotonin. It plays such as a large role in mood regulation that it's now available as a prescription, which is sometimes used to help treat depression. Folate also helps to support healthy adrenal function. Instead of taking a pill, you can get your folate fix by eating a wide variety of vegetables and beans. You may be familiar with folic acid, the synthetic form of folate found in fortified products like cereals and other grains. But most Americans eat far too many carbohydrates, which, as you know, can drain brains by spiking blood sugar. The naturally occurring folate found in vegetables is more effective and better for you than folic acid added to cereals and other carbs. Thus the better solution is to get more folate from two sources almost everyone could afford to eat more of: green vegetables and beans.

Where to get it: spinach, Brussels sprouts, kale, romaine, mushrooms, asparagus, bananas, melon, lemons, Swiss chard, broccoli, lentils, black beans, kidney beans, black-eyed peas

5. What to get: Vitamin B12: As you'll learn in the chapter on probiotics, gut bacteria have amazing brain benefits for humans. In animals, gut bacteria produce this vitamin, which we digest when we eat animal products or seafood. A vitamin B12 deficiency can cause depression, fatigue, and weakness. Some mind-body conditions that interfere with proper digestion and absorption, like Crohn's disease, can lead to a B12 deficiency. Antacids can lead to a deficiency as well since stomach acid is required for absorption of this vitamin. Older adults, vegetarians, and people who have had weight-loss surgery are at increased risk for deficiency. The CDC's National Health and Nutrition Examination Survey estimated up to 20 percent of adults over 50 have borderline low levels of vitamin B12. This may be partially because stomach acid production that is needed for absorption declines as we age. In addition to stress, vitamin B12 may also help improve sleep by resetting circadian rhythms.

Where to get it: beef, salmon, sardines, mackerel, eggs, milk, yogurt; for vegans and vegetarians, consider fortified cereals, fortified soy, or a fortified yeast like Red Star Nutritional Yeast. Vitamin B12 is light sensitive, so store fortified yeast in a cool, dark place.

6. What to get: Thiamin (also known as thiamine or vitamin B1): Like the other B vitamins, thiamin is essential in supporting the nervous system and adrenal function. It can help support the immune system when it's fighting stress while also helping to keep cortisol levels in check. Thiamin deficiencies are less common than vitamin B6 or B12 deficiencies, but they do exist and can cause irritability, nausea, and fatigue. People with Crohn's disease, alcoholics, and anorexics are at particular risk. Studies have linked low thiamin levels with poor mood.[5]

Where to get it: beef, pork, chicken, milk, oranges, nuts, seeds, wheat germ, wheat bran, rice bran, brewer's yeast, oatmeal

7. What to Get: Magnesium: Forty-eight percent of Americans don't have enough magnesium in their diet.[6] Magnesium can have a calming effect in the brain as well as the body, which can promote restful sleep, relax blood vessels, prevent muscle cramps, and neutralize acid that causes indigestion. It also protects against many major diseases like heart disease and stroke and has been used to treat many mind-body diseases like chronic fatigue syndrome and fibromyalgia. It can also help prevent cortisol spikes.[7]

Where to get it: broccoli, squash, spinach, beet greens, collard greens, Swiss chard, cashews, almonds, sesame seeds, black beans, coffee, salmon, halibut

8. What to Get: Vitamin C: Vitamin C is a vitamin cofactor that helps your body turn the 5-HTP manufactured from tryptophan into serotonin. While most people associate vitamin C with a healthy immune system, it has been shown to be effective in safeguarding your brain against stress and lowering cortisol levels. One study subjected over 100 people to a stressor. The subjects given 1,000 mg of vitamin C showed cortisol levels returned to normal more quickly with less blood pressure increases compared with those not given vitamin C.[8] Animal studies have demonstrated that vitamin C also prevented the appearance of a typical stress response like weight loss and enlargement of the adrenal glands.[9] So vitamin C helps to balance cortisol for people with typical patterns of a drained brain, and it has also been shown to help bring cortisol levels back up should your levels be too low, which can be true for atypical or extreme patterns of a drained brain like Drop Drain and X-treme Drain types.[10]

Where to get it: red and yellow bell peppers, chili peppers, acerola, papaya, guava, kale, strawberries, raspberries, oranges, melon, grapefruit, tangerines, black currant, apricots, plums, parsley, kiwi, broccoli, spinach, cauliflower, Brussels sprouts, lychee, elderberries, pineapple, garlic, limes, tomatoes

9. What to Get: Zinc: Zinc acts a cofactor that helps your body turn 5-HTP into serotonin. Getting enough is also essential for proper function of your adrenal glands. It may be lacking in many vegetarian diets since many of the richest sources are animal products, which also have zinc that is more bioavailable. Thus vegetarians may need to get slightly more zinc or increase bioavailability of the form in plant-based foods by soaking beans, grains, and seeds in water before cooking them. In our body, the highest concentration of zinc is in the brain's hippocampus, which, as you know, is the part of the brain that can help us remain resilient and also regulates our nervous system. Deficiencies aren't common but are more likely in the elderly and in those with digestive diseases like colitis or Crohn's disease.

Where to get it: oysters, beef, crab, bison, lamb, pork, turkey, chicken, yogurt, pumpkin or squash seeds, baked beans, tempeh, lentils, kidney beans, chickpeas, black-eyed peas, split peas, pine nuts, peanuts, cashews, almonds, sunflower seeds, cashew butter, natural peanut butter, tofu, fortified breakfast cereals, oatmeal, flounder, sole

10. What to Get: Choline: Choline is a nutrient that helps support brain function. It is metabolized into acetylcholine, the primary balancer of the parasympathetic nervous system. This balancer brings stress hormone levels back down after a spike. It is also important for the liver and pancreas. In fact, getting enough of this nutrient can even reduce your risk of both liver and pancreatic cancer. In terms of stress reduction, choline also helps support healthy levels of the brain balancer GABA. Higher levels of choline have been linked to decreased anxiety while low levels have been linked to increased anxiety.[11]

Where to get it: egg yolks, beef, almonds, avocado, broccoli, Brussels sprouts, cucumber, zucchini, flaxseeds, soy, shrimp, wild salmon, cod, peanut butter, chocolate

11. What to get: Calcium: Calcium is the most abundant mineral in the body, but deficiencies are common in the majority of Americans, and this can lead to anxiety. While getting enough calcium is usually emphasized to postmenopausal women to prevent osteoporosis, calcium is important for both men and women. In fact, the recommended daily allowances for calcium are the same for men and women of all ages except for a modest 20 percent increased intake recommended for women 51 to 70 compared to men in that age group. One reason that calcium deficiencies are so common is that you also need sufficient levels of vitamin D—another vitamin most people are deficient in—to efficiently absorb calcium. And since vitamin D is fat soluble, you also need healthy levels of fats to absorb enough vitamin D to then absorb calcium. The other problem is that phytic acid and oxalic acid found in some plants like collard greens, spinach, beans, and seeds can inhibit calcium absorption. But for most people eating a healthy and varied diet, these interactions are no cause for worry. One exception may be vegans since they tend to eat so many plant products containing these two acids, which may be why vegans were shown to have more bone fractures than people who consume meat and dairy.[12] One natural fix: cooking vegetables can neutralize the oxalic acid that prevents calcium absorption.

Where to get it: yogurt, cheese, sardines, milk, fortified soy milk, calcium-fortified orange juice, tofu, salmon, turnip greens, kale, cabbage, broccoli, walnuts, almonds, pecans

12. What to Get: Theanine (also known as L-theanine) and EGCG (epigallocatechin gallate): These two stress-fighting powerhouses are found in everyday teas made from the *Camellia sinensis* plant. Theanine is an amino acid, and EGCG is a flavonoid. Theanine calms the electrical activity associated with brain drain, produces brain-wave states similar to those found in people who meditate, and can help modulate the fight, flight, or freeze response. Theanine is extraordinary in its unique ability to help promote states of focus, which are usually associated with stress-inducing stimulants, while simultaneously promoting a state of calm. It can help lower blood pressure while boosting levels of brain-balancing GABA and reducing levels of brain-draining norepinephrine. EGCG also helps promote healthy levels of GABA while reducing cortisol levels.

Where to get it: Theanine is found exclusively in tea. The richest source of EGCG is also tea, but small amounts are found in some nuts like pecans and hazelnuts. Look for black, oolong, green, and white teas, which all come from the *Camellia sinensis* plant. If you're not sensitive to caffeine, enjoy a variety of these black, oolong, green, and white teas since some have more theanine while others have more EGCG. If caffeine is too activating for you, favor decaffeinated teas or white teas, which are naturally the lowest in caffeine. Black tea has the most caffeine, followed by oolong, then green, then white. Higher-caffeine teas like black tea have more theanine; less caffeinated teas like white and green tea have more EGCG. Both compounds can help to relieve stress. Avoid milk and sugar in tea. Milk and, yes, even soy milk, has been shown to blunt some of the health benefits of tea by binding to and neutralizing the antioxidants.

THE STRESS-RELIEVING POWER OF TEA

Tea making and drinking itself has inherent stress-relieving qualities independent of the active ingredients found in tea. In research conducted at City, University of London, a study divided people into two groups. Both had to complete a stressful task, and then one group got water and the other got tea. The group drinking water showed a 25 percent increase in anxiety after the stressful task, while those drinking tea saw their anxiety decrease by 4 percent. One subject talked about how the "ritual" of preparing the tea helped act a mediator of stress, and another talked about how it acted as a "partition" separating the stressful event and the time to relax.

Since tea is often made for people being looked after and a way to express care, there is also a conditioned meaning: tea means you feel cared for. Interestingly, the tea group in the study also chatted among themselves, but the group drinking water did not. This is important because social connection and shared experience help us process and relieve stress. Another study found those holding a cup of tea perceived others around them as kind and warm.[13]

Taking the time to cool piping hot tea with your breath not only protects you from burn but also can help you mindfully attune to the present moment, a stress reliever in itself.

While everyone needs to eat brain-healing fruits and vegetables, vegans and vegetarians should pay special attention to this list above. They'll need to be more diligent in getting enough stress-protective nutrition from plant-based sources. Some vitamins, like vitamin B12, are difficult to find in a vegetarian source, but alternatives do exist. Some vegans and vegetarians are at risk for vitamin, nutrient, and amino acid deficiencies that can put them at risk for drained brains and other physical diseases. Of course, the wide variety of vegetables and fruits vegans and vegetarians eat is wonderful protection against stress and other disease, as long as they also avoid too many blood sugar spikes. They must not become more *carb*atarian than *veg*etarian.

THE 80/20 RULE

Once you've completed the two-week program in this book, your goal should be to follow my 80/20 rule: 80 percent of the time, you eat these stress-relieving foods, and the other 20 percent of the time, you can let loose a bit (but within reason!). Because yes, I do understand that there are certain special occasions—from your vacation to Italy to Super Bowl Sunday—when you will just want to down that plate of pasta or a little too much pizza. An occasional indulgence is perfectly all right! In fact, sometimes saying you will "never" eat a food can increase the likelihood of you craving it.

CHAPTER 8

Eat Peaceful Proteins and Feel-Good Fats

You may have noticed that I recommended eating some things that are often included on the health-food do-not-eat list. Eggs, beef, pork—it can get confusing. And that's exactly how Nicole felt when she came to see me. Nicole was an educated working mom in her 40s who didn't know what to believe anymore. She was a self-proclaimed "health nut" and yogi who was especially anxious about what kinds of fats she was supposed to be feeding her kids. She had followed a fat-free diet in the '90s and was told "fat-free" foods like bagels were good for you. Then she did a little no-carb Atkins and South Beach Diet in the early 2000s. She'd had brief stint as a vegetarian and briefly self-diagnosed herself with celiac disease. When she was pregnant, she became more militant about toxins and was anxious about mercury.

If you're like most people, you—like Nicole—are probably anxious and confused about what kinds of fats and proteins are healthy are which are not. Decades ago, coconut oil found in processed foods and high-cholesterol egg yolks were no-no's. Now some experts say virgin, organic coconut oil is good for you while others are unconvinced, and egg yolks are good for you again. Margarine and vegetable-oil spreads made with soybean oil were supposed to be better for you than butter, but now the reverse is true. In fact, health nuts now put grass-fed butter in their coffee.

What about meat? Is it good for you or is it bad for you? Nicole had read *The China Study*, which basically said all animal products lead to disease; but then she read *The Blue Zones* and read that most of the regions of the world where they live the longest consume meat and fish. She also had recently seen meat alternatives marketed as "soy-free," which led her to question if soy was bad for you. And she was utterly confused about seafood, which was "poisoned" with mercury. However, she recently read that mainstream science has done an about-face proclaiming that the benefits of omega-3s for the brain may outweigh the risks of mercury even if it means eating farm-raised fish from time to time. And she had just heard about orthorexia—the obsession of eating healthy—and was afraid she might have it.

With all the conflicting headlines, articles, and deceptive marketing by food companies, it seems like you need a master's degree just to go grocery shopping. In this day and age with pollution affecting our oceans and industry changing our food supply, it is vital to keep up on the most current guidelines and research. Modern science is always changing, and new studies shed new light on old beliefs. Remember: some doctors used to say that smoking cigarettes was good for you. So yes, science changes as more discoveries are made. Just make sure to take each new study you see broadcast on TV with a grain of salt, because the shocking headline "Coffee Will Kill You" helps ratings, but in moderation, coffee is fantastic for the brain.

So let's jump in and use a balanced, scientific approach to deciding what kind of meat to buy at the grocery store or what kinds of oils to cook with—because they're not all created equal.

THE BASICS

So what's healthy about eating fats and proteins? In short, they contain important elements to build your body and brain. Omega-3s and omega-6s are essential fatty acids (EFAs). They are indeed essential because your body can't make them, which is why you must get them through foods. EFAs serve functions in the body like helping to transport cholesterol in the blood and aiding in bone repair. They are also crucial to your brain: getting enough of the EFA alpha-linolenic acid (ALA) can prevent inflammation in your brain.

The issue that's come to exist with the standard Western diet is that we are getting too many omega-6s and too few omega-3s, and when this balance is off, it will leave you feeling drained. And it's not just that we need to up our omega-3 intake; we need to lower our omega-6 intake. Omega-3s compete for space with omega-6s in your cells, so even if you take a high-dose omega-3 supplement every day or eat salmon at one meal, some of the benefit is actually negated by the high omega-6 levels if you eat factory-farmed meat and processed foods at the other two meals. With too many omega-6s, we experience inflammation, which leads to health problems down the road. Omega-3s are anti-inflammatory and associated with health benefits including less anxiety and insomnia, so we have to free up space within our bodies to allow omega-3s to work their magic.

Aside from omega-3s and omega-6s, fats and proteins contain cholesterol, which isn't inherently bad. In fact, in some studies, it's been shown that low levels of cholesterol have been linked with depressive symptoms.[1]

The issue is that we have to eat the right kinds of fat and protein. There are two types of cholesterol: LDL cholesterol is the "bad" version, and HDL is the "good" one. The standard Western diet often contains too much LDL and not nearly enough HDL.

A PRIMER ON OMEGA-3S

When we talk about omega-3s, we are actually talking about a few different things. There are two forms of omega-3s that your body and brain can use, and one form that has to be converted into one of the other two. The two you can use are EPA and DHA, and ALA has to be converted into these two forms. These two usable omega-3s do different things as they relate to easing drain: EPA is your "stress less" omega-3 that has been shown to reduce anxiety and ease stress, and can even help you feel less reactive or angry. DHA is your "sleep soundly" omega-3 that can help promote deep and restful sleep.

One 2003 study showed that omega-3 supplementation over the course of just a few weeks helped lower levels of the brain-draining stress hormones cortisol and adrenaline when the subjects were exposed to stress. This helped to blunt the immediate effects of adrenaline during stress exposure, as well as reduce the cortisol spike *after* the stressor. Omega-3s showed effects that directly help your nervous system.[2] Even modest amounts of the omega-3s EPA and DHA, which are both found in seafood, have been shown to decrease the amount of norepinephrine that kicks your body into fight, flight, or freeze mode.[3] The dosage of omega-3s used in these studies was equivalent to a small portion—about three ounces—of wild salmon.

Another study with stressed-out medical students found that supplementing with omega-3s containing high levels of EPA and lower levels of DHA helped to decrease anxiety by 20 percent while also decreasing inflammation. This study is significant since more and more people around the world are experiencing high levels of stress that are similar to the round-the-clock pressure medical students face.[4]

And if you're like me and tend to be a type A worrier with elements of perfectionism that carry higher risks of stroke, heart attack, anxiety disorders, and anorexia, omega-3s may even soothe you enough to help you to worry less and let go a little more. This can help to mitigate some of the stress we face in our modern world, including living in a globalized economy where more people are competing for the best jobs and spots in the best colleges. Omega-3s may even help you be less reactive or angry. One study gave a group of prisoners a fish-oil supplement, and another got a placebo. The prisoners taking the fish oil for as little as two weeks experienced a 35.1 percent reduction in violent offenses.[5] While

I'm not comparing a strung-out CEO or an Ivy League student to a prisoner, both could probably use a bit more "chill" and a little less reactivity in their lives. Another study with veterans who had a history of substance abuse and aggression, the end results of severe brain drain, had one group taking a high-EPA omega-3 supplement (2,250 mg EPA and 500 mg DHA) daily and the second group taking a placebo. The members of the group taking the omega-3s were less angry and reactive.[6]

And moving on to the idea of sleeping well, one recent study found supplementation with DHA resulted in higher quality sleep, increase of sleep duration, and fewer awakenings in the middle of the night.[7] Another found low levels of DHA were associated with more severe sleep apnea.[8] Most seafood has roughly equal amounts of EPA and DHA. The EPA can help you stress less, which can help you fall asleep, and the DHA can help you to improve your sleep overall.

The third type of omega-3, which I mentioned above, is the plant-based source. ALA is found in walnuts and flaxseeds, but remember your body must convert this type of omega-3 into "stress less" EPA and "sleep soundly" DHA, and it's not very good at this conversion. This is why the seafood omega-3 superfoods that contain EPA and DHA are even better than vegetarian superfoods that contain ALA.

As you can see from the conversion rates below, your body is more efficient at converting ALA into EPA than it is DHA. Eating foods like walnuts rich in ALA may alleviate anxiety due to the higher rates at which ALA converts into EPA, but may not be as effective in promoting restful sleep since the DHA converted from ALA is negligible—especially for men and older women. And since we produce less sleep-inducing melatonin as we age, the DHA may indeed prove to be increasingly vital to help us get a good night's rest.

Conversion rates for healthy young men:

- 8 percent of the ALA is converted into EPA
- 0 to 4 percent of the ALA is converted into DHA

Conversion rates for healthy young women:

- 21 percent of the ALA is converted into EPA
- 9 percent of the ALA is converted into DHA

Women might get twice the EPA and DHA as men because of their higher estrogen levels, which is helpful during pregnancy when estrogen soars and the baby gets lots of DHA that is essential for brain development. But older women who are going through or have been through menopause have much lower estrogen levels, and they need to make a real effort to get EPA and DHA straight from the source, no conversion required. This is why the richest source of both EPA and DHA—seafood—is the most effective way to get the omega-3s your brain needs to feel balanced, stress free, and rested.

A WORD TO VEGETARIANS

As you can see from the numbers, you need a great deal more plant-based ALA to give you the omega-3s your brain and body need. 1,000 mg of ALA sounds like a hefty dose, but that 1,000 mg of ALA is converted into just 200 mg of EPA and 100 mg of DHA in healthy young women. For healthy young men, that 1,000 mg of ALA is reduced to just 100 mg or so of EPA and almost no DHA. So for all men and aging women, you may need to supplement your intake of DHA. You can likely get all the stress-relieving EPA you need from consuming plant-based ALA. For DHA, consider a vegetarian algae supplement.

Just to break this down into easily digestible pieces:

- **EPA** is your brain's "stress less" omega-3.

- **DHA** is your brain's "sleep soundly" omega-3.

- **ALA** is the plant-based form of omega-3 that your body converts into EPA and, to a lesser extent, DHA.

A PROPER BALANCE

I mentioned before that those of us eating the standard Western diet are getting too many omega-6s and too few omega-3s. Humans likely evolved on a diet that was a 1:1 ratio of these essential fatty acids, but now most Americans get 10 to 25 times more omega-6s than omega-3s, and this shift is taking place around the world. So what has changed? Both what we eat and how we eat it.

First things first, the food we eat isn't nearly as high quality as it was in days of yore. Factory farming isn't just a cruel and cutthroat industry that's bad for farmers and animals; it also produces food that's terrible for your brain. There is a substantial difference in the omega-3 content of organic, grass-fed, free-roaming, and/or pastured meat compared with cheaper, factory-farmed, and conventional varieties. Conventionally raised beef has an omega-6 to omega-3 ratio of 7.65 to 1. Grass-fed beef brings the omega-6 to omega-3 ratio all the way down to 1.5 to 1, which means it has nearly as many omega-3s as it does omega-6s.[9] Meat from free-roaming chickens has more brain-balancing omega-3s than that from grain-fed chickens.[10] Organic milk contains 62 percent more omega-3s and 25 percent fewer omega-6s than conventional dairy, and thus the same is true for foods made from milk like butter and cheese. Eggs from chickens allowed to roam and eat nutritious grasses have more than double the amount of omega-3s than those fed an industrial diet, as well as more vitamins.[11]

The same principle is true for fish. Cheap, farm-raised tilapia fed cheap food high in omega-6s won't provide you with the omega-3 powerhouse of wild salmon free to eat their natural, nutrient-dense food.[12]

We also eat a lot more processed foods than we used to, and virtually all processed foods contain soybean oil, which is one of the biggest sources of the excessive inflammatory, brain-draining omega-6s found in most modern diets. It is found in nearly all processed foods from salad dressings to mayonnaise and, yes, even some varieties of foods that should be good for you—like hummus—made by big food companies.

The quality of the food makes a huge difference in having a balanced omega-3 to omega-6 ratio, but so does the quantity of our consumption. The standard Western diet has shifted from being whole foods to being mostly processed with a high percentage of our protein coming from meat. Meat and processed foods used to be specialty items, but now they make up the bulk of what we eat.

So what do we do to fix all these problems?

A MODIFIED MEDITERRANEAN DIET

Whether you're vegetarian, pescatarian, or a meat eater, there are ways to get the peaceful proteins and fats we now know are good for you. These proteins and fats now have decades of research behind them, and eating them is what I call a "modified Mediterranean diet." I say "modified" for a few reasons. If you're not living in a small farming village near the Mediterranean coast where the fishermen bring in the fresh catch of the day from the ocean, and the meat comes from animals grazing nearby fields, then you need to carefully modify the kinds of proteins and fats you buy at a grocery store in New York, London, or Cleveland to ensure you're getting the clean omega-3s people in Sardinia eat. Of course vegetarians and vegans can also take up an animal-product-free version of the modified Mediterranean diet with more olive oil and walnuts, while reducing their intake of soybean oil and white bread.

The basics of this diet are eat more fish, more vegetables, more fruit, more beans, more nuts, and more olive oil (and perhaps some coconut oil). As you get more protein from fish or beans, eat a more reasonable amount of high-quality meat, dairy, and eggs. And eat very little in the way of blood sugar–spiking carbs; replace them with limited amounts of healthy, complex carbs. Throw in some tea, coffee, and a splash of red wine if you drink, and you're good to go.

A modified Mediterranean diet will help you not only stress less and sleep more soundly but also be healthier in general. Study after study has linked this type of diet with a decreased risk of just about every other health condition, from dementia to cancer. With all of the rich and delicious sources of healthy fats, delectable proteins, nourishing grains, veggies, and fruits, it also tastes a lot better than militant no-carb or nonfat diets of yesteryear. The modified Mediterranean diet tastes good, will help you feel good, and keeps you healthy. Talk about a win-win.

It will also help you balance your omega-3 to omega-6 ratio and reduce the unhealthy saturated fats that are so common in Western diets.

Now let's go a bit deeper into some of the pieces of the modified Mediterranean diet.

Fish

One of the big pieces of the puzzle when aiming to raise your omega-3 levels is seafood. Seafood is the richest source of both your "stress less" omega-3 EPA and your "sleep soundly" omega-3 DHA, and most seafood has roughly the same amount of both. These high levels of omega-3s rebalance the ratio of omega-3s to omega-6s you consume, which generally shifts your brain and body from an inflammatory state to an anti-inflammatory one. "Clean" seafood is also superior to taking a fish oil supplement in many ways since the zinc, iron, selenium, and other vitamins it contains can help your body and brain optimize omega-3s. And research shows that eating fish is more effective at getting omega-3s into your bloodstream than taking omega-3 supplements.[13]

Supplements containing a very high level of the omega-3 EPA and a very small amount of the omega-3 DHA (e.g., a supplement that lists about 2,000 mg of EPA and just 300 mg or less of DHA on the back of the bottle) can be an extremely potent option for people struggling with more severe anxiety. But remember: another study found that even lower levels of the omega-3s EPA and DHA—the amount found in a small, three-ounce serving of wild salmon—also helped the body release fewer stress hormones. If you are taking omega-3s in supplement form—after clearing it with your primary care physician or specialist since there are some people who should not take them—make sure you're also getting enough seafood to help you get the natural compounds found in seafood that reduce your intake of omega-6s. And again, vegetarians can eat the plant-based omega-3 superfoods you'll find in the box on page 75 to get their stress-relieving EPAs made from the ALAs found in foods like walnuts. To get enough of the "sleep soundly" DHA, vegetarians can supplement with an algae-based supplement made with no animal or fish products.

Of course, there are so many caveats when it comes to seafood. If you're like my patient Nicole, you're told of the health benefits while also warned of the health risks of pollutants like mercury. Unfortunately, this is a reality of our polluted planet and industrial fish farming. Many of the fish we eat today are full of contaminants like mercury and aren't sustainably caught. So how do we choose? There's a good rule of thumb: always eat wild-caught, not farm-raised fish. I say it's a good rule of thumb because there are some notable exceptions. There are some farm-raised fish with high levels of omega-3s and low levels of toxins like mercury. Three of my favorites are farm-raised varieties of rainbow trout, arctic char, and coho salmon; they're also sustainable, so we aren't doing anything to harm future generations or depleting our oceans by eating them. My other favorite is something you can find next to the canned tuna in the grocery aisle: albacore tuna that's specifically labeled "troll caught" or "pole caught." While regular albacore tuna is actually higher in mercury than cheaper chunk light tuna, the pole caught/troll caught varieties are high in omega-3s and low in mercury. Chunk light tuna and albacore tuna not labeled troll caught or pole caught also aren't great sources of omega-3s. On the other hand, shrimp and scallops are generally low in toxins and fairly high in omega-3s.[14] They also tend to be easy to find whether you're eating at a Mexican joint, getting Chinese takeout, or making skewers for your family at a holiday BBQ. Of course I also love the omega-3 powerhouse of a good, wild-caught, Alaskan salmon, but this can be both expensive or hard to find in restaurants. And despite the words food companies and restaurants try to use to tell you otherwise, "fresh" or "natural" salmon doesn't mean that it's wild-caught salmon.

> **EXPERT'S TIP:** The fish-loving Japanese don't worry much about mercury for the simple reason that they often drink tea with their fish. Black coffee and green or black tea can reduce your mercury exposure by over 50 percent. This is especially important when you eat sushi, as uncooked fish will expose you to more mercury than cooked fish.[15]

To simplify matters on which fish to choose, the Monterey Bay Aquarium teamed up with the Harvard School of Public Health and the Environmental Defense Fund to come up with a fairly short list of go-to fish that are high in omega-3s, low in pollutants like mercury and PCBs, and sustainably caught. You can learn more and stay current with the latest recommendations on their website: seafoodwatch.org.

Here are the fish you want to make the focus of your brain-balancing diet:

- Albacore tuna, troll or pole caught, fresh or canned, U.S. or British Columbia
- Arctic char, farmed
- Barramundi, farmed, U.S.
- Coho salmon, farmed, U.S.
- Dungeness crab, wild, California, Oregon, or Washington
- Longfin squid, wild, Atlantic
- Mussels, farmed
- Oysters, farmed

- Pacific sardines, wild
- Pink shrimp, wild, Oregon
- Rainbow trout, farmed
- Salmon, wild, Alaska
- Spot prawns, wild, British Columbia

The list of fish you are better off avoiding is, unfortunately, just as long:

- Canned light tuna
- Canned albacore tuna (except those labeled troll or pole caught)
- Tuna steaks
- Lobster
- Carp
- Flatfish
- Bass
- Perch
- Haddock
- Hake
- Snapper
- Halibut
- Mackerel
- Roughy
- Sea bass
- Shark
- Swordfish
- Tilapia
- Tilefish

VEGETARIAN "FISH"

As a vegetarian, it's sometimes hard to get the omega-3s you need because of the lack of fish in your diet. However, other omega-3 superfoods do exist. Just remember, these contain high levels of ALA, which your body must convert to DHA and EPA in order for you to sleep soundly and stress less, and it doesn't do this very efficiently, especially in men. Vegetarian sources of ALA include:

- Walnuts
- Flaxseeds or flaxseed oil
- Chia seeds

Meat, Dairy, and Eggs

When it comes to meat, dairy, and eggs in the modified Mediterranean diet, it's all about moderation. The vast majority of people in the Western world should eat less meat in general and make it more "side" than "entrée." Doing this can be potentially life-saving to stressed-out individuals. As you know, people with anxiety are more likely to develop high blood pressure, the leading cause of death worldwide. A 2014 meta-analysis that looked at 39 different studies and trials found an association between eating a plant-based diet and low blood pressure; eating meat was associated with high blood pressure.[16] So just try to cut down. Even replacing a couple meat-filled meals a week with vegetarian bean and vegetable-based entrees is a good way to get you on the path to a healthier life.

While you're changing the *quantity* of animal products you eat, simultaneously increase the *quality*. Choose animal products that are organic, grass fed, free roaming, and/ or pastured over conventional and factory-farmed varieties. We've already covered the difference this makes in relation to balancing your omega-3 to omega-6 ratio, but in addition, they're also cleaner. Conventionally raised animal products may also contain PCBs and dioxins, industrial byproducts that have largely been banned but persist in our environment and may contribute to cancer and neurological problems.[17] Of course, decreasing your risk of major diseases like cancer is a way to prevent stress since chronic health problems are one of the worst stressors reported by people with high levels of anxiety. Grass-fed meat also tends to be a bit leaner than conventional meats, which can make it less carcinogenic, as many of the cancer-causing compounds are the result of fats exposed to heat.[18]

The leaner the meat you choose, the less you'll be exposed to these risks. Whatever type of meat you're preparing, marinate before you grill, flip it frequently, and eat it medium rare instead of well done. All of these strategies have been shown to help reduce meat's toxicity.

One of the other reasons to choose healthier, organic, and grass-fed varieties of animal proteins: conjugated linoleic acid (CLA). CLA is a fatty acid with protective health benefits. Animals that are grass-fed can produce 300–500 percent more CLA in their milk and meat compared with animals fed a conventional diet.[19]

Choosing organic dairy that contains fat is helpful in reducing stress since the soothing omega-3s are found mostly in the fat that is skimmed off in nonfat milk. Since healthy levels of calcium can reduce anxiety, you also need to make sure you get enough vitamin D to absorb calcium. But since vitamin D is a fat-soluble vitamin, you also need to consume it with fat to be used by the body. CLA also acts as a safeguard that protects you against the cardiovascular risks associated with saturated fat. Saturated fat in nonorganic dairy and conventionally raised meat has been known to increase your risk of a heart attack, but it seems saturated fat is not all created equal. CLA in *organic* dairy has been shown to offset the heart attack risk of the saturated fat it contains.[20]

Grass-fed, pastured, free-roaming, and/or organic animal products also have higher levels of the vitamins and minerals that can help your body deal with stress. Stress hormones aren't just bad for you; they're bad for animals. Conventionally raised animals with high levels of stress hormones results in tougher meat while also lowering the vitamins and nutrients it contains. These include the stress-buffering B vitamins as well as zinc, copper, chromium, vitamin A, vitamin C, and vitamin E.[21] Consumers also need to be wary of the words food companies use to trick you into buying products you perceive as healthy. Unlike eggs with the words *organic* and *free roaming*, cage-free eggs may not necessarily be better for you. In fact, animals lower on the pecking order in a "cage-free" environment may have more stress hormones than those producing conventionally raised eggs. And when stress hormones go up in animals, it can affect the nutrient content that can help *you* balance your brain as you deal with stress.

When it comes to animal products, food companies and restaurants will try and trick you into buying something that sounds healthier but is cheap for them to produce. A "fresh Atlantic" salmon does not necessarily mean that it's wild-caught salmon. "Vegetarian-fed" is misleading since many cheap industrial grains that are high in pro-inflammatory omega-6s are "vegetarian," which means the meat is higher in brain-draining omega-6s. Pastured and pasteurized sound similar but you're looking for the former when it comes to getting more omega-3s. Don't be fooled by any of the following words on animal products:

- All natural
- Vegetarian fed
- Cage free
- Pasteurized
- Fresh

If you want to relieve stress and anxiety, what you really want to do is to get more omega-3s, so look for one or more of the following words:

- Organic
- Free roaming
- Free range
- Grass fed
- Pastured
- Pasture raised

The best choice of all is when you see the words *certified humane* in addition to these terms. Some food companies can get away with labeling a product as free range if animals are given access to the outdoors. A product labeled "Certified Humane Free Range" or "Certified Humane Pasture Raised" ensures the animals are actually spending most of their waking hours outside.

While these varieties are more expensive than conventionally raised animal products, you should be eating less of them as you fill your plate with more inexpensive beans, grains, and produce. Thus, this change should be relatively budget neutral.

Beans and Soybean Products

In addition to quinoa, brown rice, and the other whole grains in Chapter 6, beans and soybean products are sources of complex carbs. They are also powerful ways to help you balance a drained brain. They do this in a variety of ways. Beans are a great source of protein, but they are also a source of fiber; and as you learned, a diet high in fiber is associated with restful, deep sleep.

Beans also have a favorable omega-3 to omega-6 ratio. This, of course, also helps your body to move from a pro-inflammatory state to an anti-inflammatory one, which helps to prevent disease and ease digestion.

In the last chapter, you learned about all the amino acids, vitamins, and minerals that help the body to combat stress and insomnia, and beans are rich in nearly all of them. For example, they contain the amino acid tryptophan, which helps your body produce balancing serotonin, and they also help your body manufacture GABA thanks to other amino acids they contain. And they're rich in vitamin B6, folate, magnesium, zinc, and calcium, which all have stress-reducing and sleep-promoting qualities. The other bonus: they're inexpensive. For meat eaters, they can be a cost-effective way to get enough protein, which will help balance your checkbook (and, of course, your general sense of health) as you eat less meat.

Foods made from soy can also help your body to stress less and sleep soundly, but there are also some complicated caveats when it comes to soy. First, let's talk about the health benefits as they relate to stress and sleep. Like beans, soy and soy products contain the amino acid tryptophan that helps your body to manufacture brain-balancing serotonin. Soy lecithin has been found to reduce stress hormone levels.[22] The natural stress relievers you learned about in the last chapter—zinc, choline, and calcium—can be found in soy products. In general, a diet with one daily serving of a product made from soybeans can help you to move away from a diet with too many omega-6s. The one soy product to stay away from at all costs: soybean oil. This is the oil I noted before that is found in virtually all processed foods.

Some things to remember about soy: cultures that have traditionally eaten soy products don't overload on them, and they tend to eat them in their natural form or fermented, which increases their health benefits. A Japanese miso soup with a few small cubes of tofu is quite different from a supposedly healthy American vegetarian diet with nonorganic, genetically modified soy protein isolate–based meat substitutes at every meal.

Processed soy products like soy protein isolate, textured soy, vegetable protein, and soy flour contain cheap ingredients that food companies use to add protein or enhance texture in all sorts of different foods. This processing can add huge amounts of isoflavones—estrogen-like structures that have been linked to infertility and altered ovarian function in animal studies—to food.[23] Soy protein isolate is of particular concern to vegetarians who regularly eat soy burgers, soy yogurt, and meat substitutes. If you do eat protein substitutes regularly, look for pea protein isolate over soy protein isolate. And favor organic and/or non-GMO soy protein isolate over nonorganic/GMO varieties. I really like the company Beyond Meat, which makes healthy and delicious meat substitutes. Their meatless ground beef crumbles look—and taste—like ground beef, and they're made from pea protein with no soy protein. Their other products are a blend of pea protein isolate and non-GMO soy protein isolate. Another one of my favorites: the vegan protein powder PlantFusion, which is also made from pea protein with no soy protein isolate. Pea protein contains a wide spectrum of amino acids, and it even contains higher levels of an amino acid that helps build lean muscle compared with the more popular whey powders.

EXPERT'S TIP: If you're a vegetarian, skip the cheap soy burgers made with nonorganic soy protein. Also stay away from veggie burgers made from blood sugar–spiking carbs, which can make you less resilient to stress while preventing deep sleep. Instead, get your protein from beans and sprouted grains, or make your own veggie burgers from black beans and chickpeas. You can also look for varieties with soy protein labeled organic or non-GMO.

Let's talk about the importance of choosing organic and non-GMO soy products. Nonorganic or non-GMO soy has one of the highest levels of pesticides of any nonorganic food; and if that weren't bad enough, over 90 percent of the soybeans in the U.S. are genetically modified.

The controversy surrounding GMOs—genetically modified organisms—could fill a whole book, so I will say simply that the only thing we do know is that we don't know how GMOs will affect human health, including the health of the brain, over the long term. And when it comes to soybeans, GMO versions are generally packed with pesticides. This is because soybeans are genetically modified to be immune to pesticides, so the crops can be sprayed without being killed. Not exactly what you had in mind when you ordered those "healthy" veggie sausages at breakfast this morning, is it?

There's also a big difference between different versions of soy. In general, favor fermented soy (e.g., tempeh) over nonfermented soy products (e.g., tofu), and favor whole soy products (e.g., tofu) over processed soy (e.g., soy protein isolate). The very best soy for both vegetarians and nonvegetarians is fermented soy, a category that includes tempeh, miso, natto, and tamari, all of which have potent anticancer properties in addition to their brain-balancing ones. Nonfermented soy—which includes all processed soy, like soy protein isolate, and textured vegetable protein—has antinutrient properties that can contribute to depression, weight gain, and fatigue. However, it's probably safe to eat a serving or two of soy protein that's labeled organic or non-GMO daily—especially when you're choosing it over factory-farmed animal products. It's clearly the lesser of two evils. Fermenting soy deactivates harmful, antinutrient processes, which is why I always choose tempeh over tofu at two of my favorite LA eateries: Veggie Grill and M Café. You'll learn even more about the power of fermenting foods as it relates to stress in the next chapter. While fermented soy like tempeh is the healthiest form of soy, whole soy in the form of tofu and edamame is your next-best choice, and these foods are fairly healthy when eaten in moderation.

SOY DOS AND DON'TS: A RECAP

- One serving of a soy food per day may help decrease stress and promote restful sleep.

- Fermented whole-soy products like tempeh, miso, and natto are better than processed soy products like soy protein isolate.

- Tofu and edamame, while not as healthy as fermented soy, are better than processed soy products like soy protein isolate.

- Organic or non-GMO soy products are better than nonorganic soy products.

Oils and Fats

There are three types of oils you'll find in my kitchen: extra-virgin olive oil, light olive oil spray, and virgin coconut oil. Olive oil has been proven time and time again in study after study to be the go-to oil for a variety of health benefits. Olive oil contains high amounts of the very best type of fat—*mono*unsaturated fat—which is associated with a healthier heart, fewer strokes, and less dementia. *Poly*unsaturated fats, saturated fats, and trans fats, which are a huge part of the standard Western diet, have been associated with a smaller hippocampus, which means a drained brain.[24] So healthier fats can help you deal with stress by preventing a shrunken brain, and they can also help you to sleep more soundly.

While olive oil is chock-full of beneficial compounds, many people misuse it by using the same type of olive oil for cooking as they do for dressings. Extra virgin olive oil isn't stable at high temperatures, so use it for dressings or cold salads. If you're going to heat it, look for olive oil that's labeled "light olive oil" or an ingredient label that reads just plain "olive oil." I love the Bertolli light olive oil spray for cooking. It's a great way to bring a little Mediterranean diet into your every meal—whether you're scrambling free-range eggs for breakfast or heating some frozen cauliflower rice for dinner.

Extra-virgin coconut oil is also safe to cook with occasionally, but there is more controversy about this oil because of the high level of saturated fat it contains. While it does have some health benefits, people with any history of cardiovascular disease may be safer sticking with olive oil. For drained individuals, a bit of extra-virgin coconut oil may potentially be helpful in improving digestion and improving the balance of good versus bad bacteria in your gut, which can help relieve anxiety (more on gut bacteria as it relates to anxiety in the next chapter). I consider it a treat in my kitchen. I use a teaspoon of it when I'm sautéing an Asian dish, and I use it to pop organic popcorn.

When it comes to other oils, there are some healthier replacements for industrial oils like soybean, corn, cottonseed, sunflower, or sesame oil. These include cold walnut oil since it contains high levels of omega-3s, macadamia nut oil, or—for high heat cooking—Malaysian palm fruit oil. The other widely available oil you'll find is canola oil, but this oil is highly processed. Despite the fact that it contains omega-3s and high levels of monounsaturated fat, which makes it similar to olive oil, these healthy fats are processed by heat which turns the omega-3s rancid while compromising the health benefits of its fats. You may not be able to detect the rancid flavor, since some food processors add deodorizers to mask the smell. GMO giant Monsanto produces genetically modified soy and canola products that are engineered to withstand high levels of pesticides, so canola oil is also dirty and should be avoided unless it's non-GMO and labeled cold- or expeller-pressed.

Again, nothing beats the health benefits of olive oil, but organic butter, ghee, or clarified butter, which have higher levels of omega-3s than conventional butter, can also be safe to eat from time to time. One recent analysis found that a tablespoon of butter a day did not have the health consequences we were warned against when it comes to this fat.[25] This is probably especially true for organic butter since it contains more omega-3s and also CLAs that can mitigate some of the heart risks associated with conventional butter.

Despite big food companies' deceptive efforts, soybean oil–based vegetable spread is not "heart healthy" nor is it healthier than butter. Soybean oil contains high levels of omega-6s. Margarine and vegetable spreads should have no place in a healthy diet. Neither should the low-calorie butter sprays I used to buy that are made with soybean oil. Say good-bye to the '90s when they thought low-fat foods were the way to better health. Now science has proven we can enjoy delicious, decadent olive oil. It will probably help you to lose weight despite its relatively high caloric content. Calories are not created equal. If it were that simple, diet soda and replacing all sugar with artificial sweeteners would help people lose weight. In reality, they're linked with weight gain.

Another note about oils: beware the word *vinaigrette*. A healthy vinaigrette is made with olive oil and vinegar, but many premade vinaigrettes are deceptively filled with sugar and draining omega-6s that crowd out balancing omega-3s. As you know, sugar and omega-6s can set you up for more stress and insomnia, whereas omega-3s set you up for restful sleep and less stress. If you're at the grocery store, read the ingredient label. You want a vinaigrette dressing that contains olive oil as the only oil and no sugar. At restaurants, avoid vinaigrettes since you can't read the label. Ask for vinegar and olive oil so you'll know what you're putting on your salad. I avoid conventional mayonnaise that's made with soybean oil. Favor mayonnaise made with all olive oil and no soybean oil. I also love Vegenaise made with expeller-pressed canola oil.

With just a few quick, easy, and delicious swaps, you'll feel less drained. Healthier proteins and fats are the building blocks of a diet that will help you cultivate balance—but they're not all that's required.

CHAPTER 9

Embrace the Power of Probiotics

My dad used to treat our home like an operating room. As a kid, I remember the latex gloves he kept all over the house and how I liked to use them as balloons. If you've ever seen *My Big Fat Greek Wedding* where the father thought Windex was the cure-all for everything from dirty windows to a skin rash, my dad had a similar obsession with Lysol. He loved to disinfect things, and there would be not one but three or four bottles in his bathroom. From his point of view, bacteria wasn't just gross; it was deadly, so he disinfected everything. When he was performing surgery, this was obviously essential, since bacteria entering the body could be life threatening, but at home?

Throughout my childhood and adolescence, he was always on the lookout for illness and prescribed antibiotics to me when he had any suspicion that something was coming on, which meant I was on antibiotics a lot. His intentions were good; they were rooted in fears about my health. In fact, there was one time where his liberal use of antibiotics probably saved my life. When I was 20, I was diagnosed with bacterial spinal meningitis the same week it killed several students at my university. Luckily my father had already put me on antibiotics days before, which kept the bacteria at bay. For years, this near-death experience actually fueled my own health anxiety. Like many of my patients, I had a genetic tendency mixed with an experience that drained me, and I succumbed to the pitfall thought pattern of pessimism. For years I wanted to go on antibiotics at the first sign of a runny nose.

However, much of the time, antibiotics aren't needed. In fact, according to the CDC, 30 percent of antibiotic prescriptions in the US aren't necessary. And overuse of antibiotics has actually created drug resistance, weakened immune systems, and an epidemic of unbalanced guts, which leads to a number of health issues, including brains that have been drained.

A WORLD INSIDE YOU

Inside each of us there is an unseen world that changes our lives in unimaginable ways. While you may instinctually think of illness when you hear the word *bacteria,* bacteria isn't necessarily bad. There is good bacteria and bad bacteria—and you have plenty of both lurking inside you. The bacteria in your gut make up a significant part of your body. In fact, the average human adult has about 1 kg—or about 35 ounces—of bacteria in their gut, with most of them taking up residence in the large intestine. This is roughly the same weight as your brain. You may hear this ecosystem in your gut referred to as your microbiome.

The good bacteria in your gut perform quite a lot of functions inside you. They help break down food. They help fight pathogens. They can even help prevent obesity.

We develop this inner ecosystem starting the moment we're born—picking up our mother's bacteria first and then dealing with everything and everyone else we come in contact with. Each interaction brings more types of bacteria into our lives—and our guts. This is important since the first few years of life are a critical period of development for the gut's ecosystem. The bacteria that the baby is exposed to sets off a response in the young immune cells that line the baby's gut. Immune cells respond by multiplying and changing. They even get "smart" through this interaction and travel through the body, and they teach other cells how to respond. They know what they're supposed to attack and what to leave alone. As the baby grows up, irritable bowel syndrome, allergies, and asthma become less likely since "smart" immune cells only attack bacteria and mutations.

But many of us have an ecosystem with high levels of bad bacteria and low levels of good ones. So how does your gut go bad? This also begins at birth. Vaginal delivery exposes a child to a mother's germs, which help an infant to start developing a healthy gut. But in the US, more babies are being delivered via C-section. And as modern moms become busier around the world, it's also common for infants to be fed with formula, which deprives the infants of breast milk and contact with their mothers' bodies—other things that promote good gut bacteria. Despite warnings about the dangers of excessive use of antibiotics, most American children have already been on three courses of antibiotics by age two. While the recommendation to physicians is now to prescribe antibiotics far less, our modern guts have often already paid the price from rounds of Z-paks and drugs that end with -*cillin*.

The irony is that many people who are anxious and shield themselves and their children from any bacteria, sterilize hands constantly, and insist on antibiotics at every turn may only be setting themselves and their children up for more—not fewer—health problems because of the effect this has on their microbiome.

The food we eat also enhances or ruins our gut bacteria ratio. Processed foods, artificial sweeteners, and a lack of fruits and vegetables can kill the good bacteria while strengthening the bad bacteria.

Growing up, our family meals consisted of a lot of processed foods. Between those and the artificial sweeteners in my drinks, I killed and disrupted what little good gut bacteria I had after multiple rounds of antibiotics. Not surprisingly, I frequently experienced anxiety and insomnia along with stomachaches and digestive problems. Sometimes the first sign that I was anxious about something wasn't a conscious thought; it was a stomachache. When I went through something stressful, my digestive symptoms would flare—sometimes leading to debilitating pain and discomfort—which led to psychological anxiety, which led to more digestive woes, including being diagnosed with gastritis, a condition associated with inflammation of the stomach lining. And so the downward spiral continued. During the worst times, I—like so many people around the world—turned to over-the-counter antacids and eventually a prescription proton pump inhibitor before turning to the natural strategies that now work wonders for me. This strategy has become increasingly important since 2016 research showed an association between proton pump inhibitors and a risk of dementia.[1]

The cause of another digestive ailment linked with drained brains—Crohn's disease—was discovered in 2016. High levels of bad bacteria interact with your *myco*biome: the fungus in your gut. They create a thin, slimy layer or "biofilm" that can adhere to different organs, including your intestines, which creates inflammation.[2] Thus steroids and immunomodulators used to treat Crohn's disease by keeping the immune system and inflammation at bay may just be managing symptoms when the "cure" will likely involve increasing the levels of good bacteria in your gut.

So as it turns out a little dirt can be good for you: playing outside, having a dog that brings in a little bit of outside, and eating leafy vegetables grown in the earth may help expose you to just enough of our natural environment. Washing your hands with regular soap and warm water is still an essential way to prevent the spread of disease, but it's not good to turn our homes into sterile bubbles where every germ is eradicated with our obsessive use of antibacterial soaps, alcohol-based sanitizers, prescription antibiotics, antibiotic-laden foods, and even toothpaste that contains the antibacterial agent triclosan. These all contribute to a disrupted gut. In 2016, the FDA finally banned antibacterial soap but not antibacterial agents in toothpaste, and the havoc that's already been done in our gut persists.

An unhealthy balance of good and bad bacteria doesn't just affect your gut; it wreaks havoc throughout your body, including in your brain. With less good gut bacteria, we are more likely to feel brain drained in its many forms: anxiety, insomnia, energy problems, and digestive woes.

YOUR SECOND BRAIN

Modern science is only beginning to realize how profound our gut is to our state of mental well-being, including our response to stress, risk of developing an anxiety disorder, or struggling with insomnia. It's no wonder our gut is called our second brain. Some scientists have even referred to our microbiome as a new organ. It's where the vast majority of one of your primary feel-good hormones—serotonin—is manufactured along with other vital neurotransmitters like stress-relieving GABA. And since developing an anxiety disorder makes you four times more likely to develop the leading cause of death worldwide—high blood pressure—these strategies that target both brain *and gut* are absolutely vital for psychological happiness, physical health, and yes, even your life itself.[3]

Psychiatrist Ted Dinan, who has been studying the connection between gut bacteria and the brain for years, refers to gut bacteria as *psycho*biotics instead of *pro*biotics because their effects are similar to psychotropic drugs like antidepressants and antianxiety medications. One of the first clues to this link between bacteria and mood was discovered almost 20 years ago. In 2000, floods contaminated the water supply of a small town in Canada with *E. coli* and *Campylobacter*. These bacteria caused physical illness in the residents immediately following the flood, but years later, many of them were diagnosed with drained brains thanks to high levels of bad gut bacteria that had taken up residence in their guts after the floods. Dr. Dinan began studying the gut bacteria of the patients in his own practice. He found that patients reporting mood symptoms like anxiety and digestive ailments like irritable bowel syndrome had guts that lacked a healthy, diverse colony of gut bacteria.[4]

So unbalanced levels of good and bad bacteria in your gut can cause anxiety, but this cause-and-effect relationship can run both ways. Being confronted with a stressful situation can lead to unbalanced levels of bacteria in the gut. When rats were exposed to moderate stressors like flashing lights at night a few times a day for six weeks, the levels of the good bacteria *Lactobacillus* were reduced.[5] Think about that for a moment. How many of *us* are voluntarily exposing ourselves to flashing lights on our iPhones at night when our circadian rhythms are telling us it's time to sleep? This is just one example of a modern stressor that may be negatively affecting our sleep—and thus affecting our gut bacteria levels. The stress hormone cortisol doesn't just make you feel stressed and exhausted; it can increase the levels of bad bacteria while reducing good ones. Cortisol also triggers the release of other chemicals that invade the gut's lining. This leads to intestinal permeability—a state that's often linked to irritable bowel syndrome, which allows harmful compounds to get through the protective wall, leading to even more harm to your health.[6]

Scientists are now using bacteriotherapy, which is the less unpleasant name for fecal transplantation, where stool from one person is transferred into the GI tract of another person. It may sound unpleasant, but it works. Scientists use bacteriotherapy to look at what changing the gut ecosystem does to anxiety and behavior. In one experiment, stool samples from human patients were transplanted into rats. The result: rats who had been exposed to the bacteria of people reporting anxiety and depression starting acting anxious. But those exposed to the bacteria of people who weren't anxious displayed no change in behavior.[7] One day, fecal transplantation may be a common way to treat anxiety and digestive disorders.

Another researcher studying rats and the effect of antibiotics that kill good gut bacteria found that many parts of the brain were negatively affected. This included many parts of the brain that are involved in feeling brain drained, including the amygdala and the hypothalamus. Brain drainers like cortisol went up, and balancers like serotonin went down.[8] A study in 2011 found that stripping rats of bacteria, which is something we do as humans when we take too many antibiotics or eat antibiotic-laden foods, led to cortisol spikes.[9] Our modern, barren guts may also be part of the reason so many people in the Western world are being diagnosed with mind-body conditions like Crohn's disease and autoimmune and inflammatory disorders.

Case in point: researchers from NYU examined the gut environment of tribe members in a remote region of the Amazon rain forest. Samples of their fecal matter were whisked back to New York City for analysis. The result: their guts had 50 percent more bacterial diversity compared with the average American. The reason: this tribe had never been exposed to antibiotics, and their diet is natural—free of the processed foods and artificial sweeteners that disrupt gut bacteria. One NYU microbiologist conducting the study noted that as cultures become more Western with more antibiotics and processed foods, there is a corresponding increase in chronic illnesses like Crohn's disease, IBS, and MS.[10] In light of other research linking psychological symptoms to bacteria levels, I would add to that list the corresponding epidemic of brain drain that plagues so many people. This epidemic is spreading around the modern world.

Another study compared children in urban Italy to rural African children. Like American children, kids in urban Italy eat a diet high in processed foods, refined grains, sugar, and factory-farmed animal protein. The African children ate diverse grains, vegetables, and beans. Again, the bacterial diversity was much lower in Italian children than in the African children.[11]

A healthy gut ecosystem can help you experience less stress throughout a busy day or trying ordeal, and it also plays a role in helping you sleep well at night. Good bacteria can increase the production of proteins called cytokines that act as chemical messengers. Cytokines modify levels of nitric oxide and growth hormone–releasing hormone (GHRH) which can help you to get restful sleep while maintaining healthy circadian rhythms.[12] In fact, research suggests that disruptions in circadian rhythms can disrupt the balance of good and bad bacteria in the gut.[13] A downward spiral can start to develop, because high levels of a bad bacteria in the gut are linked with more sleep problems and fatigue.[14]

Healthy bacteria are potent weapons against stress and insomnia because they have the ability to manufacture all your major brain-balancing neurotransmitters. These are the same neurotransmitters that antianxiety drugs like Xanax and antidepressants like Prozac aim to boost, but you can get them naturally through food. In fact, the natural form of GABA, sold as the dietary supplement PharmaGABA, is made from the bacteria *Lactobacillus hilgardii* which is used to ferment the probiotic-rich Korean cabbage dish kimchi. It releases GABA, albeit in a natural form, just like benzodiazepines like Xanax do. I find chewable PharmaGABA extremely helpful from time to time, and I can use it throughout the day without the zombie-like state that is the hallmark of addictive benzodiazepines. Let's take a quick look at the way three of your most important brain balancers are made in the gut with good bacteria:

- *Bifidobacterium* → GABA

- *Enterococcus* → serotonin

- *Escherichia* → serotonin

- *Lactobacillus* → acetylcholine, GABA

- *Streptococcus* → serotonin

So as you can see, a balanced gut is key to keeping your body—and your brain—in tip-top shape. The good news: We have the power to heal our disrupted gut every day by what we ingest. We just have to ditch processed foods while increasing our intake of probiotic-rich ones. Eat a wide variety of plant-based foods like vegetables, natural grains, and nuts. Also, only use antibiotics when you need them, choose stevia over artificial sweeteners, reserve alcohol-based sanitizers for occasional use when soap and water aren't available, and avoid toothpaste with the antibacterial agent triclosan.

PROBIOTICS OVER PROZAC

So now, let's look at how we build that good bacteria—eating probiotic-rich foods. I know it may sound too easy, but one of the most important parts of creating a healthy microbiome and balanced brain is eating probiotics daily. In 2013, the first human study proved that we can significantly reduce stress simply by eating yogurt, a probiotic-rich food—though not "light" yogurts, which are sweetened with artificial sweeteners, or those packed with added sugar. This UCLA study also proved the gut-brain connection isn't just a one-way street with the brain sending signals down to the gut; it's a two-way street where the gut can also send messages up to the brain.

In this study, women were divided into three groups. One ate yogurt with probiotics twice a day, one ate a nonfermented milk product containing no probiotics, and one ate no product. After one month, they performed brain scans on all the women. The women who ate yogurt twice daily had decreased activity in two parts of the brain that can leave people feeling drained—the insula and the somatosensory cortex—while also revealing the brain-balancing prefrontal cortex was more connected to other parts of the brain. When it comes to stress, the prefrontal cortex is vital since it can act as brakes on stress and anxiety. The women's brains weren't as "amped up" or "on edge"—like so many anxious minds are today—compared with the women who didn't eat probiotics.[15] Since the brain has a limited ability to store the serotonin precursor tryptophan, nutritional approaches like these are vital; the good bacteria in the gut can help manufacture serotonin from the tryptophan from food when the brain runs out.[16] This study was so groundbreaking that one of the authors of the study said it would lead to a whole new field of study to seek out more ways to prevent and even treat diseases like anxiety or IBS by specifically targeting this brain-gut connection.

Unlike benzodiazepines that relieve anxiety at the cost of sedation and dependence, probiotics may relieve stress while simultaneously making you sharper. In another study, subjects taking probiotics for a month were less anxious and even had an enhanced capacity to memorize material.[17] Talk about a win-win.

In the program section of this book, I'll help you to find natural sources of probiotics from yogurt and kefir to vegetable sources like fermented cabbage, along with some recipes to help you maximize the effects of probiotics to help you stress less and sleep soundly. You'll even learn how to make your own kombucha. You'll eat a different type of probiotic food every day. Like eating a variety of fruits and vegetables to get the wide spectrum of antioxidants and vitamins needed to relieve stress and insomnia, so it goes with probiotics. Even different brands of yogurt contain different types of probiotics, so even if you're someone who eats probiotics daily with your favorite brand of yogurt, it may be helpful to vary the probiotic-rich foods or even the brand of yogurt you eat from time to time. A secondary benefit: an analysis of 20 studies involving probiotics found that those people who ate a variety of different probiotics were more likely to lose weight.[18] Losing weight may then go on to help improve gut health even more, since people with lower body mass indexes tend to have healthier gut ecosystems.

Here is a list of some of the foods that contain probiotics:

- Buttermilk
- Cheese (soft varieties like Gouda, favor organic to also make sure you're getting more omega-3s)
- Dark chocolate
- Fermented milk (labeled sweet acidophilus milk)
- Kefir (dairy or coconut)
- Kimchi
- Kombucha
- Kvass
- Microalgae powder, including blue-green algae, chlorella, spirulina
- Miso soup
- Natto
- Pickles (though only the ones in the refrigerator section, not those stored on shelves in the open)
- Poi
- Sauerkraut (though only the ones in the refrigerator section, not those stored on shelves in the open)
- Tempeh
- Yogurt (make sure it doesn't contain artificial sweeteners that kill good bacteria or added sugar that negatively affects other parts of the brain)

While you can buy the probiotic-rich foods, I've listed above, there are also ways to make your own. Kefir is very easy to make, as are fermented vegetables like pickles and sauerkraut. If you start playing around with fermenting your own vegetables, there are endless options to create tasty, healthy treats at home, which is also great for vegans or those who are sensitive to dairy. I'll teach you some of these in the program section.

PREBIOTICS

There's another way to help improve your gut ecosystem besides just consuming foods with probiotics. Combine these with foods containing *prebiotics*. Prebiotics are essentially food for your good bacteria. So, once your gut gets the probiotics it needs, you need to make sure to feed them so they can multiply and thrive.

By definition, prebiotics are indigestible foods that stimulate the growth or activity of bacteria in the colon. Here are some of the best sources of prebiotics:

- Asparagus
- Banana
- Chicory root
- Dandelion Greens

- Garlic
- Gum arabic
- Honey
- Jerusalem artichoke
- Jicama
- Leeks

- Legumes
- Maple syrup
- Oatmeal
- Onions
- Red wine
- Wheat bran

PROBIOTIC BOOSTERS

Here's some other good news: the nutritional strategies you've already learned about in previous chapters also help to support a healthy gut ecosystem by acting as probiotic boosters. Foods like vegetables, fruits, beans, and high-fiber grains help create a gut environment where good bacteria thrive. Replacing sugar and flour with healthier foods like beans and vegetables doesn't just tame inflammation while supporting brain health; it has also been linked to more good bacteria in the gut. Researchers from NYU recently found an association between getting more fiber from beans, fruits, vegetables, and grains and higher levels of two types of good bacteria: Actinobacteria and *Clostridia*.[19] Diversifying your sources of fiber, like diversifying types of probiotics you eat, is important, since beans, fruits, vegetables, and grains were linked with increases of different types of good bacteria. Eating more fiber can also help you to stay slimmer, and this is vital since gut bacteria is healthier and more diverse in people with a lower body mass index.[20] In addition to preventing colorectal cancer, *Clostridia* have also been linked to the prevention of food allergies, can reverse peanut allergies in mice, and can even restore the permeability of the intestinal lining.[21] This could potentially undo damage that cortisol, which makes the intestinal lining permeable, has had on the digestive system. Of course, the strategies you will follow in this program, like eating seven servings of vegetables and whole fruits a day, more beans, and favoring quinoa over white rice, will help you to get the diverse forms of fiber that help good gut bacteria thrive which, of course, can help you feel less drained.

Another switch that will help your gut environment: getting rid of sugary sodas and diet drinks and replacing them with coffee, tea, or a nightly glass of red wine. All of the strategies in this program are designed to replace sugary, processed foods with natural foods with high levels of vitamins and antioxidants that relieve stress and promote sleep. Polyphenols are plant-based antioxidants found in some of nature's more delicious treats like dark chocolate, tea, coffee, wine, and grapes. In one study, black tea, red wine, and red grapes were shown to stimulate good bacteria in your gut.[22] Green tea also ups your levels of good bacteria while decreasing bad ones.[23] Drinking three cups of coffee a day can increase your gut's levels of the good bacteria *Bifidobacterium*, and high levels of this good gut bacteria can also prevent bad bacteria from moving into your gut.[24] If excess caffeine increases your levels of anxiety or makes sleep elusive, switch to decaf or half-caf coffee or tea that contains polyphenols but lower levels of caffeine like green, decaffeinated green, or white tea. For dessert, skip the sugary ice cream made from factory-farmed dairy and have a few bites of polyphenol-rich dark chocolate. Don't be fooled by the words *dark chocolate* on the front of a label. Make sure it also states that you're getting high levels of polyphenols by looking for brands that contain 50 percent or more cacao. The higher this number, the better. True dark chocolate will contain a number on the front or back of the bar, whereas commercial "dark chocolate" with high amounts of sugar and low levels of polyphenols won't. As you learn to appreciate the subtle richness of this natural superfood, you'll only need a few small squares to fulfill your craving as your taste buds recalibrate. When you fill your diet with the healthy fats and proteins in the modified Mediterranean diet, you'll feel fuller longer. You'll also be less tempted to eat sugary milk chocolate and other sugars that flood the brain with a short-lived surge of serotonin, because you'll be getting this soothing hormone naturally with a diet rich in probiotics, prebiotics, and probiotic boosters.

Of course, all of these healthy foods work together with another part of this program: exercise. Research has shown a group of athletes had more diversity in gut bacteria than a group who—despite being leaner—only exercised occasionally. And not surprisingly, men who didn't exercise *and* were overweight had the worst gut ecosystems of all three groups. This group also had more markers for inflammation.[25] We'll use the synergistic effect of foods along with other strategies in this program, like exercise, to restore your gut ecosystem back to its natural, stress-relieving glory.

CHAPTER 10

Jog for Joy

Mark was an accomplished, successful, and likeable man in his 50s. Until recently, anxiety, insomnia, and self-doubt were completely foreign concepts to him. His second marriage ended a few years ago, which was hard for Mark, but even more recently, a more acute and paralyzing dread had crept into his daily life. Work, an area of life usually marked by effortless success, had become more difficult. He had never taken medication before, but this new, crippling fear made two or three Xanax necessary just to make it through a typical day. The occasional Ambien Mark used to take only when traveling had become a nightly necessity.

Mark's stress, anxiety, and insomnia stemmed from complex layers in his life. He was still getting used to being single, and he was working on improving a strained relationship with his kids. He was coming to terms with the fact that there were younger, hungrier, and more successful people in his office. And his age meant that for the first time, he wasn't always the top dog—but he was still in the upper echelons of work, which meant high pressure, 80-hour workweeks, and frequent travel. Mark wasn't in terrible shape, but he certainly knew that he had begun to "let himself go." He was recently diagnosed with high blood pressure and had started to carry more weight in his midsection.

But for Mark, the biggest problem was the way his anxiety paralyzed him and made him feel out of control. It crept its way into Mark's bedroom in the morning as the sun began to peek through his curtains, and this anxiety was often joined by its emotional cousin: dread. This unfamiliar, somewhat unexplainable state made the emotions feel so much bigger than they really were. While busy, stressful days usually predicted more anxiety, sometimes easy days became "bad days" for no apparent reason. Sometimes he could white knuckle his way through with a few Xanax, but lately the anxiety would stop him in his tracks. He was routinely canceling meetings, dodging calls, and ignoring e-mails. Being drained was ruining his life.

Of course the biggest issue for Mark was the fact that work was the only way he measured his value as a human being—and he was beginning to see his work world change. This was going to be one long-term goal of our work together: we had to help him identify and embrace other areas of his life where he felt "good enough." But in the short term, we needed to figure out something to lower Mark's stress levels.

And so I prescribed a not-so-groundbreaking but oh-so-effective tool for him to use when he felt anxious: exercise. When he felt anxiety creeping in, his prescription was to take a walk around the block or a jog around the neighborhood. This would help to pull him out of the ruminative, wallowing state that was holding him back and sweeping him up into cyclones of anxiety. It helped prevent Mark from feeling out of control or feeling that "something just wasn't right" or that he "wasn't okay." Instead of stewing in his worry, he would take a contrary action—the opposite of what he instinctively *wanted* to do in that moment. By leading with the simple but meaningful action of a quick jog or even a walk, he changed his thoughts and feelings instead of allowing thoughts and feelings to dictate his actions or, in his case, a state of physical inaction. Mark learned that he had some control over his anxiety, and this eventually reduced anxiety since hope began to shine through the darkest of moments.

Chemically, exercise has the power to shut down cortisol spikes that can occur when we're paralyzed by anxiety. It also simultaneously boosts brain-balancing neurotransmitters like GABA and endorphins. Bonus: the more consistently we exercise, the more lasting and profound the boost in soothing neurotransmitters and larger the decrease in stress hormones.

Just a few weeks later, Mark was relieved when he started feeling significantly better. It may sound obvious, but to Mark exercise was profound because it helped him gain a sense of control over a feeling that made him feel powerless. Exercise didn't make the anxiety disappear completely, but it reduced it to a level where he was able to go about his day.

Exercise for Drained Brains

Exercise is one of the most potent tools to combat brain-draining stress and insomnia because of the chemicals it releases and the way it can actually help parts of the brain grow. You've likely heard of a "runner's high" and its euphoric, worry-free, and pain-relieving state. In 2008, this theory was proven for the first time. After scanning the brains of runners, researchers could see endorphins' effect on the prefrontal cortex and limbic area, two areas involved in the brain-drain process. This was not surprising, as the runners reported an increase in happiness and feelings of euphoria. The brain scans proved that the "runner's high" actually exists.[1]

More recently, science took an even closer look at this blissful response. Some scientists were skeptical that it was just endorphins responsible for a runner's high since these hormones have difficulty crossing the blood-brain barrier and thus getting to the brain. Sure enough: scientists found high levels of anandamide—also known as "the bliss molecule"—in the blood after exercise, and unlike endorphins, this molecule easily passes through the barrier and into the brain. The bliss molecule targets the brain's anxiety-relieving endocannabinoid system through exercise. This is the same system affected by marijuana, but you won't need a medical marijuana card to experience it—just a pair of sneakers. This helps us make even more sense of the runner's high and its profound ability to reduce anxiety, improve mood, and reduce pain.[2] Good news: runners don't have a patent on this high. You can also get a healthy dose of endorphins and anandamide on the elliptical trainer, in a boot camp, or from a power yoga class.

On top of these two feel-good brain-balancing chemicals, you'll also be rewarded with a hefty dose of brain-balancing GABA through exercising. Researchers measured levels of this neurotransmitter in people who exercised and compared their GABA levels to people who didn't exercise. The result? Exercisers experienced a measurable GABA boost about 18 minutes after exercising, and improvements were seen in the brain's limbic system, a part of the brain involved in emotions. But besides the short-term, measurable GABA boost immediately after exercise, researchers also studied the subjects' lives and exercise routines. They concluded that regular physical activity leads to *lasting* GABA boosts throughout the brain that can carry you through long work days and make it easier to transition into restful nights.[3] Remember: GABA is a neurotransmitter you can boost by popping a benzodiazepine like Xanax or Valium, but it can be released *naturally* and in a nonaddictive way through exercise. And unlike the benzodiazepines that have led to more and more visits *to* emergency rooms and overdoses these days, exercise keeps people *out* of them by preventing life-threatening diseases.

As your endorphins, anandamide (aka "the bliss molecule"), and GABA levels go up with exercise, brain-draining cortisol levels go down. In fact, you'll experience a truly huge reduction in cortisol levels by exercising regularly. People who were physically fit released a whopping 42 percent less cortisol throughout the day when compared with people who were unfit.[4] Being fit also helps protect your hippocampus. As you know, sugar and stress shrink this part of the brain, and so does being overweight. One study found that every two-point increase in body mass index (BMI) was linked with a 7.2 percent decrease in the hippocampal volume.[5] Of course, even healthy activities like exercise should be done in moderation since excessive exercise can actually spike cortisol levels. Done daily, about an hour is plenty to reap the rewards.

Exercise has also been shown to be a potent weapon against insomnia. Clocking just 150 minutes of exercise a week—an average of just over 20 minutes a day—was linked to a better night's sleep and feeling more alert during the day. This amount was associated with an incredible 65 percent improvement in sleep quality in the thousands of subjects in the study. People who got this much exercise were also 68 percent less likely to have leg cramps while sleeping and 45 percent less likely to have difficulty concentrating when they were tired. Just 20 minutes of exercise a day acts as a powerful alternative to Ambien that comes with a list of health benefits instead of a long list of side effects.[6]

Another study examined several different types of exercise to see if there was any difference in their ability to help you get restful sleep. The good news: All forms of "intentional" exercise in the study were associated with a lower likelihood of insufficient sleep including aerobics, biking, gardening, golf, running, weight lifting, yoga, and Pilates. People who regularly engaged in these activities were the most likely to sleep a restorative seven to eight hours a night. One surprising result: Being someone who walked a lot during the day was linked to some improvement in sleep quality, but it was the people engaging in *intentional* forms of exercise who were the most likely to get restful sleep. Just being physically active but in a nonintentional way like doing housework or engaging in childcare was actually linked to *less* restful sleep. So perhaps it's not just about the quantity of time you spend physically moving your body that helps improve sleep; the quality of that time and the headspace you're in matters as well. For parents, homemakers, or Manhattan businesspeople walking from meeting to meeting all day, this provides even more of a reason to add one precious hour of "you" time on a treadmill or in a yoga class. You're more likely to mindfully focus on the healing aspect of what you're doing in the present moment as you step out of the checklists that come with the grind of daily life.[7]

Just about any form of exercise you do has powerful brain-balancing effects. One review of several studies looking at the way exercise can help reduce anxiety found no difference between aerobic exercise (e.g., long-distance running, biking) and anaerobic exercise (e.g., interval training, sprinting, weight lifting). All types of exercise were effective at helping people feel less anxious, and this was especially true when exercise was added to other clinically proven treatments like cognitive behavioral therapy. Exercise even helped people with acute anxiety who were experiencing panic attacks or social phobia.[8] In fact, teaching oneself to tolerate physical sensations associated with exercise may act as a form of exposure therapy for people who experience panic attacks, and thus eventually make the attacks less likely to occur.[9] I recommend a gradual exposure to exercise for patients with acute anxiety or panic—starting with gentle exercise and then eventually moving to more intense forms like interval training. Slowly and surely, exposing yourself to moderate levels of stress hormones and physical sensations through exercise can help train your autonomic nervous system that it's able to rise and then return to baseline. Exercise has also been proven to be helpful for people who have been through trauma and have symptoms of post-traumatic stress disorder.[10]

While you'll start to reap immediate improvements in sleep and stress levels in just 10 or 20 minutes a day, you'll want to do more than just that for the greatest improvements in overall health and well-being. In fact, the average person needs to be spending *a lot* more time exercising. The CDC found that 80 percent of adult Americans aren't getting the recommended amounts of exercise. What's worse: even that minimum recommended by the CDC and World Health Organization is probably too low to really get significant health benefits. A 2016 study found the most significant improvements in health were found with 3,000 to 4,000 metabolic equivalent (MET) minutes of exercise per week. This number is about five or six times *more* than the World Health Organization's current recommended minimum of just 600 MET minutes and is much higher than the few hours a week of the CDC minimum. Your MET considers both the time you spend exercising and how strenuous the activity is. The current recommended minimum of 600 MET minutes per week, for example, would be achieved with either a 10-minute daily jog or a 21-minute daily brisk walk. This large analysis looking at 174 studies found that while there was a small benefit in people's physical health with this amount of exercise, significant reductions in major diseases were found with 3,000 to 4,000 MET minutes weekly.[11] The same is true for overall brain health.

You'll achieve some of your weekly MET minutes easily as you push your cart around the grocery store, walk to work, and do everyday chores. But you'll probably need to add a good 44 minutes on the treadmill or hitting the weights daily to reach that 3,000 to 4,000 MET weekly minutes to reap significant benefits in your health. By committing more time to exercise, you'll significantly reduce your risk of major illnesses like heart disease, diabetes, stroke, and cancer that become major sources of stress. Major illness was both the most commonly reported stressor and an especially troubling one with 60 percent of people in poor health reporting a "great deal" of stress according to a Harvard poll. So anytime you're preventing physical disease, you're also preventing yourself from becoming drained. On the days you don't have an hour to spare (a common complaint among busy, drained individuals), you can also use a type of interval training that only takes 10 minutes. You can also sneak in a few extra MET minutes by pacing during phone calls, taking the stairs, and choosing a parking spot that's far away from the grocery store entrance.

While *any* form of exercise you choose to do is beneficial in healing a drained brain, there are also some differences among particular types of exercise in the way they can reduce stress and insomnia. And while the best exercise is the one you'll actually do regularly, new research may make a case for varying your routine from time to time to reap the greatest benefits. You won't just be cross-training your body; you'll be cross-training your brain. Runners should do a little yoga. Sprinters should do some distance jogs. Yogis should do a few boot camps. And weight lifters should do some tai chi, because each one can relieve stress in unique ways by targeting different areas of the brain that contribute to feeling drained. So let's look at some of the different ways you can exercise.

SUSTAINED AEROBIC EXERCISE

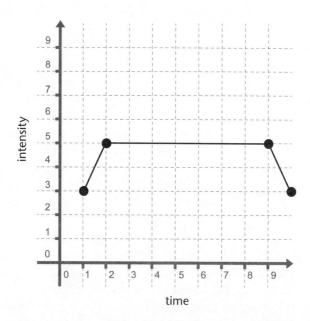

I have a confession to make: I used to hate sustained aerobic exercise like a long endurance jog or long hike on an easy incline. I used to think it was less effective than the interval training I could complete in a shorter amount of time or the yoga that was more enjoyable for me. Like many of you, I was also just doing what came easy. I've always been great at sprints but terrible at long endurance jogs. My body is genetically wired like a rabbit with fast-twitch muscle fibers; for others, endurance comes more easily. My exercise preference is also affected by my personality traits. My sensation-seeking, extroverted brain makes group interval training appealing and long jogs by myself seem boring. There's nothing wrong with focusing on your strengths, but there's also something to be said about addressing areas of weakness—especially when they can balance your brain in a unique way.

Now I've grown to appreciate a nice, steady pace from time to time. I'm glad I do, because science has shown that sustained aerobic activity is unique in its ability to increase the size of your hippocampus, which balances your brain. This type of exercise did this even better than interval training, and weight training didn't have this effect at all according to one study. Running, jogging, walking, aerobics classes, or any other form of sustained endurance increases brain-derived neurotrophic factor (BDNF), which is essentially stem cell therapy for your brain. Double or even triple the amount of new neurons have been shown to sprout this way. Improvements in this part of the brain are linked to less brain-draining anxiety.[12]

Of course this is good news for people who are stressed, have experienced trauma, or have eaten too much sugar throughout their lives since you now know how these shrink the hippocampus and thus leave you more vulnerable to stress. Instead of cracking open another bottle of beer or popping another Xanax, try a jog around the neighborhood, do 44 minutes on the elliptical trainer, take a long bike ride, or sign up for a Zumba class to help undo the damage that stress, unhealthy food, or trauma has had on the brain. As a preventive measure, this larger hippocampus will also make you more resilient and less likely to become drained in the future.[13]

Even better news: You won't have to wait months or years to start to feel an improvement. In fact, a simple walk or jog helps you to see the world in a more positive light in just 10 minutes. In one experiment, subjects were shown the dotted outline of a human. People with anxiety are more likely to perceive a neutral image as facing them since it's an indicator of threat. But after just 10 minutes of walking or jogging on a treadmill, subjects were more likely to judge the figure as facing away from them.[14]

This form of exercise is also quite soothing for many people and great for days you're feeling depleted. Sustained aerobic exercise isn't as likely to initially spike adrenaline, norepinephrine, and cortisol levels like interval training or weight lifting can, so it's a great type of exercise to choose when you're seeking immediate stress relief. A quiet afternoon jog or bike ride in nature can help you to shut off the worrying mind. So put on those running shoes or take that bike out of the garage this weekend. It will almost instantly shift your outlook and the way you see the world, and in the long term, your brain grows as your waistline shrinks.

INTERVAL TRAINING

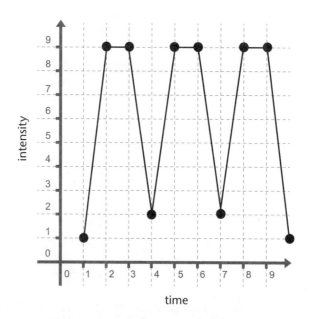

intensity / time

BENEFITS:

- less time-consuming

- more rapid improvements in physical health (e.g., reduction in body fat), which can lead to substantial and lasting decline in cortisol levels

- best at reducing high blood pressure, a life-threatening condition people with anxiety are much more likely to develop

Interval training is essentially working out for a short amount of time with bursts of extraordinarily intense exercise spliced between lower-energy movement. It's like seemingly impossible sets of box jumps or 11-mile-per-hour sprints done for a minute or two at a time. Group fitness classes around the world are using interval training to help people get into great shape in a short amount of time. I love them because they give you the "push" that's essential to power through the intense bursts of effort. I recently gave up my traditional gym membership and bought a membership at an interval training studio called

Training Mate. You get through those short moments of "I can't do this" and leave with a feeling of "I can, because I just did."

Strength training is often incorporated into interval training classes. For example, you may spend half the class on a treadmill or rowing machine and half doing weight-based resistance training. This is great because while 52 percent of adult Americans meet the aerobic activity guidelines, only 29 percent meet the muscle-strengthening minimum and, like other forms of exercise, weight lifting decreases symptoms of brain-draining anxiety and insomnia.[15] As we age, maintaining strength is vital since muscles tend to shrink as hormone levels decline.

Interval training has a few unique benefits that are particularly helpful in helping brain-drained individuals. You already know it's the second-best way to increase the size of the hippocampus after sustained aerobic exercise. The lead researcher who proved this link between aerobic exercise and neurogenesis in the hippocampus didn't discount other types of exercise. In fact, he hypothesized interval training or weight lifting probably leads to the creation of new connections between brain cells or different parts of the brain that we just haven't yet been able to prove through research. What we know now is interval training is number one when it comes to preventing and reversing hypertension, or high blood pressure. This is relevant for drained individuals, because anxious people are four times more likely to develop this condition. Hypertension is also something you want to address as quickly but safely as possible, because high blood pressure is the leading cause of death worldwide. While sustained aerobic exercise is also effective in addressing hypertension, research shows interval training is likely even more effective.[16]

Addressing high blood pressure through exercise has helped many of the patients I have treated who were particularly sensitive to the physical symptoms of anxiety. It helps you tolerate physical sensations while training your autonomic nervous system to follow the healthy pattern of a wave. What goes up can come gently and easily down. Done gradually, it can also be helpful for people who experience panic attacks. Interval training activates the sympathetic nervous system, and stress hormones are released. But remember: this short-term spike is the trade-off for long-term *reductions* in stress hormones. After a set of sprints, shortness of breath and a fast-beating heart don't mean you're having a heart attack; they're a normal response to exercise. For some people, interval training can be an alternative to benzodiazepines or beta-blockers, a class of medication sometimes prescribed to treat people who have more somatic, physical manifestations of anxiety. Unlike beta-blockers, which can interfere with restful sleep, exercise promotes it. And it's a good alternative to choose because beta-blockers have recently been linked to an increased risk of being hospitalized for a mood disorder, and benzodiazepines have led to an increasing number of ER visits and overdoses.[17] On the other hand, exercise prevents mood disorders and keeps you out of the ER.

Avoid intense interval training on days when you're feeling incredibly worked up or angry. On those days, take a yoga class or only hop on the treadmill after using one or more of the relaxation techniques I'll teach you. Here's why: being very upset and then engaging in intense exercise can triple the risk of a heart attack within the hour.[18] But don't avoid interval training altogether, because in the long run, it's one of the best things you can do to prevent heart attacks.

Interval training may also be effective in helping people to get fit more quickly, and this is vital. Remember: fit people tend to release less cortisol throughout the day and have more good gut bacteria that helps balance the brain. Compared with sustained aerobic exercise, interval training can burn fat more quickly. One study showed that in just seven sessions of interval training, whole body fat oxidation increased 36 percent.[19] With just three short 20-minute workouts a week, subjects burned subcutaneous fat more quickly than those doing sustained aerobic exercise.[20] Thus, this is a good type of exercise to use when you're short on time. It's also more effective at targeting the belly fat that we know is lethal.

Research has used different lengths of time for the "up" and "recover" lengths. You can try a version of these interval times used in research studies whether you're jogging; using weights; or on an elliptical, bike, rowing machine, or treadmill.

4 minutes high intensity, 2 minutes low intensity, repeat
2 minutes high intensity, 3 minutes low intensity, repeat
15 seconds high intensity, 15 seconds low intensity, repeat
8 seconds high intensity, 12 seconds low intensity, repeat

Looking at the numbers, you'll see some research has used long sets of high intensity with shorter low-intensity sets, shorter sets of high-intensity with longer sets of low intensity, and high and low intensity sets of equal time. You'll also see very long sets (e.g., up to 4 minutes of high intensity) and very short ones (e.g., as low as just 8 seconds of high intensity). The takeaway here is that there is no exact formula for the intervals; you just need a general up-down-up-down format throughout the workout. The length of the set will likely be determined by how difficult the activity is for you, since the point is to push you to your near-maximum potential during a high-intensity set. Again, check with your primary care physician or cardiologist to make sure there aren't any limitations before starting this or any other exercise routine.

No matter your fitness level, you can create your own interval-training routine. This can mean intermittent periods of a brisk walk alternating with a slower walk. For others, this can mean short sprints on a treadmill alternating with recovery jogs. Or you can take advantage of the interval programs on elliptical trainers or create your own with rowing machines. Weights can also be used for interval training with short bursts of maximum effort with periods of lighter intensity or cardio in between.

Interval training is a great choice on days when you feel like you're filled with energy. These workouts require brief physical bursts from your body. You may also find it easier to sleep after a grueling workout as your body will feel totally exhausted.

While most interval-training studies involve an up-and-down format for about an hour, 2016 research showed a type of interval training that may be particularly useful for busy and stressed-out individuals with even less time to spare. It's called sprint interval training. Lack of time is one of the most common reasons for not exercising regularly, so now you truly have no excuse. Sprint interval-training sessions are only 10 minutes long. Subjects who did sprint interval training three times a week for 12 weeks showed similar improvements in cardiovascular and metabolic health as the subjects who did traditional interval training. The amount of time saved was significant. The sprint interval-training group's workouts were 10 minutes, whereas the traditional interval-training group's workouts were 50 minutes. Here's a sprint interval-training format:

1. 2 minutes of warm-up with light activity

2. 20 seconds of an "all out" sprint

3. 2 minutes of light activity

4. 20 seconds of an "all out" sprint

5. 2 minutes of light activity

6. 20 seconds of an "all out" sprint

7. 3 minutes of cooldown with light activity

As you can see, there's only one total minute of intense work—three 20-second bursts—within the short, 10-minute workout. The researcher from this study also proves how tiny bursts throughout your day—like taking the stairs after lunch—can have a real effect on your overall health. The takeaway: any type of interval training can be healing for both mind and body.[21] Again, you can use a version of this with different types of workouts. If there's a choice between no workout today and this 10-minute workout, choose this one! I use it when I'm traveling and find it a great mini-workout in a tiny hotel gym. It can be part of your workout arsenal that can help you improve your fitness level, which can lead to lower levels of brain-draining hormones and higher levels of brain-balancing neurotransmitters. But remember: cross-training mind and body with a varied routine will give you the most stress and insomnia-relieving benefits.

MEDITATIVE MOVEMENT

BENEFITS:

- immediate reduction in brain drainers like adrenaline and cortisol

- immediate boost in brain balancers like GABA and serotonin

- immediate and safe reduction in blood pressure for people of all levels of physical fitness

- thickens the layers of the cerebral cortex in the brain, which helps us remain open to doing things in new ways, a key component in resilience and stress reduction

- some forms improve balance, which can reduce fears of falling

- physical improvements like weight loss combined with psychological improvements like stress reduction

- can improve quality of life for people living with mind-body conditions

I fell in love with yoga during my first class. I would drive 10 miles to take my favorite yoga teacher's classes in Santa Monica. (For those of you who don't live in Los Angeles, 10 miles means allowing for an hour or more with traffic each way.) While challenging your body, stretching muscles, and improving balance, you simultaneously strengthen your mind. Putting your mind's focus on your breath and body is a mindfulness-based practice. The whole process can take on a meditative quality.

The improvements in both mind and body become evident with just a few months of occasional practice, and the benefits seem to be particularly potent for those people who are chronically stressed. A study examined yoga's effects in a group of chronically stressed women. Half of them received no treatment, and the other half of the women received yoga classes. The classes were just 60 minutes, and they did them twice a week for a month. The improvements in the body included increased flexibility and a decrease in waist circumference. The improvements of mind included decreased levels of stress and more positive mood states.[22]

Yoga also provides stress relief that is more immediate and reliable than other forms of exercise. One study measured subjects' mood after three sessions of either yoga, body conditioning, swimming, or fencing. Only subjects taking the yoga class reported less anxiety, tension, depression, anger, and fatigue at the end of *each* class they took.[23] Different forms of yoga have been shown to be effective in reducing symptoms of OCD, phobias, and test-taking anxiety.[24]

Yoga may be even more effective than drugs in reducing anxiety. One study divided patients diagnosed with anxiety into two groups. One took the benzodiazepine Valium, while the other group did 40 minutes of yoga a day for three months. Yoga led to a greater reduction in anxiety even when compared with a hard-hitting (and addictive) drug. The overall improvement was 76.7 percent for the yoga group compared with 50 percent for the Valium group. Furthermore, a small subset of the yoga students were effectively "cured" and became symptom free after three months of practice; none of the subjects taking Valium became symptom free.[25] Another study compared six weeks of yoga to the benzodiazepine Librium and amitriptyline, an older antidepressant that is so sedating that it's sometimes used today to treat insomnia. Yet again yoga led to a greater reduction in anxiety even compared with these two heavy-hitting drugs.[26] Yoga also has been shown to increase GABA levels. One study found a boost in GABA levels after just one 60-minute yoga session.[27]

While yoga falls under the "meditative movement" category, some forms of yoga incorporate cardiovascular or interval-training elements. While traditional hatha yoga classes or energy-shifting kundalini classes don't typically burn a lot of calories, I've been to some power yoga classes that were so intense I sweat more than I do in boot camps. Others have incorporated bursts of effort that were so intense we would take a rest in child's pose between sets. I like power yoga because it's "two birds" with one workout. Your mind is meditative and learns to be calm while your cardiovascular system is challenged and revs your metabolism.

Other clinically proven meditative movements for drained brains include Qigong (sometimes referred to as or spelled Qi Gong, Chi Kung, or Chi Gung) and Tai Chi (sometimes referred to as or spelled Taiji, T'ai Chi, T'ai Chi Chuan, Taijiquan). One study looked at the effects of Qigong on people with high blood pressure, a condition common in people with untreated brain drain. After 10 weeks of Qigong, blood pressure decreased significantly. The bonus: all three of the major brain drainers—adrenaline, norepinephrine, and cortisol—went down.[28] Another study had subjects attend two Tai Chi classes a week for three months. Then they were given a mock job interview. The subjects who did Tai Chi reported 41 percent less stress.[29] One study compared Tai Chi to meditation, walking, and reading in its ability to help people recover from stress after a series of difficult tests and challenges. All four activities led to reductions in cortisol and improvements in mood, but Tai Chi led to greater reductions in adrenaline and blood pressure.[30] For people experiencing physical manifestations of brain drain, Tai Chi could be a great match. As we age, balance becomes more important in preventing falls. Like yoga, Tai Chi addresses balance, which is why research has shown that it decreases the fear of falling in older people.[31]

THE JOY OF MOVEMENT

As you can see, exercise—and movement in general—are good for the body and mind. Science has shown time and time again that the body was built to move. It's at its peak when you get up and get going, not only because it releases feel-good chemicals but also because it keeps your thoughts in the present moment, distracting you from many of the pitfall thought patterns we discussed in Chapter 3. The same is true for energy-based cognitive therapy.

CHAPTER 11

Shift Your Thoughts with Energy-Based Cognitive Therapy

Melanie experienced high levels of anxiety in her romantic relationships. Despite being successful and beautiful, Melanie sometimes felt incredibly insecure. Anytime a boyfriend didn't text her back immediately, she would imagine the worst-case scenario. She had no reason to suspect that her current boyfriend was cheating, but two of her ex-boyfriends had. Melanie's father left her mom for a younger woman when Melanie was a little girl, which spawned a deep-rooted belief that men can't be trusted.

Melanie's love life affected every area of her life. When her relationship was going well, she was a rock star at work. When it wasn't, she called in sick, missed deadlines, and forgot about meetings. A disagreement with her boyfriend would consume her, leaving her unable to do anything but worry about the problems in her love life. During these rough patches, her usually healthy confidence would take a nose dive. What was incredibly confusing and frustrating for Melanie was that logically she *knew* when she was being irrational. Despite that, she couldn't stop the emotional tsunami once it began.

"I can actually *hear* myself acting crazy," she said to me with tears in her eyes, "and yet, it's like I don't know how to stop the 'crazy train' once it's left the station."

"I can see how much you *want* to change this, but I have a feeling the surge of stress hormones makes it hard for you to act rationally. I also see how scary this is for you," I said.

"It is," Melanie said, "and confusing . . . and hopeless . . . How am I so together in other areas of my life but such a mess in my love life?"

In our next few sessions, I helped Melanie gain insight that helped her link the unconscious root of her trust issues and relationship difficulties. We discovered forgotten memories of her childhood when her father left, and this helped her feel less confused about why she reacted so strongly today. Connecting the dots often helps people understand and thus respond in a less reactive way. It helped Melanie to remain calmer, but she still needed some tools to deal with her "crazy train."

The first step was to help Melanie identify the pitfall thought patterns that were problematic in her relationships. For Melanie, the three most frequent pitfall thought patterns were pessimistic thinking, pervasiveness, and personalization.

Melanie was *pessimistic* when she considered the worst-case scenario after her boyfriend didn't text back after 45 minutes (e.g., maybe he's cheating on me and going to leave). *Pervasiveness* affected her when she allowed her love life to negatively affect different areas of her life (e.g., I'm not going into work today because of the fight we had last night). *Personalization* reared its ugly head when she pinned something not going right in her relationship on not being good enough (e.g., he hasn't proposed yet; it's because I'm not pretty or interesting enough).

Because Melanie got flooded with stress hormones as a result of fear, the effects could be seen in her body as well as her mind, so we turned to an exciting practice called energy-based cognitive therapy (EBCT).

CONTROLLING MIND AND BODY

In traditional cognitive behavioral therapy (CBT), I help patients to identify and change the seven pitfall thought patterns that we talked about in Chapter 3:

1. **Paralysis-analysis:** This type of thinking involves stewing and ruminating in anxious thoughts, preventing productive action from occurring.

2. **Permanence:** This type of thinking falsely assumes that just because something is a problem now, it will always be a problem.

3. **Personalization:** This type of thinking places the blame entirely on yourself for something not going your way.

4. **Pervasiveness:** This type of thinking allows something that is affecting one area of your life to spread to all areas of your life.

5. **Pessimistic:** This type of thinking considers the worst-case, catastrophic scenario. It dwells in the possible—not the probable.

6. **Polarized:** This type of thinking has a binary, black-or-white pattern. The words *always* or *never* are frequently found in this type of thought pattern.

7. **Psychic:** This type of thinking expects people around us to read our minds without us verbalizing what we need.

To stop these stress hormone–inducing thoughts in the tracks, energy-based cognitive therapy incorporates poses and postures from yoga and meditative movement. These physical movements change the flow of energy in the brain and body, and they can help people who get stuck in these negative feedback loops of stress and worry to disengage from them. A recent study had people hold a chopstick in their mouths while putting them through stressful tasks. Those who held the chopstick in a way that forced the facial muscles into a smile recovered more quickly.[1] Bodily based movements are helpful for drained-brain individuals, because their bodies tend to be as tense as their minds.

In these people, the sympathetic nervous system has become overly dominant. Heart rate is elevated, palms sweat, and thoughts race. A good stretch with calmer breath helps to disengage this fight, flight, or freeze response in the body, and the simultaneous cognitive reframes loosen the grip of pitfall thought patterns in the mind. This helps tilt your autonomic nervous system from a sympathetic-dominant state to a parasympathetic-dominant one. As a result, you move from fight, flight, or freeze to a calmer rest-and-digest state that's associated with more rational decision making and feeling like your best self. Stress hormones go down. Feel-good ones go up. You begin to glide through the challenges of your life with ease.

To bring EBCT into your life, it's a matter of following six simple steps:

Step 1: Identify your pitfall thought patterns.
Step 2: Use a physical pose as an antidote.
Step 3: Find the contrary evidence.
Step 4: See the right action you'd like to take.
Step 5: Revisit your brain-draining worries.
Step 6: Turn right action into your reality.

Let's look at bit more closely at what is involved in each step.

Step 1: Identify Your Pitfall Thought Patterns

Which of the seven pitfall thought patterns leave you feeling brain drained? (Go back to page 31 if you want to review examples of what these may sound like.) For many, there are a few pitfall thought patterns that tend to show up more than others. People who tend to be logical, left-brain thinkers tend to get trapped in polarized thinking, because their brains already use a black-or-white framework in the way they perceive the world. When they feel stressed out, they can become increasingly rigid, which can be problematic. Those who have recently gone through difficult times and feel hopeless may find more pessimism showing up. People who have a family history of anxiety may have lower than average levels of serotonin and GABA, making paralysis-analysis and its ruminative patterns likely. In the brain, neurons that fire together wire together. This means these thought patterns and their outcomes begin to feel normal and even automatic if you've been using them for a long time. They become your everyday reality.

Identify which three of the seven pitfall thought patterns prevent you from dealing with stress in a healthier way. Then write down the way your pitfall thought patterns sound in your head as your personal brain-draining worries. Figuring out which patterns and beliefs normally affect you will help you spot them when they take over.

Also rate how true each worry feels to you right now. If it feels like a worry is absolutely true with no chance that you could be wrong and will stay this way, write 100 percent. If you feel like this worry feels true, but some rational part of you knows it likely isn't, perhaps you'll write 50 percent. If this worry haunts you on bad days but doesn't feel all that true on most days, perhaps you'll write 25 percent. For example, when you use the pitfall thought pattern *permanence*, it feels like something you are going through right now is here to stay. If you have absolutely no hope that things could ever get better, you would write 100 percent. If you have a tiny glimmer of hope that things could get better, perhaps you'll write 95 percent. If you're mostly hopeful that things will change but still struggle from time to time, perhaps you write 25 percent next to the worry.

Here's an example of what this might look like:

THE THREE PITFALL THOUGHT PATTERNS THAT AFFECT ME THE MOST ARE: *pessimistic*, *permanence*, and *personalization*.

THEY LEAD TO BRAIN-DRAINING WORRIES THAT SOUND SOMETHING LIKE . . .

- BRAIN-DRAINING WORRY 1: I'm not okay. Something is very wrong with me. I know it. (HOW TRUE: 80%)

- BRAIN-DRAINING WORRY 2: This stress is never going to let up. I'm never going to feel better. (HOW TRUE: 99%)

- BRAIN-DRAINING WORRY 3: I'm not good enough. People leave me because something is wrong with me. (HOW TRUE: 50%)

Now write down which three pitfall thought patterns affect you the most below—or if you don't want to mark up your book, write these out in a journal:

THE THREE PITFALL THOUGHT PATTERNS THAT AFFECT ME THE MOST ARE: _____, _____, and _____.

THEY LEAD TO BRAIN-DRAINING WORRIES THAT SOUND SOMETHING LIKE . . .

- BRAIN-DRAINING WORRY 1: _____

  (HOW TRUE: ___%).
- BRAIN-DRAINING WORRY 2: _____

  (HOW TRUE: ___ %).
- BRAIN-DRAINING WORRY 3: _____

  (HOW TRUE: ___%).

Now that you've identified what you're likely to worry about, it will be much easier to start noticing, in the moment, when these thought patterns pop up. When they do, strike a pose.

Step 2: Use a Physical Pose as an Antidote

In traditional CBT, you learn techniques like picturing a stop sign when you notice pitfall thought patterns. Brain-drained individuals will benefit from physical poses because they help to interrupt the feedback loop of worry. As you know, stress and insomnia cause tension in the *body* as well as the *mind.* These EBCT poses ease tension while simultaneously boosting feel-good hormones that brain-drained individuals lack.

Each pitfall thought pattern has an antidote based in a physical move or pose. This is where the "energy" in energy-based cognitive therapy comes into play. If you consciously use a pose that physically embodies confidence, your brain will release feel-good hormones that will make it easier to *feel* confident and let pitfall thought patterns go. While I have suggested specific poses for each of the seven pitfall thought patterns, feel free to mix and match if one or more poses resonates in your mind and body. My favorite is the "half smile" antidote for a physical pose you can use anytime to disrupt the pitfall thought patterns. Each of these poses embodies positive energy states and relaxation, so feel free to learn and use all of them. Advanced yoga practitioners can experiment with other poses they'd like to use as physical antidotes. I've also suggested more discreet versions of all the poses to use in public places. After you've used the full pose at home, another option is to simply close your eyes and *imagine* your body is in this pose. This will allow you to take action even when you're sitting in the middle seat on a crowded plane.

Take the first brain-draining worry you wrote down in the last section and use the physical pose that corresponds with it.

1. Paralysis-Analysis → Tree Pose: When your mind enters that ruminative, obsessive, and worrying state I call paralysis-analysis, your brain has become stuck in a loop. Neurochemically, paralysis-analysis is like a needle that keeps replaying that one groove on a broken record. Unlike the productive outcome associated with critically thinking about a problem or engaging your imagination to seek new ideas, paralysis-analysis doesn't produce constructive or helpful solutions. Ask yourself if your line of thinking is going to *change* anything. If not, then you're not critically thinking and finding solutions; you're stuck in paralysis-analysis.

Grounding yourself to the earth taps into the faith the worrying mind has forgotten about. Paralysis-analysis is rooted in a belief that you're not going to be okay. Begin by standing with your feet shoulders' width apart and your toes facing forward. Your arms are relaxed at your sides with the palms facing forward. Now place the sole of one foot on the opposite leg—above or below the knee (not directly on the knee because this can hurt you). If this is difficult, you can place the foot on the opposite ankle while keeping the toes on the ground for support. Once you're grounded, feel the earth supporting you. Know that the universe has a way of supporting you just as gravity keeps you rooted to the earth without you having to consciously do anything. This helps turn off the ruminative worry that is rooted in the belief that you're not going to be okay. In this moment, acknowledge that you already have everything you need. If you're breathing, there's infinitely more right with you than wrong with you. Feel that energy, because you're already embodying it.

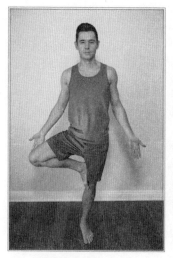 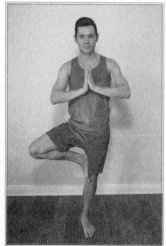

Now connect yourself to God, spirit, or your highest self. Place your hands in prayer position in front of your heart. Or take your arms up and feel the energy of God, spirit, or your highest self move through your mind and body to infuse you with a sense of faith in the world. Remain as still as you can, because stillness is the opposite of the ruminative, churning mind.

When you need a discreet version of tree pose, simply place the sole of your foot on the other foot while you're sitting in a meeting. Feel your connection to the earth like a tree rooted in soil. You can add a simple and discreet posture with your hands to this pose. Touch your thumbs to your middle fingers, and face your palms down to ground you in faithfulness and the feeling of being supported. Then flip your palms toward the sky to connect you to God or spirit. Be an open conduit for divine energy while also giving thanks for what you already have.

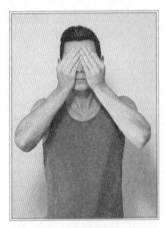

2. Permanence → Eye Cupping: When permanence rears its ugly head, it's difficult to consider the light at the end of the tunnel. It's as if you've become blind to the future. To remedy this, begin by warming your hands by rubbing them together. Physically, this heat generates relaxation in the muscles. As you rub them more and more quickly, attune to the sensation of heat that reminds you of the ever-changing nature of our universe. Also let it remind you that you have the power to change your present state. You can change the temperature of your hands in the same way that you can change how your mind is operating in the present moment. And you have the power to create a future that is different from your current state.

Once you perceive warmth, place your hands over your eyes. Cup your hand so that it's like placing an oval-shaped bowl over each eye. Allow the warmth to relax the muscles around your eyes and the tense facial strain associated with the bleak and weary state of permanence. With your eyes closed, imagine this pose is magically creating a crystal ball where you can gaze into the hope of your best future. See your best-case scenario future. This will turn off the permanence associated with stagnation and hopelessness.

This pose can be done easily at your desk and can help heal the physical strain associated with staring at a computer as well as the mental weariness of permanence. If you'd like, you can use a discreet version of this pose by simply closing your eyes for a few moments.

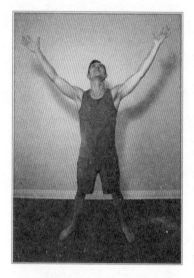

3. Personalization → Star Pose: When a runner crosses the finish line first at the Olympics, you'll often see the athlete embody a spontaneous star pose in the middle of the field. The arms go up, and the head turns upward to the sky.

While standing with your feet in a wide stance, raise your arms up into the air. Your arms and legs form an X shape. Keep your toes and palms facing forward. Turn your head toward the sky. Pay attention to the confidence and the feel-good hormones that naturally surge through your body when you embody this pose.

When you're at work, you can use a discreet version of star pose sitting at your desk. Yawn and stretch your arms toward the sky. Allow this pose to help you remember all the ways in which you are innately worthy.

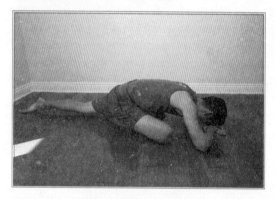

4. Pervasiveness → Pigeon Pose or Shoulder Shrugs: When pervasiveness takes over, it's difficult to prevent stress from bleeding into other areas of your life. When life hands us the most difficult circumstances, we often need to do the *exact opposite* of what our default inclination urges us to do. When we're sad, we tend to isolate ourselves or self-medicate. Seeing friends or going to the gym may be the last thing we want to do when we're not feeling our best. And yet these activities are more likely to help you to feel better than eating a gallon of ice cream alone on the couch while binge-watching TV.

Letting go of the stress we feel in the present moment can help us to move on to the next moment of our lives with a fresh and open mind. We are more able to receive everyday miracles that result from a conversation with a friend or colleague.

We tend to hold tension in our hips as we move and go through days marked with stress. Let go of this tension with pigeon pose. On a mat or soft carpet, place one leg folded in toward you with the other leg straight behind you. The more flexible you are, the more you can increase the angle of the bend in the front leg. Relax here for a few moments before moving on to the opposite side. As the tension you've been holding in your hips dissolves, notice how mental stress dissolves with it. See them melting into the earth. Letting go of this stress can help you find the equanimity you need to move forward in life with grace.

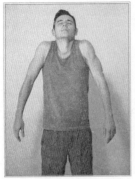
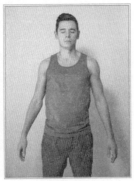

If you need a discreet version of this in the middle of work, do some shoulder shrugs. Pull your shoulders up toward your ears, and then allow them to fall down. Inhale as you bring the shoulders up, and exhale as they come down. Repeat. As they fall, imagine they are taking any physical or mental tension you may be carrying with you.

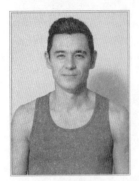

5. Pessimistic → The Half-Smile: When pessimistic thinking drags you down, you focus on the worst possible outcome. You consider the *possible* instead of the *probable*, and chances are, the worry is evident in your face and brow. Remedy this by putting a half-smile on your face. With your lips turned up, a slight smile in the eyes, and a brow that's relaxed, your brain can more easily consider the *what's right* in your life instead of the *what's wrong* or *what could go wrong*.

The half-smile is an easy-to-use antidote at any time. It's discreet. You can use it at work or on a plane. The half-smile can be added to other poses and to help remedy other pitfall thought patterns. See what changes when you adopt a half-smile for a full day. Notice if you feel differently when you put a half-smile on your face while walking into a stressful meeting. Notice how it helps you to see the bright side more easily.

6. Polarized → Spinal Twist: Polarized thinking is marked by a lack of flexibility. It's rigid and binary, and it fails to consider the 2,000 different shades of gray that lie between pure black or pure white. Remedy this with a spinal twist that can help you remain open to possibilities.

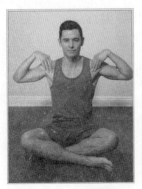
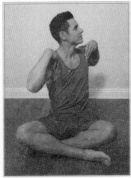
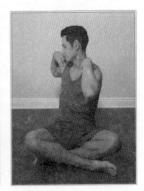

If you're flexible and at home, do the full spinal twist. Grab each shoulder with the thumb in back and the fingers in front or claw each shoulder with your fingers. Now, twist to the left on the inhale as you twist to the right on the exhale. Try to make the exhale slightly longer than the inhale, and breathe into the belly. Do this 26 times. As you go from side to side, see the entire expanse of what's around you. Notice what's in the middle. And with an open mind and heart, consciously consider all options you have in front of you to choose from. This will help you find compromise within yourself and with others.

There are a few discreet options if you need to use a spinal twist when you're at a desk or sitting at a dinner table. Simply do a few head rolls in both directions. Or use your chair and hands to help you gently twist your spine in both directions.

7. Psychic → Chest Thump: You probably remember Tarzan's signature chest thumping and signature yell: Ahhh-ayyy-ayyy-ahhh! Gorillas thump themselves to boost their own confidence while reminding others of their strength. There is an inherent power in this action. It reminds us of our courage, and it can help us reclaim our voice.

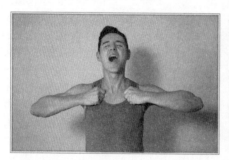 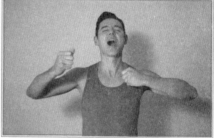

With closed fists, thump on your chest above the breastbone. You can use both hands or just one. As you lightly beat, open your mouth and let out a soothing "Ah . . ." breath. Or try letting out a laugh or even a roar. Let this physical action help remind you of your inherent power. What you have to say matters. Tarzan let the whole jungle know he was on his way. You don't have to yell like a savage, but it is vital to verbalize your point of view in a calm yet confident way. Let the out breath facilitate the movement of thoughts in your head

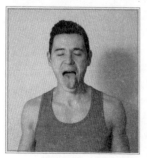 into the world. You offer a valuable point of view to the world, just as others have their own unique take. May the meeting of these differing thoughts help us learn and grow in our relationships with others. For a discreet version of this, use a version of Lion's Breath. Take a deep breath in, and sigh it out with your tongue sticking out toward your chin. As you sigh, imagine that the valid thoughts, feelings, and opinions you keep to yourself are beginning to make their way out to the world where you will be more likely to communicate them to others.

Step 3: Find the Contrary Evidence

While in these physical poses, consciously think of *contrary evidence* from knowledge and experience you already have in your life that proves your fears and anxieties to be irrational, alarmist, or flat-out wrong. This strategy is a cornerstone of modern cognitive behavioral therapy, but it is also an ancient energetic practice. Yogis may know the technique by the name *prakti paksha bhavana* as described in yoga sutra 11.33: creating a counteracting, positive thought to neutralize unwholesome ones. The physical poses of EBCT actually allow the brain to more easily access contrary evidence because of the psychological phenomenon called mood-congruent recall. When you have a half-smile on your face or enter star pose with your body, positive information "lights up" in the brain, which means you can access a happy memory more easily and quickly.

Here's an example of using contrary evidence as an antidote to a pitfall thought pattern: BRAIN-DRAINING WORRY (*personalization*): "After going through my divorce, I've decided something is wrong with me. I'm unlovable. I'm clearly not capable of staying in a relationship. I'm so weak." HOW TRUE: 100 percent. → CONTRARY EVIDENCE (while in star pose to physically help you access affirmative thoughts): "There are so many reasons why my husband and I got divorced. While there are things I need to work on, there are also things he could have done better. Both of us were at fault. Also, maybe we just weren't the right fit for each other. I have been in two long-term relationships. They fell in love with me, so I must be lovable. I am kind. I am beautiful. I'm a great mom. Maybe I'll take the lessons I've learned in my marriage into my next great relationship."

Step 4: See the Right Action You'd Like to Take

While continuing the pose, the next step is to see the action you'd like to take next. Since your body is in a pose that embodies calm confidence, and your mind has already proven your fear wrong, it will be easier to see clearly. Picture the action you'd like to take in your life in your mind's eye.

Here's an example: RIGHT ACTION: "My best friend has been trying to set me up with his colleague. I'll say yes. I'm going to act and feel more confident, talk to people more, and set up an online dating profile. I can see myself happy again. I see myself laughing."

Step 5: Revisit Your Brain-Draining Worries

Transition out of the pose gracefully as you return to your present life. Retain the energetic shifts as you return to the worry that held you back. Now that you've used a physical pose, reflected on the contrary evidence, and seen the right action you'd like to take in your mind's eye, see if the degree of belief has already started to change. Have you found even 1 percent more hope than you had before?

- BRAIN-DRAINING WORRY 1: _____
  (HOW TRUE: ____ %).

Now go back to the other brain-draining worries you wrote down. Repeat steps 2 to 4 for these worries, and see if they feel just a little less true now.

- BRAIN-DRAINING WORRY 2: _____
  HOW TRUE: ____ %).

- BRAIN-DRAINING WORRY 3: _____
  HOW TRUE: ____ %).

Step 6: Turn Right Action into Your Reality

For many people, these steps have already reduced how much they believe their worst brain-draining worries. If they haven't changed yet, that's okay. In fact, the most potent part of EBCT is taking the action that you have seen in your mind's eye and applying it in your life. It may not happen overnight, but you will eventually be rewarded when you move through your life with optimism and faith.

In the beginning, it may feel like you're feigning confidence that's not really there yet. You may feel like you're acting "as if" you're someone who believes you'll find love again or that great job. "Fake it until you make it" can be a great way to eventually help you to feel more authentically confident.

Watch and notice how these actions help you slowly change your worries and anxieties. Notice how they begin to balance and replenish your drained brain. When you are recovering from a divorce, it may take years to fully believe that you'll find love again. But when you continue to apply the *right action* you see in your mind's eye, you'll eventually love. You'll get that job. When you're having a tough time, you'll be reminded that this too will pass. When positive outcomes are realized, your brain-draining worries will become smaller, less believable versions of what they once were. From time to time, return to this chapter and revisit your brain-draining worries and see how the degree of belief has changed. They may even disappear and become forgotten remnants of your healed past. You will have set yourself free from the negative thoughts that were holding you back.

EBCT IN ACTION

So let's see how this played out for Melanie. The next time her boyfriend didn't text back right away, she noticed herself spiraling toward her "crazy train." She noticed her pessimism, her pervasiveness, and her personalization. She saw these familiar patterns pop up, so she posed. As someone who took a yoga class most evenings, Melanie loved using these familiar, physical poses.

But then she started the next step: finding *contrary evidence* to negate the pitfall thought patterns. Instead of focusing on the 45 minutes it took her boyfriend to text back, what would change if she considered the fact that he had been texting her all day long and was taking her to Hawaii for her birthday? This provided evidence that he loved and cared about her.

Then, in her mind's eye, Melanie rehearsed the action she wanted to take. Like an Olympic diver who mentally rehearses a complex sequence of twists before jumping off the board, Melanie pictured the behavior she would take in the next moment: she would simply breathe through the fear, which had loosened its grip a bit, and not text back.

The final part of the antidote is to take the *imagined* behavior and turn it into *real* action, which has the power to create even more positive change. *Right thought* leads to *right action*. It is a calmer, more rational, and healthier way to act and live. Right action does not ignore thoughts and feelings, because both are valuable *information* in our lives. Right action is *governed* by our thoughts and feelings without being *reactive* to them. Drained brains become balanced ones.

The result: Instead of sending accusatory texts when she hadn't heard back from her boyfriend right away, Melanie waited without reacting impulsively. A few minutes went by, and he sent a text apologizing for not getting back to her right away. He had been stuck in a meeting at work.

These changes created a dynamic that made her boyfriend feel more excited about being with her, and in the long run, it also meant he wanted to spend even more time with her. For him, it was a relief to be given credit for the trust he had earned. This also made *him* feel good enough as her partner. The first few times she used this strategy, it felt difficult. But it got easier every time she made the decision to go down this unfamiliar path.

When we don't address pitfall thought patterns, they can create self-fulfilling prophecies that turn irrational fears into realities. For Melanie, constantly accusing her boyfriend of things he didn't do was creating a relationship filled with conflict. When couples fight more often than they get along, relationships are likely to end.

Now Melanie had changed her pitfall thought patterns, which resulted in a change in her actions. Her relationship improved, and the feedback she got from improving her relationship eventually resulted in fewer pitfall thought patterns in the first place. This turned a downward spiral of insecurity into a snowball effect of confidence and love.

You can change your life, too. Use EBCT as an antidote whenever you notice a pitfall thought pattern. This is a fluid process. It becomes more potent every time you use it.

CHAPTER 12

Sleep Better with Cognitive Behavioral Therapy for Insomnia

Jessica is a professional woman in her early 40s. She's also one of the 50 to 70 million Americans who struggle with chronic sleep disorders. And according to the CDC, 83.6 million American adults are sleeping less than 7 hours per night, increasing their risk of many diseases.[1] Like many people who struggle with insomnia, Jessica had tried everything from melatonin to herbal remedies to prescription sleeping aids. When she realized none of these was actually helping her overcome insomnia, she began to worry that this would become a permanent problem, which, of course, only drained her brain while making the insomnia worse.

Our constantly connected, smartphone–tethered ways may have some bearing on Americans getting an average of six and a half hours of sleep on weeknights, which is less sleep than all but one of the other countries surveyed in a major poll. American women fared especially poorly, with 67 percent reporting having trouble sleeping multiple times a week.[2]

THE STRESS-SLEEP CYCLE

Sleep restores frazzled, run-down, and drained brains. Of course, the times when you are desperate for a good night's sleep may be the times it's most elusive. Another problem: Many of the ways people commonly deal with insomnia make problems worse in the long run. When we're stressed and have difficulty sleeping, we're tempted to reach for alcohol, processed carbohydrates, benzodiazepines, and sleeping pills. Processed carbohydrates and alcohol may knock us out initially, but they disrupt deep, restful sleep. Benzodiazepines and sleeping pills cause dependence and rebound insomnia, so a short-term fix becomes a long-term problem.

Most people think of the hormone melatonin when they think of sleep, but the stress hormone cortisol also plays a vital role in natural sleep rhythms. To help you sleep, melatonin levels rise as cortisol dips. In the morning, cortisol rises as melatonin dips. Of course this is how nature designed balanced brains to work. However, this process goes haywire in drained brains.

We are born without a 24-hour circadian rhythm. As we're exposed to the natural light of the world, we soon develop one. In healthy infants, cortisol begins to follow a healthy rhythm: low at night, high in the morning. Ideally, sleep and activity patterns line up with the sun rising and setting to the delight of parents who get to sleep through the night.[3] Even as children, sleep patterns affect cortisol levels, and those cortisol levels influence behavior. Young children with fragmented sleep patterns have cortisol levels that spike higher than those who sleep through the night. These children are more likely to become upset in response to minor stressors and display behavioral difficulties.[4]

Alignment with these natural rhythms isn't just vital for sleep; it's vital for our overall health. Blood samples revealed that just one week of insufficient sleep affected over 700 genes.[5] Perennially high levels of cortisol wreak havoc in the body and play a role in mind-body conditions like irritable bowel syndrome. Insufficient melatonin levels at night are problematic as well and have been linked to cancer. Female night-shift workers, who have perennially low levels of melatonin thanks to exposure to artificially light environments at night, have a 70 percent increased risk of breast cancer.[6] A review of several studies including over one million people found that people who sleep too little (e.g., six hours) or too much (e.g., 10 hours) face a greater risk of death.[7] Thus, aiming for that sweet spot of about eight hours of sleep per night is ideal.

Sadly, our modern, stressful lives get in the way of these natural sleep rhythms. In fact, high levels of stress can actually annihilate circadian rhythms. Not surprisingly, soldiers in a stressful, five-day boot camp experienced cortisol and adrenaline spikes that negatively affected performance. The surprising part was that this acute stress response *extinguished* their circadian rhythms, and these rhythms weren't fully restored even after five days of rest.[8]

Drained individuals often experience events that feel as stressful as a soldier's boot camp, and their brains pay the price. Even a full weekend of rest won't be enough to fully restore the natural sleep-wake cycle after excessive amounts of stress.

So stress can lead to insomnia, and insomnia can also lead to stress and anxiety. Chronic insomnia is a risk factor for developing an anxiety disorder.[9] Being sleep deprived during the day makes minor stressors feel grueling, and this keeps cortisol levels high all day long. Levels of leptin, the hormone that helps you feel full after eating, go down when circadian rhythms are disturbed. When stress is constant or untreated trauma is present, cortisol levels can eventually bottom out and cause fatigue, as happens in the worst forms of drained brains. While you don't want cortisol levels too high, you also don't want them perennially low since a small rise of this stress hormone in the morning helps you to wake up and give you energy.

When sleep remains elusive for a long period of time, the brain shrinks. This, of course, can make you less resilient and unable to deal with stress. In one study, adults aged 20 to 84 had their brains scanned. They had a second scan three and a half years later and were asked about their sleeping habits. A rapid decline in volume was seen in the poor sleepers' brains.[10] This shows that a problematic stress-sleep cycle could eventually lead to Alzheimer's disease and other forms of dementia. Lack of sleep also prevents your brain from reaping the full benefits of your brain's "wash cycle." During sleep, channels between neurons expand up to 60 percent, which allows cerebrospinal fluid in. All that extra space between neurons allows the fluid to flush out plaques that fog the brain and spike dementia risk.[11] In older adults, cortisol interacts with those plaques in the brain. Those with high levels of cortisol decline more rapidly than those with lower levels of the stress hormone.[12]

Sleep might also reinforce brain cells; a 2013 study showed that while mice slept, their brains were making more myelin, the brain cells' insulation that allows the electrical current of happiness to flow freely.[13]

A University of Pennsylvania experiment found that people who slept about six hours a night for multiple nights in a row had the same performance deficits as people who had been totally deprived of sleep for two nights. Even more alarming: when subjects were asked to report their subjective experience of sleepiness throughout the study, they were largely unaware of their deficits.[14] Not sleeping enough can also affect your body's ability to regulate stress hormones and lead to high blood pressure. This is problematic for stressed out, brain-drained people. Remember: people with anxiety are four times more likely to develop high blood pressure, the number one cause of preventable death in the world. So not getting enough sleep isn't just difficult to deal with; it can be life-threatening.

Hopefully this research motivates you to reprioritize sleep. For many people, this means making significant changes in their lives. However, this information can also make some people excessively worried about sleep, which can lead to insomnia and more anxiety. In fact, research shows insomniacs tend to have more unrealistic expectations about their sleep requirements, and they have stronger beliefs about the negative consequences of insufficient sleep.[15] The Stanford Sleep Medicine Center found insomniacs overestimate the time it takes them to fall sleep by 30 minutes while underestimating their total time sleeping by an hour. While the effects of sleep deprivation are scary, take them with a grain of salt. Doing so will allow you to apply one of the most helpful insomnia strategies, and it's a surprising, counterintuitive treatment: getting *less* sleep on purpose in the short-term to promote *more restful and efficient* sleep in the long run.

CBT-I: THE NATURAL TREATMENT

Cognitive behavioral therapy for insomnia, or CBT-I, is the natural way to treat insomnia so we can balance our brains and remain resilient in the face of stress. It also helps restore the 24-hour cycle of melatonin and cortisol so you feel refreshed when you wake up and tired at night. In 2016, the American College of Physicians recommended CBT-I as the initial treatment—instead of medication—for adults with insomnia.[16] This group is the largest medical-specialty organization in the U.S., so this about-face was an important decree for health professionals and patients alike. They're encouraging CBT-I while trying to reverse the overprescribing and overconsumption of sleeping pills that have become increasingly problematic.

One of the great things about CBT-I is that it works equally well for different types of insomnia. It works for people who have trouble falling asleep and staying asleep, and those who wake up too early. It's even effective in reversing dependence on sleeping pills. One study recruited 100 people with insomnia. Of these, 18 reported problems falling asleep, 18 reported trouble staying asleep, and 64 reported both. Their insomnia was fairly severe. The vast majority had used sleeping pills, and some were dependent on them. They'd been experiencing insomnia for an average of 10.7 years. They attended an average of about eight CBT-I sessions, and the results were impressive. In just a few months, they reduced the time it took to fall asleep from an average of about an hour down to 30 minutes. There were similar improvements in staying asleep and waking up too early. More time was spent sleeping, and less time was spent lying awake in bed. CBT-I even helped insomniacs dependent on sleeping pills either reduce or eliminate their use. Over the course of treatment, there was an overall 59 percent reduction of medication intake. Better yet: almost half of the drug-dependent insomniacs were drug-free at the end of the treatment.[17]

A review of 59 other studies of CBT-I produced similar results. More than 2,000 subjects received an average of about four or five sessions. Some subjects even self-administered the therapy without any face-to-face sessions with a professional. The average time it took to fall asleep improved by 41 percent while the time spent waking up too much or too early improved by 45 percent. Unlike sleep medications, which stop working after you stop taking them (and make insomnia worse in the long run), a short course of CBT-I results in lasting improvements. Follow-up data showed the improvements of insomnia symptoms were stable for months after treatment.[18] Remarkably, CBT-I can even help people fall asleep faster than prescription sleeping pills.[19]

All of this is great news because we've come to realize over the past few years that women don't metabolize these medications as quickly as men. Some medications remain in women's bodies after eight hours of sleep, and this can lead to grogginess and delayed reaction time. In 2013, the FDA recommended lower doses of Ambien for women after studies showed that 15 percent of women still had enough Ambien in their blood to impair their driving eight hours after taking the nonextended release 10 mg dose. For the newer extended-release Ambien, that number jumps to 33 percent of women.[20] Ambien is also problematic for seniors, since cognitive impairment and falls can result. Research shows for people over 60, the benefit of the medication probably does not outweigh the risk.[21]

According to the U.S. Substance Abuse and Mental Health Services Administration, Ambien comes with other dangers, too. ER visits for adverse reactions to Ambien climbed 220 percent from 2005 to 2010. Most patients were women, and the most common age group was 45 to 65.[22] Researchers also identified an association between Ambien and both cancer and death in 2012, though they couldn't conclude that the relationship was a cause-and-effect one.[23] Belsomra, the prescription sleeping pill that received FDA approval in 2014, doesn't seem like it is going to be the solution to the world's sleep woes. It's the first orexin-receptor antagonist to be approved for insomnia and works differently from Ambien or similar drugs like Lunesta and Sonata. Belsomra side effects may include next-day alertness, sleep walking, and suicidal ideation.[24]

The good news: You already have a leg up since you'll be using other principles I've already described in this book that work synergistically with CBT-I. For example, probiotics and omega-3 DHA will help you to manufacture sleep-inducing GABA and serotonin, which insomniacs may be lacking. Eating a wide variety of vegetables and whole fruits can help regulate cortisol levels. Replacing brain-draining sugar and flour with high-fiber meals improves the quality of your sleep. Engaging in exercise helps to keep relaxing GABA levels high, and remember, this is the same neurotransmitter that benzodiazepines like Xanax and sleeping pills like Ambien boost. The difference: you'll be getting this neurotransmitter in a natural, nonaddictive way while enjoying the "side effect" of a wide variety of health benefits.

THE PIECES OF CBT-I

Some CBT-I strategies are common sense. Keep your room dark and quiet. Avoid caffeine in the afternoon. Cool the room down when you sleep. But this program takes things one step further. There are three different levels of CBT-I to treat everything from minor to major sleep problems. The simple CBT-I strategies in level 1 are enough for some brain-drained individuals to make a significant difference in their sleep-stress relationship in a matter of days. Others with more significant sleeping problems will need more time, but the beauty of the personalized CBT-I in this program is that it's flexible. It's more cost effective than CBT-I sessions or apps that can cost hundreds or thousands of dollars. I've included seven days of a sleep journal as part of the program in the back of this book, which will be sufficient for people with minor sleep problems. If you have significant problems, make several copies of the sleep journal before writing in it so you can use it over the course of weeks or months. Once you learn this flexible version of CBT-I, you can come back to it if you should ever have problems in the future.

If your goal is to reduce or eliminate your dependence on sleeping pills, consult your prescriber to help come up with a schedule to taper the medication gradually. This tapering schedule will likely depend on the severity of your insomnia, the type and dose of medication, and how long you've been using it. If you are taking sleeping pills on a regular basis, you may need to use the CBT-I program for six to eight weeks. Most of the patients I've treated with CBT-I find the most success if they continue taking their medication with no change for the first seven days of the program. Then they reduce the drug by 50 percent in week 2, reduce another 50 percent in week 3, and then discontinue the medication altogether in week 4. For example, someone taking 10 mg of Ambien on a nightly basis would keep taking 10 mg every night in week 1 of the CBT-I program. Then the dose would be reduced to 5 mg in week 2, 2.5 mg in week 3, and then no medication in week 4. However, every person's goals and medical history are different. Some people with long-term insomnia may respond to a more gradual taper. Do you want to stop taking sleeping pills altogether? Do you want to go from using them four to five nights a week to one to two times per month? Work with your prescriber to come up with a tapering schedule that takes your goals, the type and dose of medication you take, and the severity of your insomnia into consideration.

There are some people for whom CBT-I will not work. For example, CBT-I does not work for people who have sleeping problems resulting from sleep apnea. If you snore loudly, wake up gasping for breath, or wake up with a very dry mouth, you may benefit from an overnight sleep study to see if you have sleep apnea. Local sleep specialists can administer this test in clinics, and there are now in-home studies available, and it is usually covered by insurance. Getting diagnosed and treated for sleep apnea is important, because untreated sleep apnea has health risks. For example, it can triple your risk of stroke.[25]

CBT-I also does not work well if sleeping problems are the result of another untreated physical or mental illness, such as a urinary tract infection or major depression. In these cases, treat the illness first. CBT-I can sometimes be beneficial as an add-on treatment after the primary problem has been diagnosed and treated. Also, CBT-I does not directly treat restless legs syndrome. That being said, some of the strategies you'll learn, like progressive muscle relaxation and self-hypnosis, can be added to CBT-I to help manage symptoms of this condition that makes it difficult for people to sleep.

IMPLEMENTING CBT-I

CBT-I involves a series of specific steps to help you sleep more easily, soundly, and efficiently. The strategies I'll outline here prime your brain for the low cortisol/high melatonin state that promotes restful sleep.

Level 1: For Minor Insomnia

These simple steps in level 1 of CBT-I may be enough for some people with minor problems to improve their sleep quality. If these fixes don't do enough to improve your sleep, you'll proceed to levels 2 and 3 after completing level 1.

Step 1: Set a Stable Bedtime and Wake Time: Remember, your circadian rhythms of melatonin and cortisol are designed to create a daily symphony of wake and rest. The high-melatonin, low-cortisol evening and low-melatonin, high-cortisol morning are designed to function in a 24-hour rhythm that corresponds to natural light. One of the simplest and easiest ways to help your sleep-wake cycle get back on track is to set a bedtime and wake time you can adhere to on a regular basis—yes even on weekends. Going to bed and waking up at different times on weekends has been called "social jet lag" and may affect about two-thirds of the population. By doing this, you experience effects similar to taking a transatlantic flight every weekend and returning every Monday.

When you're figuring out what times will work for you, consider your obligations on both weekdays and weekends. Consider the people you live with and their schedules. If you are a night-shift worker or work very early or very late, consider a time that works for your job as well as allowing time to see your family and friends. If necessary, have a conversation to decide on a bedtime and wake time that you, your significant other, and/or other family members can agree on. One of the most important principles of CBT-I is setting a consistent wake time you can adhere to seven days a week. The ultimate goal is eight solid hours of restful sleep per night, but it also means getting out of bed at your target wake time even when you didn't sleep well.

If you're someone who sleeps in until 10 A.M. on the weekends but wakes up at 6 A.M. to go to the gym on weekdays before work, decide on one time or the other. In an ideal world, you would simply wake up around 6 A.M. on the weekends since that would also allow for your circadian rhythm to align itself with natural sunlight. There are benefits to this strategy. One study proved waking up early and exposing yourself to natural light early in the morning—when blue light is at its highest—has been linked to lower body mass index. (Daytime light exposure needs to be at a level that is difficult to achieve with indoor lighting.)[26] However, other factors like frequent work events and dinners may require you to work late, which can make this difficult. If you can't see yourself waking up that early on the weekends, then perhaps it would be better to change your morning workout routine into a lunchtime one. This option would allow you to sleep in later on weekdays so your new, consistent wake-up time is around 8 A.M. every day of the week. While you want to choose a time you can stick to on a regular basis, you also don't want to become extremely rigid, since this can lead to anxiety about sleep. A bit of flexibility is inevitable from time to time. Try to get up at your new wake time even when you didn't get to bed at your prescribed bedtime. Even though you may be slightly tired for one day, this will prevent your sleep-wake cycle from shifting, which can potentially zap your energy for weeks. However, try to keep these times stable through this course of CBT-I since the goal is to reset and restore your sleep-wake cycle. It's sometimes helpful to begin this process on the weekend or on a day where you don't have anything important to do since you may experience some daytime sleepiness in the first few days when beginning this program. Avoid driving during this time if you're not sleeping well, and don't compensate by drinking too much caffeine since this will prevent a reset of your sleep-wake rhythm that night. Stay busy with light activity or a walk outside to keep yourself awake on these days.

Also limit naps. In fact, don't take them at all if you don't need them. If you do, limit them to one short nap of 20 to 30 minutes. If you find you need naps often, try scheduling them at a set time of the day. This allows your brain to prepare for this ritual, which will help you to fall asleep quickly and reap the benefits of this short time. The best time for most people is after lunch when your sleep-wake cycle takes a small dip. If you're exhausted, a 20-minute nap at 3 P.M. is better than an extra-large coffee. A short nap won't disrupt nighttime sleep as much as a hefty dose of caffeine in the afternoon and evening. Just make sure the naps aren't long, because they disrupt the recalibration of natural sleep-wake rhythms. Remember: The goal of CBT-I is to help your body and brain rediscover what it's like to naturally become sleepy at bedtime. Long or frequent naps and afternoon caffeine can disrupt this recalibration.

My bedtime is: _____

My wake time is: _____

Note: Ideally, these times should be roughly eight and a half hours apart. This allows for eight hours of sleep, the amount of time most brains need for optimal health while allowing for about 30 minutes to fall asleep. If you still find yourself tossing and turning all night, we'll modify these times later in the program.

Step 2: The 60-Minute Wind Down: Now take your target bedtime and subtract one hour. This is when your 60-minute wind down begins. This wind down is essential, because it's priming your brain and body for sleep. If you have children, you know how important a wind down is for helping them sleep. Your kids may need a bedtime story before bed, but your adult brain needs its own wind-down strategies. Just because *you* and your conscious mind want to go to bed right now doesn't mean that all the other parts of your brain and body agree with you. This wind-down time primes brain and body for rest.

My target wind-down time is: _____

So what do you do during this wind-down period?

- COOL: Since your body cools down as it enters sleep, help facilitate this process by turning the thermostat down a few degrees at wind-down time. If you have a programmable thermostat, you can make this change automatic. Another way to relax your muscles and drop your body temperature is taking a warm shower or bath. When you get out, your body temperature will drop as the water evaporates from your skin. You want to be a few degrees cooler but not cold. If your feet get cold in bed, put socks on. Another way to cool your body is to exercise in the afternoon. Research suggests that as your body temperature drops after the spike that occurs during exercise, sleep improves.[27] (Morning workouts have also been linked to better sleep, but this is likely due to light exposure and movement helping to realign your circadian rhythms as opposed to the cooling effect of afternoon workouts.)[28] If possible, move moderate to intense exercise from evening sessions to morning or afternoon ones, since they can warm the body for hours and make sleep difficult.

- DIM: Turn off all electronics. This includes your TV, cell phone, and computer. If you charge your cell phone in the bedroom, find a new home for it in another room. Invest in a simple $10 alarm clock for the bedroom. Electronics emit higher levels of the blue light that is particularly potent in suppressing melatonin production. Newer LED and compact fluorescent light bulbs emit more blue light than traditional, incandescent bulbs. Use incandescent light bulbs on dimmers at night, or look for LED lights that have been specifically manufactured to reduce the blue light for nighttime use. There are now several brands that make these, and they're significantly more affordable than they were a few years ago. GE's Align PM LED bulb is engineered to reduce blue light, and it's dimmable. It uses just seven watts of energy and costs about $20 per bulb. While they cost more up front, they last longer and cost less to run.

- **PREP:** Get ready for the day ahead of you. Take a moment to make an inventory of everything you need to do the following day. This preparation can help prevent the *Oh, shoot I forgot about . . .* thoughts that cross your mind just as you're about to enter a restful sleep state. Do a brain dump. Write down the things you need to remember so your brain can let go. Get your clothes ready for the following day. Put your briefcase and the documents you need to take with you by the door. This preparation allows your unconscious mind to sleep deeply by preventing anxious dreams and waking up too early.

- **RITUAL:** Are there any rituals that you enjoy before bed? Enjoy a cup of chamomile tea and a good book to calm you. Say a prayer or meditate. Make yourself a delicious "bedtime latte" with saffron, which has been shown to improve sleep. See my recipe below. Take a natural melatonin supplement. Natrol's fast-dissolve melatonin is helpful for people who have trouble falling asleep. If you have trouble staying asleep, try their time-release version. Light a candle as you get ready for bed. Use all your senses to help different parts of your brain and body prepare for rest. Paint your bedroom a soothing color or hang pictures that fill you with a sense of calm. Lavender has been shown to help promote rest. Rub a drop of lavender essential oil in your palms and inhale, find a lavender spritz that calms you, or put a few drops in a presleep bath or shower. Your brain will begin to pair this smell with sleep. Make these rituals things you can take with you so your brain doesn't panic if they're not available. Put a spritz of lavender on your travel eye mask, or put a few bags of your favorite evening tea in your suitcase. This will help you to create a wind-down ritual you can use anywhere. If there is a pose from EBCT that resonates with you and any anxieties that prevent sleep, use it before you climb into bed.

BEDTIME LATTE

Heat 1 cup of your favorite type of milk (coconut, almond, or organic dairy) on the stove or in the microwave. Add 1/2 teaspoon turmeric, 1/2 teaspoon black pepper, 1/2 teaspoon cinnamon, and 5 threads of saffron.

- **HEAD START:** The true preparation for sleep actually begins hours before bedtime. Reduce or eliminate caffeine after lunch. If you are desperate for a caffeine boost in the afternoon to get through your day, switch to half-caf, decaf, or green tea. Green tea has about one-third of the caffeine of coffee. Eat a dinner and evening snack that contain vegetables, whole fruits, grains, and probiotics that promote restful sleep while helping your body manufacture soothing hormones like GABA and serotonin. Avoid blood sugar–spiking processed carbs that have been shown to disturb restful sleep. Limit alcohol to one serving per night. If you have a newer phone, open the settings and change the light preferences. iPhones have a new setting that will automatically reduce the blue light emitted each evening. Wear sunglasses in the afternoon and evening if it's sunny out to reduce your exposure to evening light. Orange-tinted ones are especially good at this, since they block blue light. When you get home in the evening, dim the lights and avoid bright, fluorescent, or LED lighting (except ones that have been manufactured to reduce blue light). Exercise regularly. Quiet, meditative movement like hatha yoga or Tai Chi can be a great pre-bedtime workout; they both increase GABA while reducing cortisol levels. A stroll in nature is great, too.

Step 3: Go Time: Now that it's time to head to your bedroom and crawl in bed, make sure that you're ready.

- **PAIR YOUR BED AND SLEEP:** Your brain needs to be reminded what your bed is for: sleeping and sex. If you watch TV or work on your laptop from bed, your brain is paring your bed with states of activity, productivity, and wakefulness. There is one exception to this for some people. If reading a book that calms you for 15 or 30 minutes in bed under dim light makes you sleepy, then you are creating a sleep ritual that helps prime your brain for sleep. If you find yourself reading for longer periods of time and/or experience difficulty falling asleep or staying asleep, then don't read in bed.

Find a nice chair in the living room to read in, and make this part of your 60-minute wind-down routine. One common problem is many people try to compensate for a night of poor sleep by going to bed early the following night. By doing this, you're getting in bed before your 24-hour sleep-wake cycle is ready to initiate sleep. You're likely to spend more time lying awake in bed than if you wait for your set bedtime. You're draining your brain when you're trying to balance it. Again, lying awake in bed is pairing your bed and wakefulness.

- **LIGHTS OUT:** Make sure your bedroom is as dark as possible. Light disturbs sleep and suppresses melatonin production. This is more important as we get older, because melatonin production declines with age. Keeping our exposure to light low can maximize declining melatonin levels. Invest in blackout shades or a good eye mask. If you're not used to wearing one, it can feel strange at first. Eventually, your brain will pair the feeling of the mask and sleep. In fact, it will begin to feel strange when you're not wearing one.

- **QUIET TIME:** Make sure your bedroom is as quiet as possible. If there is constant or intermittent noise where you live, use earplugs or a sound machine. My favorite sound machines are the Marpac Dohm ones, which cost about $50. I find the steady, rich sound of the actual fan in this device to be better than cheaper ones that use a white-noise recording. However, if you're a frequent traveler: remember that you're pairing this sound with sleep, so you may want to consider that if you choose to use it at home. Of the apps I've tried, I like Sound Machine. If you travel frequently, pairing the sound of a fan with sleep can eventually make it harder to sleep without it. Earplugs are fantastic because they're easily portable. Just like eye masks, they sometimes feel strange at first. Eventually they'll become familiar and part of your sleep routine. Another easy strategy: switch your central heating and cooling system so that the fan is continuous as opposed to shutting on and off throughout the night. The quiet "whoosh" of this sound can help block out noises that can interrupt sleep while helping to purify the air. You can recreate this sound in most hotel rooms by setting the fan mode from "automatic" to "on."

- **BE REALISTIC, NOT PERFECTIONISTIC:** Perfectionistic expectations get in the way of good sleep. Expect that it will likely take you about 30 minutes to fall asleep. This is the average amount of time that insomniacs took after being successfully treated with CBT-I. Falling asleep in less than 10 minutes every single night is rare. Also, remember that people struggling with sleep tend to overestimate the amount of time it takes them to fall asleep. So when it *feels* like you've been lying there for 30 minutes, it may have only been 15. Keep calm. The way you'd introduce yourself to a friend's dog is the way you should greet sleep. Put your hand out gently, and let him come to you.

- **TRYING BY NOT TRYING:** One of the most helpful strategies is to avoid "trying" to fall asleep. In many ways, your brain is like the 10-year-old child who wants to do what you tell him or her *not* to do. If you let go of expectations, the onset of sleep may surprise you after just a few minutes. Adopt a mindful, curious, childlike mind-set that finds pleasure in noticing the physical sensations in your body like the air on your cheek and how nice the pillow feels under your head. Shift from "doing" mind to "being" mind. The more you actively try to force sleep to happen, the more you are pairing the feelings of frustration and anxiety with your bed and nighttime. If you find yourself lying in bed and it feels like it's been a long time or you're getting anxious, don't panic. Without judgment or frustration, simply get out of bed and do some light activity in another room under dim lighting until you find yourself becoming sleepy. Sleepiness is like surfing. You can paddle out into the ocean ready to surf, but then you have to wait for a wave. Sometimes the wave is just a few feet away. Other times you'll have to wait a bit for the next set to come in. Just read, knit, or do some light cleaning until you can feel the wave of sleepiness approaching. This strategy keeps anxiety at bay while maintaining a strong pairing between bed and the initiation of sleep. If you have to do this two or three times, that's okay. This may result in one night of just five or six hours of sleep, but it's actually setting your brain up for eight restful hours the next night—and for the long term. One optimistic way of reframing a lack of sleep one night is to focus on how *restful*, *easy*, and *deep* your sleep is likely to be the next.

- **STOP CLOCK-WATCHING:** With all of the previously mentioned focus on time, common sense may say perhaps you should keep your alarm clock handy all night to calculate minutes. But clock-watching creates anxiety that interferes with sleep. It's actually better to turn your clock around or put it under your bed. If you wake up in the middle of the night, don't look at it. Looking at the clock at night creates anxiety about getting enough sleep. This makes sleep more elusive. If you're the type who panics about waking up in time and frequently checks the time in the morning, then get two clocks with loud alarms so you can sleep soundly without anxiously checking the time.

Level 2: For Moderate Insomnia

For people who have a bit more significant sleep problems, you can add these steps to the ones covered already.

Step 4: Relax: Add a relaxing technique to your sleep routine. In later chapters, I'll teach you how to practice clinically effective relaxation techniques, including diaphragmatic breathing, progressive muscle relaxation, autogenic training, and hypnosis. Once you learn them, you can do them in bed, which will help prime your brain and body for restful sleep. Find the one that works best for you. People with knots in their stomach may find the tense-and-then-relax format of progressive muscle relaxation more effective since this can help dissolve tension. Others with pain or stiff muscles may find autogenic training easier since no movement is required. Hypnosis can help you to distance yourself from your greatest sleep fears. As you learn these techniques, you can even combine them in novel ways to help you sleep. Your brain will learn to pair this activity with the onset of sleep.

Step 5: Reframe: This process is similar to the work we did in the last chapter. We're going to identify your biggest sleep worry and then change it using the strategies you learned from EBCT.

- **IDENTIFY YOUR BIGGEST SLEEP WORRY:** Do any of these worries—or a similar version of them—sound familiar? They represent versions of the seven pitfall thought patterns as they relate to sleep:

  1. Paralysis-analysis: This type of thinking involves stewing and ruminating in anxious thoughts which prevent positive change (e.g., restful sleep) from occurring. For example, "What did that mean when my colleague said that today? Maybe he doesn't like me. I wonder if he resents that time last year when I got assigned to the project he wanted. Or I wonder if maybe he knows something I don't. Am I getting fired? My mind is racing. How will I be able to sleep?"

  2. Permanence: This type of thinking falsely assumes that just because something is a problem now, it will always be a problem. For example, "I'm an insomniac today, which means I'll be an insomniac tomorrow, next month, and next year. These problems are here to stay."

  3. Personalization: This type of thinking places the blame on you for negative circumstances or outcomes. For example, "My sleep difficulties are just another example of how undisciplined and lazy I am. What's wrong with me? Other people don't have these kinds of problems with sleep."

4. Pervasiveness: This type of thinking allows something that is affecting one area of your life to spread to all areas of your life. For example, "If I don't sleep well tonight, I'm going to skip yoga tomorrow and cancel my dinner plans."

5. Pessimistic: This type of thinking considers the worst-case scenario. It dwells in the possible—not the probable. For example, "If I don't get eight hours' sleep tonight, I'm going to botch that presentation and get fired. I won't be able to afford my mortgage if I lose my job. Where will I live? How will I eat?"

6. Polarized: This type of thinking has a binary, black-or-white pattern. The words *always* or *never* are frequently found in this type of thought pattern. For example, "If I don't always get eight hours' sleep every single night, I just can't function."

7. Psychic: This type of thinking expects people around us to read our minds without us verbalizing what we need. For example, "Why is my husband still watching TV? He should be able to tell by looking at me that I'm ready for bed. Doesn't he know how important tomorrow is for me?"

Write your most draining sleep worry below. It may be one of the ones listed above, your own personal version of one, or an entirely different worry. First, identify which pitfall thought pattern affects you most. Then write down the way this pitfall thought pattern sounds in your head as your own, personal sleep worry. Next to the worry, write how true that feels to you right now. Remember, 100 percent means that you know for certain that this worry is absolutely true. For example, people who believe they'll always be insomniacs with absolutely no hope of ever changing would write 100 percent; but if they have a tiny glimmer of hope, perhaps they'll write 97 percent. If you think it's probably true or true most of the time, perhaps you'll write 65 percent next to the worry. If it probably isn't true but can be once in a while, perhaps you'll write a 25 percent next to the worry.

Give it a shot here:

THE PITFALL THOUGHT PATTERN THAT DISRUPTS MY SLEEP THE MOST IS: _____

_____.

THIS LEADS TO A SLEEP WORRY THAT SOUNDS SOMETHING LIKE . . .

SLEEP WORRY: _____ (HOW TRUE: ___%).

- **CHANGE YOUR THOUGHTS, SEE YOUR SUCCESS:** Once you have identified your sleep worry, overcome and change it using the strategies you learned from EBCT. First, use a physical pose. Second, find the *contrary evidence* from knowledge and experience you already have in your life. Third, see your success in your mind's eye. Here's an example:

    SLEEP WORRY: *pessimistic:* "If I don't get eight hours of sleep tonight, I'm going to botch that presentation and get fired. I won't be able to afford my mortgage. Where will I live?" → CONTRARY EVIDENCE (while using the half-smile physical antidote): "Throughout my life, there have been plenty of times I haven't gotten eight perfect hours of sleep. I've managed to get through plenty of stressful days, meetings, and situations on less-than-ideal sleep. I may not have been at my absolute best, but I wasn't fired as a result. My relationship didn't end. I made my mortgage payment. I got through the day." → MIND'S EYE: "I can see myself getting through my presentation tomorrow with ease and grace. I feel well-rested. I have a smile on my face, and I feel good about myself. My colleagues are looking at me, and they're impressed with the work I do. In fact, this confidence is so powerful that I see myself performing well no matter how tired or alert I may be at that moment."

REVIEW OF EBCT POSES

1. Paralysis-analysis → Tree Pose

2. Permanence → Eye Cupping

3. Personalization → Star Pose

4. Pervasiveness → Pigeon Pose or Shoulder Shrugs

5. Pessimistic → The Half-Smile

6. Polarized → Spinal Twist

7. Psychic → Chest Thump

Take your sleep worry and write the contrary evidence you already have in your life. After using a physical pose (described on page 116), reflecting on this contrary evidence, and seeing your future in your mind's eye, how true does it feel now?

- CONTRARY EVIDENCE: _____

- SLEEP WORRY FROM ABOVE: HOW TRUE: _____%

For many people, this process significantly reduces how true this worry feels. This reframing is the *cognitive* part of cognitive behavioral therapy. Your sleep worry becomes less powerful, and it may bother you a little less. This helps to ease sleep worries, fears, and anxieties that prevent restful sleep.

This next level will allow you to use the *behavioral* part of cognitive behavioral therapy. You will create an experiment where your new, future experience will continue to counteract your sleep worry.

Level 3: For Acute Insomnia

The following steps can be added for those people who have more significant sleep problems or have not responded to the interventions in levels 1 and 2. These steps begin to significantly alter the sleep-wake cycle for those people who may need a harder reset. This step is sometimes challenging in the beginning, because it involves a period of partial sleep deprivation; however, this short-term discomfort leads to lasting gains.

In addition to steps 6–10, below, I will sometimes prescribe cranial electrotherapy stimulation (CES) at this point if a patient has not responded to the interventions in CBT-I levels 1 and 2. CES employs a noninvasive, FDA-approved device that can be used at home to treat both insomnia and anxiety. This device sends a tiny amount of electricity through electrodes placed on the earlobes or neck, which the patient will feel as a slight tingle. An average session increases levels of endorphins by 98 percent, serotonin by 50 percent, and melatonin by 25 percent. It also reduces cortisol by 18 percent.[29] One recent study found significant improvements in sleep after just five daily treatments, and studies have found this at-home device to be quite effective for anxiety as well.[30] Side effects are rare and tend to be very minor. The protocol involves daily use for the first month followed by maintenance treatment a few times a week. While you can use the device while reading or watching TV, you can also combine it with other practices you'll learn like meditation. For more information on CES and how to purchase one, see my website: drmikedow.com.

Step 6: Calculate Your Sleep Efficiency: In the final phase of CBT-I, people with the worst cases of insomnia will use a strategy where they will paradoxically sleep less in order to make themselves tired enough to sleep more. This involves temporarily moving your sleep and wake times, and then strategically shifting them to achieve easy, deep, and restful sleep. In order to use this strategy, you will need to determine your sleep efficiency, which is a simple calculation of how much time you spend in your bed *sleeping* compared with how much *total* time you spend in your bed. Obviously, the goal is to be sleeping nearly the entire time you're in bed. The only exceptions here, which are left out of this calculation, are (1) up to 30 minutes of reading *only if* this activity helps you to sleep and (2) sex. The basic equation is this:

Step 1: Number of Minutes in Bed (A) – Number of Minutes Awake (B) = Total Time Asleep (C)
Step 2: Total Time Asleep (C) / Total Number of Minutes in Bed (A) = Sleep Efficiency Expressed as a Decimal
Step 3: Sleep Efficiency as Decimal X 100 = Sleep Efficiency Percentage

So if your bedtime is 11 P.M. and your wake time is 7:30 A.M., this means you were in bed for a total of eight and a half hours or 510 minutes. (Remember, don't include time up to 30 minutes of reading or sex.) So A = 510.

If it took you 45 minutes to fall asleep and you woke up once for about 60 minutes, then you were awake for 105 minutes. So B = 105. (NOTE: Remember that insomniacs tend to overestimate these times, so consider this finding when making calculations. It's best to estimate instead of calculating this number exactly, because looking at the clock all night prevents restful sleep.)

Now subtract B from A, and you get 405 as the Total Time Asleep. So C = 405.

Now, divide the amount of time you are actually sleeping by the time you were in bed: 405/510. This gives you 0.7941. Multiply by 100, which means move the decimal point over two places, and you get 79.41 percent.

You spent just over 79 percent of the time you were in bed sleeping, which means you have just a bit of work to do. Healthy sleep is a sleep efficiency of 85 percent or more. Great sleepers often have a sleep efficiency around 90 percent. If your efficiency is 85 percent or more and you're sleeping a healthy eight hours, then you're in good shape. There's no need to proceed to the next step.

Unhealthy sleep is a sleep efficiency less than 85 percent. Many people who struggle with insomnia have sleep efficiency numbers around 65 percent. If you still need to up your sleep efficiency, you can move on to the next step.

Here is a simple worksheet to help you use this formula. Use this to calculate your own sleep efficiency.

Step 1:
Number of Minutes in Bed Last Night Was ____ (A) minutes
Number of Minutes I Spent Awake in Bed Last Night Was ____ (B) minutes

Calculate **Total Time Asleep** *by Subtracting B from A:*

_____(A) −_____(B) = _____ (C)

Step 2:
Calculate **Your Sleep Efficiency** *by Dividing Total Time Asleep by Number of Minutes in Bed:*
_____ (C) / _____ (A) = _____ *SLEEP EFFICIENCY EXPRESSED AS DECIMAL*

Step 3:
Now, move the decimal two places to the right:
My Sleep Efficiency Is _____percent.

* Healthy sleep is a sleep efficiency above 85 percent.

Step 7: Setting a Paradoxical Intention: If you're still struggling with falling asleep, staying asleep, sleeping too much or too little, or have a low sleep efficiency, here's where we begin to introduce a concept called paradoxical intention. If you struggle with insomnia, you probably fear not sleeping well and the consequences of sleep deprivation. When you wake up and can't fall back to sleep, anxiety can take over. In this step, you're going to set an intention to not get enough sleep—on purpose. The goal is to make yourself so tired that you actually do sleep when you get into bed. This helps reset your circadian rhythm while pairing sleeping and bed strongly in your brain.

Doing this also creates a real-life experiment that gives you the opportunity to prove your sleep worries completely or partially wrong. Here's an example: SLEEP WORRY: *pessimistic:* "If I don't get eight hours sleep tonight, I'm going to botch that presentation and get fired. I won't be able to afford my mortgage. Where will I live?" → SETTING A PARADOXICAL INTENTION: "This weekend, I'm going to move my bedtime later and get up earlier. My worry is that I can't function without eight hours of sleep, but I have a lot to do this weekend. I'll create an experiment to see if I can prove this worry wrong. By doing so, maybe I'll also show myself that I may not be my *optimal* self with less than eight hours of sleep, but I probably also won't do so poorly that I get fired. Perhaps this worry will feel significantly less true by doing so."

Step 8: Sleep Compression: Sleep compression is how you go about putting that paradoxical intention into practice. In this step, you'll gradually "compress" your sleep, which results in a sleep efficiency boost. You will sacrifice total time spent in bed to increase the percentage of time you spend *sleeping while you're in bed*. Here's how you do it: Reduce your time in bed by 30 minutes per day until you notice your sleep efficiency improving. Some people prefer to move their bedtime 30 minutes later, but others may want to make their wake time 30 minutes earlier. Others prefer to split the difference, with a 15-minute change on both ends. Whatever method you choose, make sure your wind-down time still begins 60 minutes before your bedtime. The maximum sleep compression in this program is five hours between bedtime and wake time, but very few people will need to compress their sleep this much.

Don't drive or engage in any activity that could be dangerous during sleep compression. There is usually a spike in car accidents the Monday after the beginning of Daylight Saving Time, which tells us that even mild sleep deprivations or sleep-wake cycle shifts can result in delayed reaction time.[31] Potentially dangerous activities like climbing on your roof to clean out the gutters or operating heavy machinery should be avoided during this step as well. Since you may encounter daytime sleepiness during this step, keep yourself busy. Go outside for fresh air to avoid falling asleep.

Continue compressing your sleep until your sleep efficiency number rises to 85 percent or above. Then keep these bedtime and wake up times stable until they stay at or above 85 percent for at least three days. People experiencing severe insomnia may want to keep these times stable for up to two weeks before readjusting the time. Once your sleep efficiency is consistently at or above 85 percent, move on to step 9.

Check out a couple of examples of implementing sleep compression:

- **EXAMPLE 1:** Carol set a bedtime of 11 P.M. and a wake time of 7:30 A.M. in level 1. However, her sleep efficiency was only 80 percent. This is just slightly less than 85 percent, so she used sleep compression to improve efficiency. Carol decided to move her bedtime to 11:15 P.M. and wake time to 7:15 A.M. Her sleep efficiency went up to 85 percent by the second day using these new times. She kept this time stable for three days before moving on to the next step.

- **EXAMPLE 2:** George set a bedtime of 10 P.M. and a wake time of 6:30 A.M. He'd been struggling with insomnia for years and had always found it difficult to fall asleep. George took 2.5 mg, a relatively small dose, of Ambien nightly. His initial sleep efficiency was 65 percent. On day 1, he moved his bedtime to 10:15 P.M. and his wake time to 6:15 A.M. There was no change. On day 2, he moved his bedtime to 10:30 P.M. and his wake time to 6 A.M. His sleep efficiency went up to 70 percent. At this point, George decided to move his wake time only since his wife liked to be in bed by 10:30 P.M. and had difficulty when he came to bed late. On day 3, his bedtime was 10:30 P.M. and wake time was 5:30 A.M.; sleep efficiency went up to 75 percent. On day 4, he kept his bedtime at 10:30 P.M. and moved his wake time to 5 A.M. There was no change. On day 5, his bedtime was again 10:30 P.M. and his wake time was 4:30 A.M. George's sleep efficiency actually dipped to 70 percent. On day 6, his bedtime was still 10:30 P.M., and his wake time was 4:00 A.M. His sleep efficiency rose to 80 percent. On day 7, he moved his wake time to 3:30 A.M. On this day, his sleep efficiency was 90 percent. Since George's sleeping pill dose was small and the goal was to eliminate dependency, he and his prescriber decided George would stop using the drug when sleep efficiency improved. On day 8, he stopped taking Ambien. His sleep efficiency dipped to 80 percent on days 8 and 9. But by day 10, his sleep efficiency went up to 85 percent. George kept these times stable for one week. During this program, he let his wife drive since he knew his reaction time was impaired. Also, George began to feel very sleepy and had to stay active to avoid dozing off during the day. He was surprised at how easily he could fall asleep and was looking forward to the next step of this program, since he wanted to spend more time in bed. Even though he was tired, George was also happy that he no longer associated his bed with tossing and turning.

Step 9: Sleep Expansion: After your sleep efficiency has remained at or above 85 percent for three days for mild insomnia and up to two weeks for severe insomnia, slowly begin to expand your sleep back to the target bedtime and wake time you set in level 1. You'll add sleep more gradually than you took it away. This helps keep your sleep efficiency high, which keeps bed and sleep securely paired in the brain while allowing you to shift your sleep-wake cycle as needed.

As you begin to expand your sleep, you'll do it in 15-minute increments. Consider your new bedtime and wake time, and decide whether you want to add the 15 minutes to the bedtime or wake time to hit your target times. People with very mild sleep problems can add 15 minutes back per day; those with severe problems should add sleep time by 15 minutes back per week. Ideally, you can add time until your bedtime and wake time are eight and a half hours apart. If this is not possible for you with your work and family duties, get as close to this number as possible. Should you ever struggle again, you can simply return to step 8 and repeat the compression/expansion process.

There's no need to panic if you have one or two days where your sleep efficiency dips below 85 percent. If this dip is consistent, just return to step 8 and repeat this process. For some people, this could be information that you may want to move through this program more slowly the second or third time around. Let's look at how Carol and George expanded their sleep times:

- **EXAMPLE 1:** After three days with a bedtime of 11:15 P.M. and wake time of 7:15 A.M., Carol moved her bedtime back to 11 P.M. and her wake time to 7:30 A.M. She monitored her sleep efficiency, which was now averaging 90 percent. With less anxiety around sleep, she eventually saw her sleep efficiency average 95 percent.

- **EXAMPLE 2:** George began slowly adding 15 minutes to his wake time each week. Since the last few days of sleep compression left him with a bedtime of 10:30 P.M. and a wake time of 3:30 A.M., it took him a few months to reach his target bedtime of 10 P.M. and his wake time of 7:30 A.M. He moved his wake time by 15 minutes at first and then adjusted his bedtime during the last few days. His sleep efficiency was now above 85 percent most days.

Steps 8 and 9 in this sleep-improvement process can be practiced in a fluid way, and you can return to them whenever your sleep-wake cycles are off or when you notice you're not sleeping well. Some people may move on to step 9 too quickly and see their sleep efficiency go back down. If this happens, simply return to step 8. You'll learn how quickly your brain and body respond to this process, which will help you know how quickly you can move through this process should you need it in the future.

Step 10: Reassess Your Sleep Worry: Return to your sleep worry to see how your experience has continued to change it. Let's return to the former example. In this case, let's say the EBCT strategies may have shifted how true this worry feels—from 95 percent to 75 percent. However, this person needed even more potent experiences to draw upon. This last step of CBT-I provided the information that serves as concrete evidence the fear is too alarmist.

SLEEP WORRY: *pessimistic:* "If I don't get eight hours sleep tonight, I'm going to botch that presentation and get fired. I won't be able to afford my mortgage. Where will I live?" →
MY EXPERIENCE HAS TAUGHT ME: "During sleep compression, there was a week where I was only sleeping about 5 hours a night. I went to work every day. I may not have been at my best, but I got through my responsibilities and duties fairly well. My pessimistic, catastrophic fear that I would be fired and lose my house did not become a reality. Now I'm actually sleeping more soundly than ever before. With eight restful hours, I'm performing better than ever at work." → HOW TRUE THE SLEEP WORRY FEELS NOW: 5 percent. While the sleep worry may still be there in some form, it's just a passing thought. There's no need to believe it or to take the thought or fear too seriously.

In this case, notice that the person combined EBCT with the last step of CBT-I so that now the degree of belief is only 5 percent. The worry may still surface occasionally. However, it's not distressing since only 5 percent of you believes it could be true. As a result, the thought quickly disappears and doesn't cause any significant distress.

Let's use this strategy for you. Return to your sleep worry on page 139 and see how the last step of CBT-I has changed how true it feels.

- SLEEP WORRY: _____ (Previously ___% true)

    MY EXPERIENCE HAS TAUGHT ME: _____

    - NOW THIS WORRY FEELS ___% TRUE

Use this CBT-I program whenever you experience significant difficulties with sleep. The stress reduction strategies in later chapters work synergistically with this program and may help you to sleep even more soundly. Sleeping soundly is yet another piece of the brain-balancing puzzle. It is also the last piece of the big fix for brain drain. If you make the lifestyle changes outlined in the last seven chapters, your brain will be well on the way to balance. In the next section of the book are even more tools to help you bring balance to your brain. These are simple, in-the-moment tools you can add into the healthy routine you've created up to this point.

PART III

THE BRAIN DRAIN SUPER FIX

CHAPTER 13

Relaxation Therapy

There are many forms of relaxation therapy you can add to your brain-balancing toolbox. Let's start with the simplest one to learn. In 1975, Harvard cardiologist Herbert Benson, M.D., published a groundbreaking book called *The Relaxation Response*. At the time, it was still somewhat controversial to claim practices like meditation had health benefits that could be as powerful as prescription medication. Using the mind to change the brain and body was still "alternative." In a televised interview, Dr. Benson taught Barbara Walters how to do something novel at the time: how to relax. Even more incredible: this simple response required no Valium or other benzodiazepines that were popular at the time. As Dr. Benson says, you can "use the mind like you would use a drug." His drug-free practice was incredibly simple and could be learned in minutes.

Dr. Benson advocated for health care to add self-care as a third piece to the approach of treating illness with pharmaceuticals and surgery or other medical treatment. In fact, he believed that self-care should be the biggest piece of treatment. His approach involved natural treatments like relaxation therapy, nutrition, and exercise, which are, of course, integral parts of The Drained Brain program. The other pieces, pharmaceuticals and surgery, should be used only when necessary.

To create his method, Dr. Benson studied practitioners of Transcendental Meditation and knew there were physiological benefits that could improve disease in addition to spiritual ones. Meditation turned on what he dubbed the "relaxation response." With a simple and gentle intention to relax from the mind, the parasympathetic nervous system's rest-and-digest response can become activated. Stress hormones and blood pressure go down, helping people with heart disease or hypertension. People with other diseases can benefit as well, since the course of diseases like cancer are influenced by stress.

Dr. Benson provided a valuable endorsement for spiritual practices, and America listened since he was a mainstream Harvard cardiologist. He told people prayer, meditation, chanting, yoga, Tai Chi, breathing exercises, guided imagery, Qi Gong, and progressive muscle relaxation all elicit "the relaxation response." This wasn't a new invention. In fact, he said, "We claim no innovation but simply a scientific validation of age-old wisdom." While he touted the measurable health benefits of these practices, he also endorsed the spiritual element behind them. Dr. Benson believed that belief and faith are crucial to health since belief "can definitely counteract the harmful effects of stress . . . Believe in what you're doing to counteract the stress. Believe in relationships, and if you're of a religious nature, believe in the protective aspects of God. That's good for us because it gives us hope, and that hope is a very wonderful way to cope with many of the stresses in everyday life. Now I'm not saying that we should all believe in God. I'm saying if your belief system is to incorporate God, and that kind of spirituality, that's wonderful. If you're not religious, then use another belief system in which you have faith, and that belief can also help you counteract the harmful effects of stress."

Decades later, Dr. Benson's advice still holds true. A few claims in his groundbreaking book have been disproven—like the discredited recommendation that margarine is good for the heart and eggs are bad for it. However, his principal claims of the mind's power over brain and body are truer than ever. In fact, in 2008 Dr. Benson was involved in research that proved that our ability to relax may be even *more* potent than originally thought. This research was the first compelling evidence that eliciting the relaxation response changed gene expression in both short- and long-term practitioners. The researchers found that this simple practice had anti-inflammatory and antioxidant effects in subjects who used it for just 20 minutes a day.[1]

Eliciting the relaxation response for 10 to 20 minutes once or twice a day has the power to improve your mood, reduce your risk of disease, and positively influence the expression of your genes.

RELAXATION THROUGH MANTRA

Dr. Benson's instructions to bring about the relaxation response involved using a mantra to shut off the thoughts of an active mind. The word *one* is an example of a simple mantra you can use. It's a user-friendly version of mantras used by Transcendental Meditation practitioners.

Here's a simple way to practice the relaxation response that Dr. Benson taught. It's very short and easy to memorize. You can also go to my Facebook page to watch a video if you'd like to practice it with me (www.facebook.com/drmikedow).

- Find a comfortable seated position and close your eyes.

- Relax your muscles, starting with your feet and allowing the relaxation to spread all the way up to your head.

- Breathe easily and comfortably through your nose, and mindfully become aware of the breath.

- Attach a mantra like the word *one* to your breath as you say this word to yourself on each inhale and exhale. You can also choose another soothing word if you'd like.

- Maintain a passive attitude so that relaxation unfolds at its own pace.

- Continue for 10 to 20 minutes.[2]

In week 2 of The Drained Brain program, you'll use this and two other forms of relaxation therapy to see which of them you'd like to add to your long-term brain-balancing toolbox. All forms of relaxation therapy elicit what Dr. Benson dubbed the relaxation response, so all of them provide similar benefits. The best practice for you to keep in your toolbox is the one you will do regularly.

RELAXATION THROUGH PROGRESSIVE MUSCLE TECHNIQUE

The second form of relaxation therapy is progressive muscle relaxation, which is especially helpful for people with insomnia and any physical conditions involving pain or tension like headaches. It uses the release of physical tension as the "way in" to achieve mental tranquility. As you feel the difference between a state of tension versus relaxation, you become acutely aware of where you're carrying physical tension.

This protocol was published by a Chicago physician named Edmund Jacobson decades before Dr. Benson's book, and it is used as an add-on to standard treatments of digestive disorders and hypertension.

You can use progressive muscle relaxation lying down if you'd like, and this makes it a perfect addition to cognitive behavioral therapy for insomnia that you learned about in the last chapter. For insomnia, use the practice in bed since it can prepare your brain and body for restful sleep. You can also use this practice during the day in a seated or lounging position to dissolve tension and stress. Because it can affect heart rate (usually for the better), it's recommended that you check with your primary care physician or cardiologist before using it if you have a serious heart condition.

Here's a simple version of progressive muscle relaxation. You can memorize it easily, or you can also see and hear me reading this script on my Facebook page (www.facebook.com/drmikedow) if you'd like to do it without needing to memorize it:

- Begin by finding a comfortable seated or lying down position and closing your eyes.

- Inhale through your nose for a count of 5. At the same time, flex your feet and tense your calf muscles. Notice the feeling of tension in this part of the body.

- Exhale through your nose for a count of 10 while releasing and feeling all the tension dissolve. Notice the difference between tension and total relaxation.

- While inhaling through your nose for a count of 5, squeeze your leg muscles as you straighten your knees. Notice the feeling of tension in this part of the body.

- While exhaling through your nose for a count of 10, release and feel all the tension dissolve. Notice the difference between tension and total relaxation.

- Inhale through your nose for a count of 5. At the same time, squeeze your buttocks together. Notice the feeling of tension in this part of the body.

- Exhale through your nose for a count of 10 while releasing and feeling all the tension dissolve. Notice the difference between tension and total relaxation.

- While inhaling through your nose for a count of 5, squeeze your abs as if you're doing crunches. Notice the feeling of tension in this part of the body.

- While exhaling through your nose for a count of 10, release and feel all the tension dissolve. Notice the difference between tension and total relaxation.

- Inhale through your nose for a count of 5. At the same time, squeeze your back muscles by squeezing your shoulder blades toward each other. Notice the feeling of tension in this part of the body.

- Exhale through your nose for a count of 10 while releasing and feeling all the tension dissolve. Notice the difference between tension and total relaxation.

- While inhaling through your nose for a count of 5, make fists with both your hands, straighten your elbows, and contract your biceps and triceps. Notice the feeling of tension in this part of the body.

- While exhaling through your nose for a count of 10, release and feel all the tension dissolve. Notice the difference between tension and total relaxation.

- Inhale through your nose for a count of 5. At the same time, raise your shoulders and tense your neck as you bring your chin to your chest. Notice the feeling of tension in this part of the body.

- Exhale through your nose for a count of 10 while releasing and feeling all the tension dissolve. Notice the difference between tension and total relaxation.

- While inhaling through your nose for a count of 5, tense your jaw, wrinkle your nose, and squeeze your eyes even more closed. Notice the feeling of tension in this part of the body.

- While exhaling through your nose for a count of 10, release and feel all the tension dissolve. Notice the difference between tension and total relaxation.

- Inhale through your nose for a count of 5. At the same time, raise your eyebrows as you feel tension in your forehead and across your scalp. Notice the feeling of tension in this part of the body.

- Exhale through your nose for a count of 10 while releasing and feeling all the tension dissolve. Notice the difference between tension and total relaxation.

Once you've used this protocol, notice where you physically carry the most tension. You can use a shorter version of this practice at your desk if you find your tension is mostly in your face or shoulders. If you carry tension in your abdomen and suffer from digestive problems, tense and release this part of the body several times a day with the breath when you notice tension beginning to grow. Reverse the practice if you'd like by starting with the forehead and scalp and work your way down to the feet and calves. You can also slow the practice down. Instead of one exhale to the count of 10, extend the length of the release portion of each muscle group. Add a few relaxed inhales and exhales between each muscle group as you make the practice longer.

After you have mastered progressive muscle relaxation and its tense-and-release format, you can eventually move on to release-only relaxation. This is also an alternative for people with paralysis or for whom the tensing of muscles may be too painful. On the inhale, bring your awareness to a muscle group without tensing. On the exhale, release the muscle group and feel any and all tension dissolving.

RELAXATION THROUGH AUTOGENIC TRAINING

The final form of relaxation therapy is called autogenic training. This protocol was developed around the same time as progressive muscle relaxation by a psychiatrist in Germany named Johannes Heinrich Schultz. Whereas Dr. Benson studied practitioners of Transcendental Meditation to create his protocol, Dr. Schultz noticed that patients treated with hypnosis would enter a relaxed state with limbs that felt heavy and warm. He took advantage of this phenomenon to create his protocol.

Like the other forms of relaxation therapy, it's simple to learn. Dr. Schultz recommended using it for 15 minutes in the morning, at lunchtime, and in the evening. You can use autogenic training lying down during the day or before bed, or use it in a reclined or seated position. A 2002 meta-analysis looked at 73 studies using autogenic training. It found autogenic training improves mood, cognitive performance, and quality of life. It's effective in treating or managing symptoms for a long list of diseases including anxiety, asthma, depression, headaches, heart disease, hypertension, insomnia, and pain.[3] If you have a heart condition, diabetes, high or low blood pressure, or untreated and/or severe mental illness, it's recommended you check with your primary care physician or specialist before using it.

Like the other two forms of relaxation therapy, autogenic training balances drained brains by shifting the activity from sympathetic nervous system dominance to parasympathetic nervous system dominance. Remember, a balanced brain is mildly parasympathetic dominant with short-lived sympathetic nervous system activation when stressors are present. A balanced brain also easily recovers from sympathetic nervous system activation and short-term spikes of stress hormones, shifting easily back into the rest-and-digest response of the parasympathetic nervous system. If your brain is drained, this practice is yet another tool to add to your brain-balancing toolbox.

Here's a simple version of autogenic training. Say these phrases silently to yourself in a comfortable seated or lying position. You can also click on the video of me on my Facebook page if you'd like to use it without memorizing it (www.facebook.com/drmikedow):

- I am completely calm.

- My arms are heavy. (six times)

- I am completely calm.

- My arms are warm. (six times)

- I am completely calm.

- My legs are heavy. (six times)

- I am completely calm.

- My legs are warm. (six times)

- I am completely calm.

- My heart beats calmly and regularly. (six times)

- I am completely calm.

- My breathing is calm and regular. (six times)

- I am completely calm.

- My abdomen is warm. (six times)

- I am completely calm.

- My forehead is pleasantly cool. (six times)

- I am completely calm.

You can use the following sentence if you need to wake from the relaxation therapy and return to an alert state. If you'd like to stay in this relaxed state (e.g., when using this practice in bed before sleep), skip this last phrase:

- Arms firm, breathe deeply, open eyes.

In week 2 of The Drained Brain program, you'll have the opportunity to use all three relaxation therapy protocols in one day. After you see which ones you like best, you can use them whenever you need them. But let me assure you, with these three potent and clinically proven forms of relaxation in your toolbox, you'll be able to naturally balance your brain whenever you'd like.

CHAPTER 14

Pranayama

Pranayama—also known as "breath control" or yogic breathing—is a potent balancer for drained brains. One of the simplest breathing exercises you'll learn in this chapter, Diaphragmatic Breathing, is a clinically proven strategy for reducing anxiety.[1] And Sudarshan Kriya Yoga (SKY), which uses sequences of pranayama practices including Bellows Breath and chanting *om*, has been shown to reduce levels of the brain-draining hormone cortisol while improving mood.[2] It works quickly, too. One study showed that it balanced levels of cortisol after just one session, and another showed that it improves the quality of sleep.[3] Pranayama can even help you to have a profoundly spiritual experience and feel at one with God or the divine. Psychiatrist Stanislav Grof created his protocol Holotropic Breathwork to help patients attain nonordinary states of consciousness without needing to take a hallucinogenic drug. One study found 82 percent of subjects reported a "transpersonal" experience, and another found it reduced subjects' fear of dying.[4] This type of breath work uses a form of breathing similar to the Bellows Breath practice you'll learn.

Pranayama even works in the most serious cases of drained brains. In patients hospitalized with a mood disorder, electroconvulsive therapy (ECT)—one of the heaviest hitters in treating severe mental illness—was only *slightly* more effective than pranayama. Pranayama was also nearly as effective as prescription antidepressants and was so effective the researchers deemed it an alternative "first line treatment" for acute mental illness.[5] Of course, pranayama comes with the added bonus that you don't have to go under general anesthesia as you do with ECT or tolerate a long list of side effects as you do with prescription medications. You just have to breathe.

Pranayama's benefits, like the rest of the Drained Brain program, are thanks to its ability to rebalance your autonomic nervous system. As you know, the autonomic nervous system takes care of your "automatics" like breathing, digestion, and heartbeat—even when you're asleep. But unlike other functions controlled by the autonomic nervous system, breathing can be done in a voluntary *or* involuntary way. Using pranayama is like a pilot disabling "autopilot" mode and navigating a plane manually instead.

First let's take a look at what happens to the breath when it's running on the "autopilot" mode of everyday life. When the autonomic nervous system shifts into a sympathetic nervous system–dominant state, the release of stress hormones moves the breath up toward the chest, speeds it up, and makes it inhalation dominant. These shallow, rapid breaths can potentially give your muscles the energy they would need for a quick getaway from a tiger. But in drained brains, this response isn't temporary, and the breath remains shallow all day long. And of course it's not just tigers that trigger this response; it's the stress of everyday life. The result: you're robbed of the energy you need and are left feeling anxious, panicky, and depleted. Since you didn't discharge this energy by running from a tiger, you're stuck in this problematic psychological and physiological state.

What *should* have happened is a return to the parasympathetic-dominant, rest-and-digest state thanks to brain-balancing neurotransmitters. When this happens, the breath automatically migrates back down to the belly area, slows down, and is exhalation dominant. You no longer need extra oxygen to run from that tiger—or deadline—that's chasing you. Your breath should also naturally transition to this easy state when you fall asleep. For people with insomnia, the relaxing breath exercises you'll learn in this chapter are a great add-on to the CBT-I program you learned in Chapter 12. They can shorten the time it takes to fall asleep.

As you know, the "ideal" state for balanced brains is one of mild parasympathetic nervous system dominance with short-lived, occasional waves of sympathetic nervous system activation—only occurring when a stressor is encountered. Your breath should be like Goldilocks. Your breath doesn't stay "too high" as it does in people with untreated anxiety disorders. It doesn't stay "too low" as it can with the use of excess benzodiazepines or extreme fatigue. The breath—along with the general response of your autonomic nervous system—finds the sweet spot that's "just right" with the flexibility to rise or fall as needed.

Pranayama can also help you become an "energy wizard" as you learn to manipulate your nervous system without needing caffeine or processed carbohydrates to take it up or down, respectively. The brain learns it can easily move into the activated state of fight, flight, or freeze and return to a calm state of rest-and-digest by using the sequences you're about to learn. Think of these practices as interval training for your breath, which helps you efficiently deal with life's stresses without depleting your energy reserves. Your energy levels will soar once the breath and nervous system learn to easily recover from activated states.

These breath sequences are even effective for people who get "stuck" in sympathetic nervous system dominance with atypical and severe presentations of drained brains.

Pranayama can help heal PTSD and its associated footprint of high norepinephrine but low cortisol levels—also seen in people with adrenal fatigue or exhaustion. Pranayama practices were shown to be effective in reducing the symptoms of PTSD in survivors of the 2004 tsunami in Asia.[6] It works on other brain-balancing neurotransmitters as well. Oxytocin levels rise; cortisol becomes balanced.

For people experiencing mind-body brain drain or more bodily based presentations of anxiety, Pranayama can act as a pathway to influence affected nervous system functions. It can change your heart rate, improve immune function, and aid digestion. This reminds us that the brain-breath connection is not a one-way street. While most of us allow the nervous system to determine the speed and depth of our breath, we can also use the breath to influence the state of the nervous system.

We can also take advantage of the phenomenon of respiratory sinus arrhythmia (RSA), the naturally occurring variation in heart rate that corresponds to your breath. Your heart rate will increase ever so slightly on inhales and decrease on exhales. By changing the length of these two parts of the breath, you can change your heart rate. Moving your breath from shallow breathing into deep belly breathing with a longer exhale can convince the brain that danger has passed and it will revert to a parasympathetic-dominant state through stimulation of the calming vagus nerve that wanders from your brainstem to your body's organs. Conversely, inhale for two seconds and exhale for one second to nudge the brain into a sympathetic-dominant state. This can speed your heart rate while focusing the mind.

Let's take a look at how you can use Pranayama to balance your drained brain. There are eight breathing practices in the chapter. I've split them up between calming and activating practices so you can use them for as long as you need them. You should only have to do them for a few minutes to begin to feel a shift, and short practices are also helpful when time is limited. That being said, use them for longer periods of practice when you have the time since a longer practice will help you reap more of the rewards.

CALMING BREATH

If you find yourself feeling anxious or overwhelmed, try out one of these simple breathing exercises to convince your body that it's time to move toward parasympathetic activation of your nervous system. If you want to supercharge the balancing of these practices, you can do them while wearing the cranial electrotherapy stimulation device I discussed on page 141. I personally find this combination to be incredibly calming.

Diaphragmatic Breathing

Diaphragmatic Breathing is one of the simplest ways to help a stressed-out mind back into a parasympathetic-dominant, rest-and-digest state. The diaphragm is located at the base of your lungs. The diaphragm and abdominal muscles help you to breathe and can be used together to powerfully empty the lungs. Diaphragmatic Breathing has other benefits and can strengthen the diaphragm itself. Breathing becomes more efficient with more oxygen reaching all your body's cells. If this practice is difficult for you at first, keep using it. As the muscle strengthens, this practice will become easier.

- Lie down with a pillow under your head and one under your knees. This is the easiest and most comfortable way to use Diaphragmatic Breathing.

- Place one hand over your upper chest and the other hand below your rib cage over your belly.

- Inhale through your nose. Keep the hand on your chest still, and breathe into the belly so you feel the hand on the belly moving out.

- Exhale through your mouth. Again, the hand on your chest should remain still. The hand on the belly should now move toward you. Contract your abdominal muscles to push all the air out. Take slow and steady inhales and exhales.

- Practice this for several minutes a few times a day.

This is the simplest way to do this practice. You can do a more advanced, weighted version to strengthen the muscles by doing this practice lying down with a heavy book over your belly. Or you can do it while sitting in a chair or standing. Any of these methods will help strengthen your diaphragm and calm you down in the process.

One thing I love about this process is that you can use it to help you figure out how stressed you are in the moment. When you begin to feel stressed in your daily life, check in with your breath by placing one hand on your chest and the other on your belly. Which hand is moving? If the hand on your chest is moving, this is a clue that the sympathetic nervous system has become dominant. Gently correct this by using the Diaphragmatic Breathing exercise you just learned. Move the breath into the belly so that only the lower hand moves as the hand on your chest remains motionless. Eventually, you can perform this process without using your hands at all. You can become mindfully aware of where the breath is moving simply by paying attention to it. Notice how high or low the breath is riding right now. Note the speed of inhales and exhales while you're going about your day.

Try using this practice while lying in bed as an add-on to the CBT-I protocol you learned since it can help your body and mind relax, drifting effortlessly into sleep as the parasympathetic nervous system is activated. Eventually this type of breathing can become your default way of breathing. The result: less stress and sound sleep.

3:6 Breathing

Since the sympathetic nervous system tends to be inhale dominant and the parasympathetic nervous system tends to be exhale dominant, nudge your autonomic nervous system into a parasympathetic-dominant state by making your exhalation longer than your inhalation. Once you've mastered Diaphragmatic Breathing, add 3:6 Breathing to it. Or do 3:6 Breathing on its own. This exercise is helpful for brain-drained people if they can catch the sympathetic nervous system activation early—before it has spiraled out of control into acute anxiety or a panic attack. Wherever you may be, simply use 3:6 Breathing. This and other calming breath practices are particularly helpful to use in the evening for people who have altered levels of melatonin and cortisol. Remember, cortisol should rise in the morning as melatonin dips. In the evening, cortisol should dip as melatonin rises. CBT-I and other strategies you've learned can correct the timed rise and fall of melatonin and cortisol if they're out of sync. Use 3:6 Breathing in the evening, and help your brain bring cortisol levels down in the evening. You can also reverse 3:6 Breathing into 6:3 Breathing at other times when you need more energy and activation. Interestingly, 3:6 Breathing also trains the tongue to gently rest at the top of the mouth with the mouth closed when breathing or at rest, which can help relax the mouth and jaw during the day. It's also associated with other health benefits, such as reducing your risk of gingivitis.

- With your mouth closed, place your tongue so that it's gently touching the roof of your mouth just above the gum line or, if it's more comfortable, touching the back of your front teeth.

- Breathe in through your nose to a slow three count. Pause for a moment at the top.

- Breathe out through your nose to a slow count of 6. Pause for a moment, and feel this transition point fully. Notice how there's no need to immediately gasp for your next in breath.

- Repeat.

As you continue to use this practice, you may notice your breath beginning to slow down even more. When you start using this practice, you may notice the three count takes about three seconds and the six count takes about six seconds. As you begin to calm down, the slow three count of the inhale may begin to take 5 seconds and the slow six count may begin to take 10 seconds. There's no need to watch the clock. Your breath will begin to gradually slow down as the parasympathetic nervous system becomes more and more activated through this practice. Pranayama is a skill and a practice. The more you use it, the more effective it becomes. It also works synergistically with the other principles of the Drained Brain program, so combining it with EBCT and lifestyle changes will begin to supercharge your results.

Try combining 3:6 Breathing with Diaphragmatic Breathing, breathing the three counts into your belly and exhaling for six, pressing the breath out with your diaphragm.

Chant "Om"

Om is said to be a mystic syllable. It's said to be the sound of the universe, and it's been shown that this sound can actually synchronize biorhythms.[7] It appears at the beginning and end of Sanskrit texts and prayers, and many yoga classes will "seal" or end the class by chanting it three times. Attach your own spiritual or religious meaning if you wish. The major religions of the world all have a word that sounds like *om*—shalom, amen, and salaam—so you could even substitute a word from your faith. Or you can simply use the phonetic vibration as a secular meditation as you attune to your sense of sound. *Om* is usually pronounced as three separate sounds: "ah," "oh," and "mm."

- In a comfortable seated position on the floor or in a chair, begin by taking a deep inhale into your belly for three seconds.

- For "ah," relax your mouth. The sound should originate in the belly.

- For "oh," your lips should make a circular shape. Picture the sound moving into your heart.

- For "mm," close the lips and feel the vibration of the sound and the buzzing in the head. This sound should last longer than "ah" and "oh" and continues until you've run out of air. In that moment, pause. Feel the peace of the silence for a moment.

- Take another deep breath, and repeat "om" two more times.

- Notice how the exhale and the corresponding buzzing of "om" means the exhale is much longer than the inhale, exerting a calming effect on the nervous system.

Mantra Breath

Mantra Breathing is simply breathing slowly and saying a word or phrase to yourself on the inhale and another on the exhale. On the inhalation, the word or phrase should represent what you are breathing in and embracing. On the exhalation, it should represent what you are letting go of. Make these words or phrases special to you. They can have spiritual or religious influences. Or they can be physical or psychological goals. Here are some examples:

- peace/stress
- "I'm okay."/worry
- gratitude/pessimism
- God/ego mind
- love/fear
- relaxation/tension
- connection/separation
- hope/hopelessness
- faith/doubt
- confidence/criticism

- loving-kindness/resentment
- joy/depression
- kindness/anger
- "Breathing in, I know that I am perfect as I am."/"Breathing out, I let go of self-doubt."
- "On this in breath, I feel all the love I have in my life."/"On this out breath, I let go of resentments that hold me back."

One of the great things about Mantra Breathing is that you can add it to pretty much any other breathing technique. You could do Mantra 3:6 Breathing. Or you could do Mantra 3:6 Diaphragmatic Breathing.

Ujjayi Breath

Many yoga classes use Ujjayi Breath to accompany physical poses. It's an extremely calming practice for the nervous system, and the audible sound helps you mindfully stay focused on the slowing breath. It's especially helpful when you feel angry or agitated. *Ujjayi* means "victorious" in Sanskrit, so you may hear this referred to as Victorious Breath.

- Begin by exhaling with your mouth open like you're going to fog a mirror. Feel the way your throat opens, and hear a sound that resembles the ocean.

- Now, keep your throat open and your mouth relaxed, but close your lips gently. Inhale through the nose, and feel the air making contact with the back of the throat. On the exhale, feel the warm air in your nasal passages.

You should hear an audible sound on both the inhale and the exhale which may remind you of Darth Vader or the ocean.

- Like Diaphragmatic Breathing, begin by filling the belly. Second, fill the lower rib cage. Finally, fill the chest and then the throat. This is slightly different than the instructions for Diaphragmatic Breathing where you keep your chest still. For Ujjayi Breath, you're taking an extremely deep breath and are maximizing your capacity by using the belly, chest, and other parts of the body.

- Use a timer at first. Slow the breath down, and make the in breath and out breath equal lengths. Begin by using seven seconds on the inhale and seven seconds on the exhale so that you slow your breathing down to about four breaths per minute. If possible, see if you can slow the breath even further to reach up to 15 seconds for the inhale and 15 seconds on the exhale to bring your breath down to two breaths per minute.

Moon Channel

The sympathetic and parasympathetic nervous systems are governed by different parts of the brain; the former by the left prefrontal cortex and the latter by the right prefrontal cortex. In the kundalini yoga tradition, Pingala and Ida are two energies that intertwine up the spine. Each represents an opposing energy. Pingala energy is on the right and has the activating energy of the sun. It's associated with the sympathetic nervous system and its fight, flight, or freeze response. Ida energy is on the left and embodies the calming energy of the moon. It's associated with the parasympathetic nervous system and its rest-and-digest response.

When you feel yourself becoming activated with stress, try Moon Channel Breathing to move to a calmer, Ida energy state.

- With your right hand, fold your index and middle fingers into your palm.
- Exhale normally.
- Close your right nostril with your right thumb. Inhale through your left nostril.
- Close your left nostril with your right pinky and ring finger. Exhale through your right nostril.
- Repeat.

If the hand position noted here is too awkward, you can always just alternate your thumb and index finger, like you're plugging your nose. This is also more discreet if you're doing this at your desk or somewhere else in public.

You can supercharge Moon Channel breathing by combining it with Diaphragmatic Breathing and/or 3:6 Breathing. It's another great combination.

ACTIVATING BREATH

If you're looking for a little extra energy—throwing your body a bit more toward the sympathetic nervous system rather than the parasympathetic—try one of these activating practices. These are helpful to use first thing in the morning to get you going. They can also help correct the 24-hour cycle of melatonin and cortisol levels by creating a gentle lift of cortisol levels in the morning when a slight increase is actually helpful.

An important caveat for people with panic disorder and PTSD: I recommend these activating breath practices as *part* of a treatment plan. If you have untreated PTSD, panic disorder, or acute anxiety, begin by using the calming breath practices. You can add the activating breath practices after psychotherapy results in symptom improvement.

Sun Channel Breathing

This is simply the opposite of Moon Channel Breathing. It is a mildly activating practice you can use when you notice that midafternoon energy slump. Continue using the thumb and then pinky and ring finger. Again, you can also use your thumb and index finger if this is too challenging.

- Exhale normally.
- Close your left nostril with your right thumb. Inhale through your right nostril.
- Close your right nostril with your right pinky and ring finger. Exhale through your left nostril.
- Repeat.

Supercharge Sun Channel breathing by adding 6:3 Breath. Inhale to the count of six and exhale to the count of three. The long inhale and shorter exhale results in even greater sympathetic nervous system activation.

Bellows Breath

Bellows Breath, or Bhastrika Breath, is an advanced breath practice and is the most activating breath practice you'll learn. When used correctly, you're contracting the muscles so powerfully it feels as though you've just completed an abs class.

There are some people who should not use Bellows Breath. If you are pregnant or have high blood pressure, untreated trauma, uncontrolled panic attacks, cardiovascular disease, epilepsy, or a hernia, do not use Bellows Breath. You can use a mildly activating practice, like Sun Channel Breathing or Sun Channel Breathing with 6:3 Breath for moderate activation. Also, it's best to do Bellows Breath on an empty stomach, and don't eat immediately after using it.

This practice is great for a post-lunch energy boost or before a big game. It's also helpful for people with certain low-cortisol brain-drained footprints like those seen in adrenal fatigue or PTSD to use first thing in the morning. You can also use it to combat jet lag. Just don't try it before bed since the activation will prevent restful sleep.

- Sit in a cross-legged position or in a chair with your spine straight.

- Take a deep, cleansing breath.

- Inhale through your nose, and puff your belly out.

- Exhale through your nose, forcefully pushing the air. Use the diaphragm and abdominal muscles together to push your belly button inward toward your spine with every exhale.

- With every inhale, your belly button should move away from the spine.

- Speed your breath so that you are taking one second for the inhale and one second for the exhale. You may wish to use a clock with a second hand or a phone with a stopwatch when you learn this practice to learn the pacing. Stop if you feel dizzy or light-headed. Begin with 5 or 10 breaths. If this is comfortable, eventually work your way up to one minute of practice with 30 breaths.

ADVANCED PRANAYAMA SEQUENCES

Now that you've learned several variations of breathing, put them together in novel ways. Here are a few suggestions. Once you have learned these practices, try combining the ways that work for you. You can use very short breath practices if you have 20 seconds before a meeting starts, or when you have time, do a 15- or 30-minute breath sequence.

The Cleansing Heart

This is a centering practice that helps you to let go of negative emotions. It can be used when you're feeling disconnected from others or your spiritual center. Allow the energy to touch your heart while it calms your nervous system:

- Use Diaphragmatic Breathing for 10 breaths with equal inhales and exhales. Place your right hand over your heart and your left hand on your belly. Physically move the breath into the belly; this hand will be the only one moving. As you keep the hand over your heart still, imagine the breath giving you anything you need in this moment.

- Add Mantra Breathing as you silently recite a word or phrase to yourself on the inhale and a word or phrase on the exhale for 10 breaths. Imagine that your heart is inhaling something you need and letting go of something that's not serving you. If you use this before bed, try inhaling "peace" or "rest" and exhaling "stress" or "doing mind."

- Chant "om" three times to seal the practice, taking whatever you intended to cultivate with you.

The Crouching Tiger

This is an extremely activating sequence that ramps your energy up to prepare you for action like a big race. It can also be used anytime you need a big boost of energy. Avoid using this sequence in the evening before bed. Don't use this full sequence if you are one of the people who should avoid Bellows Breath outlined in the section above. If you are one of these people, a modification would be to only use the first three of the four practices below, and make the third practice here 25 breaths instead of 10:

- Five slow Ujjayi Breaths as you feel the inherent energy of your mind and body

- Sun Channel Breathing with even inhales and exhales for 10 breaths

- Sun Channel breathing with a 4:2 pattern (four seconds per inhale, two seconds for the exhale) for 10 breaths

- Bellows Breath for 15 breaths

Breathing Loving-Kindness

If you need to find compassion, patience, or forgiveness in your life, this practice culti-vates loving-kindness. Use it before walking into a work or family gathering with someone who has irritated you. Remember that people who treat others poorly are ones who haven't yet been blessed with the gift of healing from all the people who hurt them. Use this prac-tice to cultivate gratitude for the love you have in your life.

- Use Diaphragmatic Breathing for 10 breaths with equal inhales and exhales. Place your right hand over your heart and your left hand on your belly. Physically move the breath into the belly as the hand on your heart becomes motionless. Feel the loving-kindness that resides in your heart. Ask it to awaken if it's a little dormant right now.

- In your mind's eye, you will now visualize a series of people (or, if you'd like, animals) for five breaths each.

  1. Begin with the image of someone who is easy to love. There is little or no conflict in this relationship. Feel an energy of loving-kindness radiating from your heart for five slow breaths. Silently recite, "May you be happy and peaceful."

  2. Now visualize someone you love who is slightly trickier. There has been some conflict with this person, but for these next five breaths, you radiate the same loving-kindness you had for the first person. Silently recite, "May you be happy and peaceful."

  3. Now see a person who is difficult to love or have kindness toward. With five deep breaths, radiate loving-kindness from your heart and see it wrapping this person in this energy. Silently recite, "May you be happy and peaceful."

  4. Finally see yourself. Shine the same intensity of loving-kindness you had for others onto yourself for 10 breaths. See yourself bathing in the energy radiating from your heart. Silently recite, "May I be happy and peaceful."

- Return to normal breathing as you take note of the state you have just cultivated. Take it with you, and allow the loving-kindness to put a slight smile on your face and wrap you in an armor that shields you from difficult people you may encounter. Remember: you are lucky to be blessed with this gift. If there are people in your life who are not yet enlightened, send a silent wish that they are blessed with this gift soon.

The Sleeping Lion

This practice can be used to help facilitate sleep. You can either do it before bedtime or while you're in bed:

- Use Diaphragmatic Breathing for 10 breaths with equal inhales and exhales.

- Now add 3:6 Breathing to this practice for 10 breaths.

- Now add Mantra Breathing as you silently recite a word or phrase to yourself on the inhale and a word or phrase on the exhale for 10 breaths.

- Chant "om" three times to seal the practice, taking whatever you intended to cultivate with you.

The Healing Warrior

This sequence is fantastic for drained brains because it activates the sympathetic nervous system and then comes gently down back into parasympathetic activation. It helps to teach the body and brain how to recover from periods of activation so you don't get stuck in them and end up feeling brain drained.

- Use Diaphragmatic Breathing for five breaths with equal inhales and exhales.

- Add Ujjayi Breath for five breaths with equal inhales and exhales.

- Use Sun Channel Breathing for five breaths with equal inhales and exhales.

- Continue with Sun Channel Breathing with a 6:3 pattern for five breaths. Inhale for six seconds, and exhale quickly for three seconds.

- Do Bellows Breath for 30 breaths.

- Repeat the above steps once.

- Chant "om" 3 times.

To hear these and other pranayama sequences, head over to my Facebook page. Breathe with me!

CHAPTER 15

Self-Hypnosis

Like meditation and other forms of relaxation, hypnosis can produce an altered state of consciousness. In hypnosis, this state is often called a "trance." Trance is not an unusual state. In fact, people frequently enter into a trance in everyday life. If you've ever found yourself in a blissful daydream or completely engrossed in a beautiful movie, that's a type of trance. You're not worrying, and some part of you has "left" the stress and worries of life. Drs. Herbert and David Spiegel, the father/son, Columbia/Stanford psychiatrists who wrote the hypnosis manual *Trance and Treatment*, believe that having the ability to daydream or become engrossed in a film is actually a predictor of being hypnotizable.[1]

Clinical hypnosis works by putting you into a balancing type of trance: one where the parasympathetic nervous system and its rest-and-digest response becomes dominant. Drs. Herbert and David Spiegel say hypnosis can facilitate this "changing of the guard" from sympathetic to parasympathetic nervous control. When in this hypnosis-facilitated state, you are relaxed and become more open to suggestion—a helpful quality if you want to achieve goals or give up unhealthy behaviors. Of course, this can also help to balance a drained brain that is sympathetic nervous system dominant, stuck in too much fight, flight, or freeze.

Hypnosis is not a new discovery by any means. It was used by ancient Egyptians. It has been part of the process for healing and spiritual growth by shamans. In the 18th century, a German physician brought hypnosis into the field of medicine. You may already be familiar with him; the word *mesmerized* comes from his last name: Mesmer. Around that time in Germany, a mathematician created a theory: a force called "animal magnetism" was responsible for disease, and thus treatment would have to alter this magnetism. Dr. Franz Mesmer drew on this theory and claimed hypnosis was a cure for any illness due to its power to affect magnetism. While hypnosis can work wonders on anxiety disorders and insomnia, it obviously won't cure smallpox or meningitis. It also has nothing to do with a magnetic field between doctor and patient. Clearly Dr. Mesmer was wrong on many counts, but he did inspire Etienne Félix d'Hénin de Cuvillers, who correctly attributed the healing aspects of hypnosis to the *mental* process involved—not magnetism. He also was the first person to use the word *hypnosis*, which was derived from the ancient Greek word *Hypnos*, the god of sleep.

Decades later, English ophthalmologist Dr. James Braid made the word *hypnosis* popular. Dr. Braid made an astute observation that staring paralyzed the eye muscles and created an unusual state of the nervous system that he believed was in between being awake and being asleep. Although he did not fully understand the neurological explanation of the phenomenon, Dr. Braid's eye fixation technique worked to create hypnotic trance in patients. You'll use a type of eye fixation in the simple self-hypnosis technique you'll learn in this chapter.

In the 19th century, there were two famous schools in France with opposing opinions on hypnosis. One thought it was part of the disease, the other part of the cure. The Paris School believed hypnosis was a mental disorder and related to hysteria, a then-popular, now-defunct diagnosis. On the other hand, the Nancy School in Nancy, France, believed that hypnosis was a physiological state that could be induced in healthy individuals and used to heighten a natural tendency to respond to suggestions. Sigmund Freud was one famous Nancy School student who used hypnosis with his patients but, of course, became better known for his trademark treatment: psychoanalysis.

In the 1900s, the influential American psychiatrist Milton Erickson made hypnosis popular. Hypnosis was endorsed by the American, British, and Canadian Medical Associations in the 1950s, and in 1995, the National Institutes of Health (NIH) recommended hypnosis as a treatment for chronic pain.

Of course, Las Vegas showmen have taken advantage of how hypnosis can almost magically alter the brain, which also tarnishes the public's perception of it if they think of it solely as a show trick. But what if this "brain magic" could actually be part of a treatment plan to treat debilitating illnesses?

Recently hypnosis has received renewed respect from researchers at some of the most prestigious institutions. One of the most interesting studies comes from Dr. Amir Raz, a former professional magician who is now the Canada Research Chair in the Cognitive Neuroscience of Attention at both the Department of Psychiatry at McGill University and the SMBD Jewish General Hospital and did much of his research at Cornell. His study validated hypnosis's ability to "change focal brain activity in a way no drug we have can do." In hypnotizable individuals, hypnotic suggestion alters brain activity and overrides involuntary processes. Dr. Raz believes these findings prove hypnosis could be effective in difficult-to-treat mental illnesses, including impulse control and eating disorders.

The study used functional magnetic resonance imaging (fMRI) and event-related potentials (ERP) to measure activity in subjects' brains, providing concrete evidence to validate hypnosis's clinical claims. It found highly hypnotizable individuals undergo dramatic changes. Imaging showed the anterior cingulate cortex, a part of the brain that lights up when a widely used psychological test called the Stroop test is given, was turned off in subjects' brains. You've probably seen a version of the Stroop test where, for example, the word *green* is printed in red, and the word *yellow* is printed in blue. Trying to name the ink colors and not the printed word is difficult, because it activates cognitive conflict in the brain. While the subject was in a hypnotic trance, Dr. Raz's voice told the subject that the actual words he or she would soon see would be "gibberish" and be like "characters in a foreign language"—but he or she would be able to see the colors quite easily. A post-hypnotic suggestion was given so this would remain true even when the person was no longer in trance and the Stroop test was then administered. Later, the highly hypnotizable subjects could suddenly name the colors instantly, but the subjects who were resistant were still slow to name the colors.[2] Since hypnotic influence over these brains persists even after the trance ends, it validates hypnosis as a treatment that has value in changing our everyday responses or behavioral choices.

While there are some people who are highly hypnotizable, it's important to realize that it can be an innate talent but, for most, also a learned skill. Michael Phelps clearly has a knack for swimming and quickly began setting national records. That being said, any swimmer can get better with practice. According to Stanford psychiatrist Dr. David Spiegel, 10 to 15 percent of adults are highly hypnotizable, 20 percent are resistant, and the rest are in between. Translation: there's an 80 percent chance that hypnosis will work for you—especially if you use it consistently.

HEALING WITH HYPNOSIS

I have to admit, I was a skeptic going into my first professional hypnosis training, which was also my first personal experience with hypnosis. A few studies had me intrigued. I had read one study in which subjects with high blood pressure were divided into two groups. The group receiving hypnosis had both short-term and long-term improvements in blood pressure.[3]

Hypnosis has also been beneficial in treating severe cases of irritable bowel syndrome. A groundbreaking study published in *The Lancet* divided patients with severe IBS, a difficult-to-treat condition that is often unresponsive to medication, into two groups. One group received hypnotherapy and the other received psychotherapy with placebo pills. While the group receiving psychotherapy with placebo pills improved somewhat, the group receiving hypnotherapy showed dramatic improvement in all IBS symptoms. Furthermore, the group receiving hypnotherapy remarkably had no relapses during a three-month follow-up.[4]

Hypnosis works synergistically with other clinically proven treatments like ones you've learned in this program. A recent study divided subjects with disturbances in mood into two groups. One group received cognitive behavioral therapy, and the other received CBT combined with hypnosis. These two clinically valid treatments work synergistically with each other. While both groups improved, the group receiving hypnosis in addition to CBT had greater improvements in anxiety and depression. These improvements were stable at 6- and 12-month follow-ups.[5]

Hypnosis has even been shown to be an effective treatment in some of the most serious cases of drained brains. Being diagnosed with terminal cancer is certainly associated with brain-draining symptoms like acute anxiety and fear. In one study, terminal cancer patients were divided into two groups. Some patients received standard care that included cognitive psychotherapy and pain management. The second group received four sessions of one-on-one hypnotherapy in addition to standard medical care. Anxiety and mood were then measured by the Hospital Anxiety and Depression Scale. After just four sessions, the patients who were treated with hypnosis reported less anxiety and better quality of life.[6]

Another study, a joint effort between The Ohio State University's Department of Psychiatry and the Department of Molecular Virology, Immunology, and Human Genetics, showed how self-hypnosis—the tool you'll use in this chapter—can measurably improve the immune system by balancing the brain. The lead author of the study said hypnosis was akin to "hitting the reset button" when subjects were faced with anxiety and distressing thoughts. Since the sympathetic nervous system's fight, flight, or freeze response depresses the immune system, the researchers measured T cells in subjects' blood, a marker of immune response. For their subjects, researchers used medical and dental students facing their exams—a highly stressful event with serious consequences that could mimic stressful events drained people face in their everyday lives. T cells went up in the subjects who practiced self-hypnosis and went down in those who did not. The more frequently the subject practiced self-hypnosis, the better the response of his or her immune system.[7]

Even with all of this research, I still secretly predicted I wasn't going to be an enthusiastic believer in the power of hypnosis. Even if I did believe in its clinical value, I predicted that I personally would not be a hypnotizable person. I thought I knew too much about therapy in general and would probably just be analyzing the process and theoretical underpinnings too vigorously to "let go." My mind is always running, thinking, and planning. Then I was hypnotized for the first time.

To my surprise, I went easily into a deep and wondrous trance. It wasn't pretty, since I also looked like a drooling rag doll, but I can tell you *it felt incredible*—almost like a "high." I now truly understood why psilocybin (the psychoactive compound in "magic mushrooms") was being used to treat anxiety in patients with cancer; psilocybin and hypnosis both shut off the activity in the brain's cingulate cortex. I felt a deep state of relaxation devoid of worry that I had only occasionally reached with thousands of hours of meditation practice.

Hypnosis uses the power of the mind to heal the body, and this is helpful for people with mind-body ailments. As you know, people with anxious, drained brains are much more likely to develop high blood pressure, the number one cause of preventable death.

One of my professors was a lovely dentist from Virginia with a sweet voice that reminded me of my loving mom. What struck me is the language in hypnosis scripts we studied were quite similar to the meditation scripts I often use in my practice. To me, the difference was the warmer tone of voice she used and word choice that contained more positive feedback that more easily bypassed my rational, adult, perfectionistic mind that's always judging. It felt like this hypnosis professor was speaking to a seven-year-old version of myself as she said, "That's perfect . . . You're doing great. I wonder if you'll feel even more relaxed on your next breath . . ." Yes, I *did* feel more relaxed! How did she know? How did all the judging, planning, and worrying melt away so quickly? In that first minute undergoing hypnosis, I became an enthusiastic believer in the treatment.

SELF-HYPNOSIS

Like other forms of psychotherapy, hypnosis can be more effective when you use it one-on-one with a licensed health-care professional who is also certified in hypnosis. While the use of titles like "physician" or "psychotherapist" require a license governed by state boards, the title "hypnotherapist" (in and of itself with no other professional title) does not. Having a license also makes it more affordable to the patient since a physician or psychotherapist who is also a hypnotherapist can potentially bill insurance; an unlicensed "hypnotherapist" cannot. If you're interested in tackling deeper issues, find a licensed health-care professional who is also certified by the American Society of Clinical Hypnosis (ASCH) or the Society for Clinical and Experimental Hypnosis (SCEH). These advanced certifying boards only train licensed health-care professionals in fields of psychology, medicine, and dentistry to add hypnosis to their vast clinical expertise; you can find a local provider on their websites (www.asch.net and www.sceh.us).

There is also a simple form of self-hypnosis designed to help you relax and balance your brain. You can use it to achieve a deep state of relaxation in just a few minutes during the busy day, or use it lying down in bed if you have trouble dealing with an anxious mind before bed. You can also go to my Facebook page to see and hear this in video form:

> Begin by settling into a comfortable seated or lying down position in a place that's safe, comfortable, and quiet. Place one of your hands in front of you with your palm

facing away from you. Begin with your fingers pressed gently together. Your elbow is bent so that your hand is at eye level.

Now fix your gaze on your middle finger with your eyes still open. You may notice that after some time, the finger will go in and out of focus or perhaps the eyes become tired. Notice any interesting sensations in your hand. I wonder if you've already begun to notice any changes associated with your intention to relax. You may notice tension has dissolved in the shoulders or neck, or perhaps your body begins to feel lighter. You may even feel a slight tingling or warming sensation throughout the body. I don't know what exactly you'll experience, but that's not important. All that really matters is you enjoy this time, because you deserve to rest.

As you become more and more comfortable and relaxed, the fingers will begin to spread. I don't know which finger will move first. Maybe it will be the index finger. Maybe it will be the pinky, or maybe they'll move at the same time. As soon as the mind is ready to deeply relax, then the hand will begin to move closer and closer to your face. That's right. Good.

You feel the eyelids becoming heavier as your hand moves toward you. Heavier and heavier. Closer and closer. As soon as you're ready to relax even more deeply, the hand will make its way to your face, the eyes will close fully, and the hand finds its way to a comfortable position.

The next five breaths will take you down into an even deeper state of relaxation. As you're descending into this peaceful and calm state, you may notice the body feel like it's floating in the air like a feather. I wonder if the body will even begin to feel like a rag doll as a wonderful ease spreads. Every sensation you notice and feel in this moment takes you to a deeper state of rest and relaxation.

Breathing easily in a wonderful and relaxed way, you may even wish to imagine that every breath is spreading a calming energy through every cell and organ in your body and brain. You may wish to see a color of your choosing in your mind's eye. Your mind, your body, and your spirit are all becoming so calm and so comfortable. Spread this peace throughout the body from the toes to the top of the head. That's right. Perfect.

This calming energy may even feel like a pleasant type of daydream. I wonder what easy, relaxed, and comfortable sensations you will feel. Linger here.

(If you use this practice to fall asleep, stop the meditation here and allow yourself to drift to sleep whenever you're ready as you take whatever time you need to do so. If not, continue.)

Really notice the quality of this sensation. In the future, you'll be surprised by this calm energy returning to you during situations that previously made you feel stressed. You'll feel comfortable and relaxed.

Now allow the next five inhales and exhales you take to be refreshing, invigorating ones, bringing a balanced energy to every cell in your body. Each breath is bringing you back up into a fully awake state. As soon as you're feeling fully alert, then the eyes will open. When that happens, you'll feel an urge to move and stretch your limbs. You'll go about the rest of your day with a relaxed confidence you need to move through it with grace and ease.

Self-hypnosis is a simple way to shift your body from that sympathetic-dominant state to the parasympathetic state and balance your hormones in the process.

CHAPTER 16

Kindness, Gratitude, and Connection

You've learned fundamental ways to cut brain-draining "negatives" like sugar and pessimistic thinking from your life, and you've learned about ways to relax. Now it's time to take the brain balancing to a whole new level with soulful "positives." Some of the most powerful fixes for a drained brain include kindness, gratitude, and connection. They may come from the heart, but these spiritual fixes also rebalance feel-good neurotransmitters and stress hormones in your brain.

KINDNESS

Cultivating kindness—or engaging in what researchers call "prosocial behaviors" have a miraculous ability to neutralize stressors you face. Stressors are like withdrawals you make from your bank account, and brain-balancing activities and foods are like deposits. Make more deposits than withdrawals, and your brain is balanced. This can be especially helpful when the stressors you may be dealing with are out of your control—choosing to add a little more kindness to your daily life is something you can always do.

The miraculous power of kindness to balance drained brains has been proven by scientists. In 2015, Yale researchers had subjects note all the stress they were experiencing in several different areas of their lives including relationships, finances, and health. They also noted how many times they helped others each day. Kind behaviors could include even small acts like holding a door open for someone. Subjects reporting high levels of stress who didn't help others much felt more negative emotions and fewer positive ones. In other words, they had drained brains. However, subjects reporting high stress levels who helped others reported their mood was unaffected—which also meant they had more balanced brains. Remarkably, they had experienced just as much positive emotion as people who didn't have much stress in their lives. Kindness was like a vaccine against stress with feel-good brain-chemical boosts they could immediately feel.[1]

This research is particularly useful for people who are drained since they inherently tend to be busy with 80-hour work weeks, the responsibility of taking care of an ailing parent, or energy-consuming life transitions. They may not have 40 hours a week to spare as a volunteer right now, but they may have a few hours or minutes. Remember: this study found even small acts like the four extra seconds it takes holding a door for someone had a positive effect. No matter who you are or what your current circumstances are, you can *always* find small ways to help others. Do what you can with what you have now. Perhaps it's volunteering a few hours a week delivering meals or fostering dogs on weekends for a rescue group. If you can't afford to donate money this year, donate belongings to charity. Donate blood. Write a thank-you note to someone who has made a difference in your life. Take a friend who's having a rough time to lunch, or give her a call. Tip your coffee barista. Committing kind acts for others will balance a frazzled and overwhelmed brain.

In the Drained Brain program, you'll optimize the brain-balancing effects of kindness in a scientifically proven way. In a research study, one group of subjects performed five acts of kindness spread over the course of a week. Subjects in the second group performed all five acts in one day. Remarkably, only the group who performed the generous acts in one day displayed a significant boost in well-being. This may be the result of the brain's tendency to adapt to a "new normal." Just one single act of kindness may feel unremarkable. But stack those five kind acts in one day and you've undone the psychological phenomenon of "hedonic adaptation." It means you'll receive a noteworthy boost you can really feel.[2] This boost creates a positive feedback loop, and that makes you more likely to make this a regular occurrence in your life.

In day 12 of the Drained Brain program, you'll embark on a "day of kindness." The five acts of kindness you'll commit in a single day will improve your well-being while inoculating you against stress. You'll be "drunk" on kindness. It's a spiritual, brain-balancing strategy you can continue for the rest of your life. Perhaps Sundays become your new "day of kindness," where there's a very conscious intention to help others. Of course, the other side effect to this strategy is that you'll be helping others in an hour of need. You balance *your* brain with the act of kindness, and the recently divorced friend you took to lunch gets a little brain balancing as well. Like the ripples of a pebble dropped into a lake, kindness radiates outward from your heart and into the world.

GRATITUDE

Another act that comes from the heart and works its way up to your brain is gratitude. A gratitude practice takes advantage of the psychological phenomenon of selective attention. By choosing to consciously take note of something, it will begin to feel as if there is more of whatever it is you're looking for—and fewer of things you're not. This "superpower" can be used for good or evil—creating a balanced brain or a drained one. If you look for evidence of why you're lucky and blessed, you'll find it. However, the opposite is also true.

You may have noticed this phenomenon when you're thinking about making a big purchase like a car. If you're considering buying a Prius, you suddenly notice all the Priuses on the road. The number of Priuses did not change, but it *feels* like they're suddenly everywhere. The same goes for blessings in your life. Use selective attention right now as you look around the room while you say the word *green* to yourself. Notice how your eye is drawn to the everything that's green around you. Now replace the word *green* with the word *blessings* as you think about your life. This simple trick begins to train the brain to look for what's right in your life instead of what's wrong.

This, like kindness, is contagious. If you've ever been around someone who embodies a true attitude of gratitude, you can feel their energy. There's a woman named Alicia who works at the American Airlines lounge at JFK airport in New York, and I go out of my way to chat with her every time I'm there. As much as I try to practice gratitude, I caught myself feeling sorry for myself after work required me to take four cross-country flights in four days. To say I was a "little" jet-lagged was an understatement.

Alicia is from Argentina, and I asked her if she was going home for the approaching Christmas holiday. She said, "Not this year, but that's okay because you know what . . . to me, *every day* is Christmas! We are so lucky to be alive *every day, mi amor*!" Her attitude shot through my heart like an arrow. Here I was in this beautiful lounge with comfy couches, great views, big-screen TVs, and lots of free food, yet I was saying to myself, *Oh, poor me!*

In that moment, I used selective attention to refocus my attention on what's right in the present moment. Alicia's vigorous attitude of gratitude reminded me how important it is to cultivate this attitude each and every day—with the big things and the small ones. Instead of paying attention to how exhausted I was, perhaps I should pay attention to the fact that I was flying for a job I love. I get to help people lead happier and healthier lives for a living! I was killing time in this nice lounge because my good friend Jeremy had bought me a pass the year before as a totally unexpected Christmas gift. Perhaps I should pay attention to all the love I had in my life. You can even use gratitude to find simple blessings like the fact they were serving veggies and hummus—one of my favorite brain-balancing snacks.

Paying attention to specific blessings is a clinically proven, brain-balancing way to maximize gratitude. The power of specificity will supercharge your gratitude. It's great to think, write, or pray, "I'm grateful for my friends." But getting specific about what you love about your life and examining it will help you see your blessings more clearly. What exactly are some of the blessings you've never stopped to notice? Why are you grateful for this? What would your life be like if you *didn't* have this blessing? "I'm grateful for my friends" becomes, "Today I'm grateful for the fact that I get to see Kathy tonight, *because* I wouldn't have made it through my divorce without the gift of her friendship and support. I'm so glad I've been making an effort to see my friends more." Getting specific and reflective can turn your life into a scavenger hunt, and the object is to look closely to find as many blessings as you can. Seek, and ye shall find.

Here's something you can be grateful for: We'll use the power of combination therapy by using kindness and gratitude together. Like helping others, the brain tends to become immune to the effects of gratitude if it's something you *have* to do every day. You want to keep gratitude—at least the structured, intentional, journal-based variety—something you *get* to do. Science reveals that this is the most effective way to balance your brain. A study divided subjects into two groups. One reflected on their blessings three times a week. The other was instructed to do so once a week. The subjects who reflected on their blessings once a week had more profound boosts in well-being. Having a day of gratitude in a week can make this attitude feel more special.[3] Perhaps this is why so many religious traditions have one day a week specifically dedicated to spiritual growth and thanksgiving. This intentional, weekly reflection may eventually begin to shift your overall perspective throughout the week. You may even begin to have a global attitude of gratitude like my friend Alicia does. Embarking on a "day of gratitude" one day a week for the rest of your life is a fantastic tool you'll have to keep your brain in balance.

CONNECTION

Connection is another practice that buffers us from the effects of stress hormones when making our way through turbulent times. It's been suggested that women are more likely to use a healthier alternative to the typical fight, flight, or freeze response: tend and befriend.[4] As hunters and gatherers, it was in a mother's best interest to create bonds for the sake of her child, just as men needed to take swift action with animals they hunted. If the child's father was killed by a tiger, friendships would ensure mother and child would still be provided with food and protection. Responding to stress by "tending and befriending" boosts the brain balancer oxytocin while simultaneously lowering levels of the brain drainer cortisol.[5]

This tend-and-befriend response also gives human beings an evolved alternative to the primitive response of the sympathetic nervous system. Otherwise you only have three choices to choose from: (a) determine you're stronger than an enemy and *fight*, (b) determine you're not powerful enough to win and take *flight*, or (c) realize that you're not strong or fast enough and *freeze* in fear. Wouldn't it be nice to have an evolved and peaceful alternative to these three animalistic responses? Wouldn't our world be a better place if more people learned to respond with a tend-and-befriend response when facing difficult times?

Human beings were meant to connect to others. Instead of making an excuse and canceling a dinner with a friend, go. The more you don't feel like going, the more important it is to resist the urge of canceling because you're "busy" binge-watching Netflix.

Your brain was wired to seek connection before you were able to speak. Your body learned to self-regulate its nervous system through touch and eye contact with your caretakers. Mothers release oxytocin when they breastfeed, and you can get oxytocin as an adult by cuddling with your significant other or even a pet. Oxytocin can increase hormones that aid in digestion.[6] The amygdala, an overactive part of a drained brain, is less reactive to stress when high levels of oxytocin are present.[7] Oxytocin can even potentially prevent PTSD from developing. One study administered an intranasal dose of oxytocin to people who had experienced trauma within the past few weeks. This brain-balancing hormone helped to lessen future risk of post-traumatic stress.[8] Luckily, you don't need to carry around an inhaler to get an oxytocin boost; you just have to connect with loved ones in your life.

Connection can even potentially prevent mental illness from developing thanks to the intersection between our genes and our environment—also known as epigenetics. In an animal study, a psychiatrist from Johns Hopkins and his team found that cortisol spikes associated with social isolation triggered a cascade of problematic behaviors like fearful behaviors. However, this was only true in mice with genetic predispositions to traits associated with mental illness. Elevated cortisol—a result of isolation—was shown to trigger a cascade of responses and negatively affect levels of feel-good hormones that *did not return* to normal once activated by stress. Genetics loaded the gun, but environment pulled the trigger as the gene became "expressed" and the human equivalent of a mental illness took hold.[9] The takeaway: connection has the power to correct cortisol levels, and this can even prevent a cascade of neurotransmitter imbalances that can turn into a diagnosable mental illness. This is especially true for developing brains and anyone with a family history of mental illness. It also reminds us that an ounce of prevention can be worth a pound of cure, and this is very true when it comes to stress.

Like connecting with other human beings, relationships with animals can balance your brain as well. Anyone who has spent 10 minutes with me knows how much I love my dog, Rocco. I adopted him 12 years ago after a local pound deemed his shattered leg too expensive to fix and was going to euthanize him. He has provided me with unconditional love on days where I faced disappointment, setbacks, or heartbreaks. Generally, it is my belief that we should favor beagles over benzodiazepines and pranayama over Paxil in all but the most severe cases. Even in acute cases, using natural strategies like connection can reduce the amount of prescription medication needed to treat a mental illness.

I believe in the healing power of connection so deeply that I certify dogs as psychiatric service animals or emotional support animals for my patients with severe anxiety disorders. When specifically trained, a psychiatric service animal can perform specific tasks to help a person with a disability due to mental illness. Patients with severe panic attacks benefit from deep pressure therapy where a dog is trained to provide a calming effect by providing bodily pressure to minimize the duration of a panic attack. Psychiatric service animals can even be trained to interrupt self-harming behaviors or to fetch a bag containing medication. These wonderful animals are protected by federal law by the Americans with Disabilities Act, the Fair Housing Amendments Act, and the Air Carrier Access Act. Emotional support animals, on the other hand, do not need to be trained for specific tasks, but they still can have a benefit for people with a mental illness as a reasonable accommodation during travel.

Some of the most effective and safest "medicine" we have doesn't come in an orange bottle. Using Xanax to treat panic attacks can result in dependence and has also been linked to a troubling rise in overdoses. Animals, on the other hand, are linked to health benefits in addition to the love they provide. One study showed heart attack patients with dogs were a staggering *eight times* more likely to be alive a year later than those who didn't have a dog and also had higher measures of heart rate variability—a measure of the heart's ability to handle stress.[10] Just a few minutes of petting an animal has been shown to boost levels of the brain-balancers serotonin and oxytocin while reducing levels of draining cortisol.[11] Animal visits in an acute-care facility resulted in decreases of the brain-draining stress hormones adrenaline and norepinephrine.[12] If you have the space, lifestyle, and financial resources to give an animal a good life, check out the rescue animal locator at petfinder.com. You can search by zip code, size, and age of pet you'd like to adopt with pictures and descriptions of animals that need homes. That's how I found my beloved Rocco and the newest edition to our family: Emmett.

In week 2 of the Drained Brain program, you'll do something that helps you to feel more connection on the same day you're embarking on a day of kindness and gratitude. Ditch the phones and take your significant other on a romantic dinner date. Have a bonding conversation with a close friend. Take your dog to his favorite park, and give him 20 extra minutes of belly rubs that evening. Take your daughter to a play, movie, or concert. Since this is also the day where you'll be drunk on kindness and gratitude, you'll also be more likely to express your love and feel close to each other. Your brain learns it has an alternative to resorting to choosing between fighting, taking flight, or freezing in fear. It tends and befriends with love instead. You'll balance your brain while your heart runneth over.

CHAPTER 17

Mindfulness

Mindfulness is the act of consciously becoming aware of what's happening in the present moment. It's devoid of the usual patterns of judgment, clinging, or wanting things to be different than they are. It favors single-tasking over multitasking, because mindfulness also means paying attention to one thing at a time. Traditional mindfulness meditation can help people to find a stillness and presence that's lacking in modern lives. Sitting on a cushion quietly and observing the present moment leads to a state of peace and keeps anxiety at bay.

Mindfulness isn't just about attaining a "Zen" state. It's clinically proven to treat a wide variety of mental illnesses. Researchers have combined mindfulness with traditional cognitive behavioral therapy into effective protocols I use in my practice: mindfulness-based cognitive therapy (MBCT) and dialectical behavioral therapy (DBT). Energy-based cognitive therapy is a mindfulness-based practice as you become aware of your body and mind in poses and mental tasks. These protocols are incredibly effective in helping my patients to feel less drained.

However, you don't have to visit my private practice, your local hospital, or a yoga studio in order to be mindful. In fact, you can turn many everyday activities into a practice in mindfulness. Whether you're in yoga class, taking a bike ride, eating, or taking a shower, simply pay attention to the sensations you're perceiving in the present moment with your five senses. If you're not doing anything in particular, simply become *aware* of your awareness. If you're thinking, notice what thought is floating into your conscious awareness right now. Then notice when that thought floats away. Notice how this simple change has the power to subtly but powerfully transform your everyday life.

MULTI- VERSUS SINGLE-TASKING

I find that one of the best places to begin with mindfulness is to step away from multitasking. Most people assume that they'll get more done if they are doing many things at once, but in reality, multitasking is just rapid single-tasking. A 2009 study showed that subjects trained to do two things simultaneously did indeed increase the speed of processing and therefore got better at "multitasking"—or so it appeared. But brain scans revealed that while it appeared the subjects were multitasking, they were really switching between tasks so rapidly that it gave the *illusion* of doing two things simultaneously.[1]

So if we aren't really doing more than one thing at once, it makes sense that we're actually using more time than if we were to complete one thing in a focused way before beginning another. In a 2001 study, it was shown that as the complexity of tasks grew, subjects began to waste more time switching between them. Task switching can actually lead to a *40 percent decrease* in efficiency, which can add stress and lead you toward brain drain.

The study also found that multitasking led to subjects' brains becoming overloaded, so they couldn't filter out irrelevant information.[2] This is yet another form of stress that can add to your anxiety and feelings of being overwhelmed.

Mindfully "single-tasking" won't just help you feel less frantic and more focused; it will also help you become more efficient so you can finish tasks more quickly, thus avoiding brain-draining stress.

THOUGHT STREAM MEDITATION

As I already mentioned, you can apply mindfulness to any area of life—walking, doing dishes, even tying your shoes. But every once in a while, I find it helpful to dedicate specific time to focus on staying in the present moment. One of my favorite ways to do this is a meditation called the thought stream meditation. It's based on one of my favorite teachings from mindfulness pioneer Jon Kabat-Zinn.

You can do this at any point in your day—all you need is a quiet and comfortable place where you won't be disturbed and 12 minutes. To do this, read the meditation below a few times so you know exactly what is expected of you. Then set a timer for 12 minutes. Begin by closing your eyes, and then walk yourself through the meditation in your mind. If you finish the instructions before the timer goes off, rest in the mindful silence you have cultivated and relish the beauty of the moment. If the timer goes off and you haven't completed the practice yet—or if you find yourself wanting to meditate for longer—take all the time you need or want. You can also head over to my Facebook page to see and hear me guiding you through it.

Imagine yourself sitting by the side of a peaceful river. The river represents the thoughts and feelings in your mind. For the next 12 minutes, spend some time just watching what's in your river at this moment. Without any judgment . . . without trying to slow the river down or speed it up . . . just watch your river.

And while you're at it, notice the difference between *you* sitting next to the river and the *river* itself. Most of the time, we have a tendency to overidentify with our thoughts and feelings. We believe that we are our thoughts and feelings, and we forget who we really are. But we're so much *more* than our thoughts. Feelings come and feelings go. They're useful information to help guide our lives. But we also must remember who we are and not feel imprisoned by them.

This happens when we proverbially *jump into* our river. When you notice you've "jumped in," simply find your way out of the river and feel yourself back on the side of the bank.

You'll be left with the feeling of peace when you sense that part of you that is you. It's the part of you that always has been and always will be. It's the part of you that is connected to all living beings.

Now that you've learned the basics of mindfulness, let's apply it to two areas of life that often cause people stress: worrying and working. At first glance, worrying and working seem to be antonyms of mindfulness and the stress-relieving states it can create. Yet applying mindfulness to these two areas is particularly helpful for people with drained brains. Having a drained brain means you probably worry a lot or are a very busy person—or both.

THE MINDFUL WAY TO WORRY

Now that you've learned the basics of EBCT which will be part of the core the Drained Brain program, you have a potent remedy for the pitfall thought pattern *paralysis-analysis*. Chronic worriers frequently struggle with this pattern. EBCT can help you disengage from the circular pattern of ruminative and distressing thoughts. One add-on strategy that can reduce paralysis-analysis even more is called stimulus control. Research has shown it to be an effective way to manage brain-draining worry and anxiety.[3]

I call stimulus control *the mindful way to worry*, because you're doing one thing—and only one thing—at a time. That's an attribute of mindfulness. You're either consciously worrying *or* you're deciding not to worry while you choose to do something else in the present moment.

Perhaps you've tried to keep worries at bay by doing something to "zone out" like binge-watching TV, but there's still a little piece of your brain that knows the worry hasn't gone away. The same is true for any type of self-medication, from drugs to alcohol to shopping to food. Trying to not worry as we try to distract ourselves isn't an effective long-term strategy. The problem for most people is that telling themselves *not* to worry is like saying, "*Don't* think of a pink elephant." Chances are, it's impossible *not* to think of a pink elephant at least once.

In some ways, the mindful way to worry appeases that part of the brain that wants to do the opposite of what you tell it to do. The trick is counterintuitively *indulging* the brain in a prescribed "worry time" each day. This strategy gives the brain a sense of relief, because it will get the opportunity to engage in the kind of thinking that may have become familiar and hard to get rid of completely.[4]

The trick is to worry *mindfully,* and here's how you can do it in three simple steps.

Step 1: Pick Your Worry Time and Place: Pick a time of day when you will worry, and make it consistent. This will teach the brain that it will get its chance, and it will eventually begin to "hold" worries in your subconscious until you've reached your prescribed worry time. At worry time, invite worries into your consciousness. This also helps the brain reduce connections it previously made between worry and the time of other activities like dinner with your family. For most people, I recommend finding a time in the afternoon or evening. This will allow any worries that come up throughout the day to get their chance to return later in the same day. However, some people who struggle with personal worries during the workday may find morning a more suitable time.

Pick a neutral worry place. You don't want your brain to associate worry with your desk at work, and you don't want it to associate worry with your bedroom, either. Find a neutral place in your home like the kitchen counter or living room. You could even do this in your parked car before you walk in your home or office. This can create an energetic barrier between stress and a place you want to either focus or relax. It can help you to truly leave worry "at the door."

Typically, 30 minutes is the prescribed length of time for worrying, but I have found that some people only need 5 minutes. The amount of time needed varies from person to person. Self-proclaimed worrywarts may need the full 30 minutes, but others with less anxiety may find a few minutes to be sufficient.

Step 2: Become Mindful of Worry When It Surfaces: Throughout your day, realize *when* you are worrying as quickly as possible. In the moment you *realize* that you're worrying, congratulate yourself. You've just become mindful by becoming aware of what is happening in the present moment, so it's a good start. The problem with worry is that most of us enter into the pitfall thought pattern *paralysis-analysis* and its ruminative state for seconds or even minutes before we realize that it has taken our attention away from the task at hand. It's like reading a book while you're thinking about something else. Your eyes may have been scanning letters and words, but you realize that you haven't actually *read* anything when you get to the bottom of the page. You've wasted time by trying to do two things at once and have to start the page over. So it goes when you worry while also doing something else. Sometimes it takes us a long time before we even fully realize we're worrying. By paying attention to the present moment, you can catch the worry as quickly as possible when it surfaces outside the prescribed time. In time, you'll become even faster at mindfully becoming aware of worry as soon as it surfaces. This, in and of itself, is an effective long-term strategy in healing a drained brain.

When you catch yourself worrying, gently say to this part of your brain: "I see you. I'll come back to you later." Your brain is more likely to release the worry because it knows it will get a chance to return to the subject. Then gently bring your focus back to whatever you were doing. You may find it helpful to ground yourself in the present moment with physical sensations. Feel the way your fingers feel on the cool plastic keypad of your laptop, hear the buzz of the air conditioning, or notice the color of the eyes of the person across from you. Attuning to your five senses can bring your mind back to the here and now by disengaging from worry that tends to be future oriented.

Step 3: Turn Unproductive Worry into Constructive Worry: The difference between the state of paralysis-analysis and thinking critically about a problem is that the former doesn't solve or change anything while the latter leads to a solution. Once you've reached your prescribed worry time and are in your worry place, learn to worry in a different way.

Begin by creating a worry journal. It can be anything from a simple notebook to a leather-bound journal. If writing is physically painful or difficult, you can also try saying worries out loud. Most people don't write or speak their worries. They're off in their heads engaging in a state that's like daydreaming—only it's filled with negative thoughts. Of course this state drains the brain by flooding it with stress hormones.

Write or speak without editing in a free-flowing format. Consciously remain immersed in worry. Remember, you're mindfully doing one thing—and only one thing—at a time. Thus, this is a time to stay in this state. When your mind tries to take you into positive states of gratitude or neutral planning, nudge it back into worry. (Spoiler alert: this new way of worrying sometimes teaches your brain, "This is uncomfortable and tedious! I don't *want* worry! Maybe I'll do it less often.")

While writing in this free-flowing way, also consider these questions: What am I going to *do* about this worry? What are *solutions* to this problem? Eventually, this can transform paralysis-analysis into the type of thinking that leads to changes—as opposed to keeping you stuck.

As you use this strategy, you may find that you only need to use it once in a while or for a shorter amount of time. Your brain will naturally begin to stop hijacking your thoughts with unproductive worry, because it eventually learns that you have the power to solve your problems in a graceful, solution-focused way. When that's true, what would be the point of worrying so much?

THE MINDFUL WAY TO WORK

When doing a mindfulness meditation anchored on thoughts as you did in the thought stream meditation, you focus on the sensations of one aspect of your experience: your thoughts. By the same token, it's possible to focus your attention on one *task* at a time.

When used together, combining the mindful way to worry with the mindful way to work can radically change your life. If you are someone who is stuck in an unfulfilling job, you probably daydream about the life you want to create for yourself. This, of course, means that you're not being mindful. You're daydreaming when you should be working. Remember: mindfulness means doing only thing at a time and paying attention while you're doing it. If you're someone who is happy with what you're doing with your life, these strategies can even add a sense of quiet enjoyment to tedious tasks. Many mindfulness classes give a homework assignment to mindfully wash the dishes; mindfulness can transform something that was perceived as a negative experience into a neutral or positive one.

For people who want to make changes to their lives, there may be a low-grade misery associated with going into work on Monday morning or a feeling of wanting something "more." But if I asked you to rate your actions in manifesting this life for yourself on a scale from 0 to 10 (with 10 being "I'm doing *whatever* it takes and pulling out *all* the stops" and 0 being "I'm doing nothing to actively change my situation"), can you honestly say you're at a 10? If not, these strategies will help you get there. If you're already there, these strategies will help you to keep doing what you're doing in a calm and steady way.

These strategies can also help you do what you *have* to do until you can do what you *want* to do. To have the resources to make big changes in your life, you may need to significantly increase your productivity. This could allow you to work harder in your current job to put extra money away so you will have the resources to start the company of your dreams. The exercises you'll learn will also help you stay focused on what's truly important to you, and this will mean that someone with a full-time job can find the 20 hours a week to start *creating* the life he or she sees. Using a vision board or guided visualizations are fantastic tools, but you also need to create the stepping-stones to manifest that dream life. In fact, some of the most successful people in the world integrate mindfulness-based productivity tools in their work philosophy. You can, too.

Consider Warren Buffett's famous 25–5 Rule. The successful CEO once had his private pilot, Mike Flint, list his top 25 career goals. Then Buffett instructed Flint to circle the top five most important goals. Buffett asked Flint what he would do about the 20 things that weren't the most important. Flint replied they were almost as important as his top five goals, and he would work on them intermittently. This is where Buffett corrected Flint.

"No. You've got it wrong, Mike. Everything you didn't circle just became your Avoid-At-All-Cost list. No matter what, these things get no attention from you until you've succeeded with your top five."

How much unnecessary stress, inaction, and even insomnia is your long list of too many goals causing in *your* brain? Are the items on it draining your brain or balancing it? What would happen if you only focused on your most important ones, completing them, and *then* concerning yourself with what goal you wanted to tackle next? Could this possibly even bring an element of mindfulness to your work? Could it help you to supercharge your productivity, reduce stress, and balance your brain?

Writing your own, personal 25–5 will help you be mindful of the overall, "big picture" focus of your life's work. You'll have a chance to complete it in the program section of this book.

Armed with this "big picture" strategy to frame your goals, let's look at a mindful strategy that will supercharge your everyday tasks in service of these larger goals. Another wealthy and successful businessman, Charles Schwab, once sought the advice of a productivity expert named Ivy Lee. Ivy shared the following strategy with Charles's executives. There was no up-front fee for his consultation. Ivy told Charles he could send a check in three months for the amount he thought it was worth.

Ivy instructed Charles's executives to write down the six most important tasks for the following day at the end of the current workday. These six tasks were to be prioritized by level of importance from most to least important. At the beginning of tomorrow's workday, focus *only* on the first task. Finish it, and then move on to the next task. If you don't finish all six, simply move the unfinished tasks to the next day's list.

Three months later, Charles was so happy with his company's increased productivity that he wrote Ivy a check for what would be worth almost a half-million dollars today. The simple strategy can be learned in minutes, but the results are indeed powerful and can save thousands of hours of lost productivity.

Research has proven the effectiveness of this strategy. A recent study gave people a warm-up task followed by a brainstorming task. When subjects were prevented from finishing the warm-up task, they performed worse on the brainstorming task. Because the first task was uncompleted, it was still stuck in the brain's active memory.[5] You can heal your drained brain by remaining focused on the task at hand. You'll prevent it from wasting energy on unfinished tasks, and you'll have more energy to give to what you're doing in the here and now. You'll have a chance to use a version of this mindful list-making strategy in the program section of this book.

COLOR YOUR WAY TO BALANCE

The final mindfulness practice in this chapter takes you right back to being a kid—a time when you were not generally plagued by worry. Coloring has become unexpectedly popular. Even publishers and booksellers were surprised by the sudden adult coloring book craze. All of a sudden, they topped bestseller lists in Europe and the U.S. Even brands like Crayola wanted a piece of the action, launching a line of coloring books and colored pencils for adults in 2015.

Research has validated the stress-relieving effects that keep so many enthusiasts coming back. One study began by creating an anxious state in three group of students that would mimic a draining stressor people face in everyday life. One group colored mandalas: round frames filled with geometric patterns that are also a spiritual representation of the universe. A second group colored a plaid design, and the third was given a blank page to color. The group coloring the blank page did not experience any reduction in anxiety while the other groups did. Researchers concluded, "structured coloring of a reasonably complex geometric pattern may induce a meditative state that benefits individuals suffering from anxiety."[6] A follow-up study found mandalas outperformed *both* blank pages and plaid patterns in terms of anxiety reduction.[7] Thus, there's a clinically valid reason you'll color mandalas filled with small, geometric patterns as part of the Drained Brain program.

Remember, drawing and coloring are not the same in terms of stress relief. When you have a blank, 8 1/2" x 11" canvas it may actually cause you more stress. It may have too much in common with your task-oriented, decision-filled, grown-up life. Your drained brain thinks, *What should I draw? Hmm . . . Oh gosh, there are millions of choices. Well, I guess I'll draw . . . a butterfly. What do the shapes of monarchs' wings look like again? I don't remember what their eyes or ears are supposed to look like, either. Hmm . . . this is harder than I thought. Ugh. This doesn't look* anything *like a butterfly. I better start over! I'm not very good at this.*

Luckily, adult coloring books have done all that hard work for you. There are also adult coloring book apps like Colorfy. Even Disney has one. You can sit back, relax, and take part in the luminous, vibrant show. Escape your everyday state of "doing mind," where tasks need to be completed to serve a timely cause. Enter into a state of "being mind," where you can do something at your leisure simply for the sake of doing it. This can activate a mindful, meditative state as purple, peach, and periwinkle peacefully fill a page. Your mood may dictate your choice of color, and this expression may be just what you're needing in this moment.

The small, repetitive motions themselves may also have a healing quality. After all, spiritual practices like the use of prayer beads involve repetitive physical motions.

The beauty of this brain-balancing activity lies in its simplicity. The best way to learn more about this mindfulness tool is to arm yourself with some colored pencils and a coloring book.

PART IV

YOUR TWO-WEEK PLAN

CHAPTER 18

Program Overview

Now it's time to take everything you've learned and apply it to your life—and brain—over the next two weeks. In week 1, you'll make core lifestyle shifts that create a foundation to build upon—like the solid base of a tree. I'll guide you through implementing fundamental shifts in diet, exercise, and sleep—along with energy-based cognitive therapy (EBCT) to change your general outlook—to help relieve your frazzled, fatigued brain. In this first week, your stress hormone levels will begin to drop as feel-good neurotransmitters start to rise.

In week 2, you'll use the brain-balancing tools you learned about in Part III to take these results to the next level. Think of these tools, like meditation, coloring, and so on, as branches extending from that stable trunk you created in the first week. Practicing these tools throughout week 2 will help you understand which make you feel best, and then you'll be able to turn to them as a first aid kit to use whenever life presents you with a new and draining stressor. Of course, the basic changes you've made to your life also lead to long-term decreases in stress hormones, boosts in feel-good ones, and a bigger brain—which means stressors will actually feel more manageable and less draining in the future.

WEEK 1: THE BASIC BRAIN BALANCER

- Change your **diet** and **exercise** to go from drained to balanced.

- Liberate yourself from the seven pitfall thought patterns through **energy-based cognitive therapy** to go from pessimistic to resilient.

- Apply **cognitive behavioral therapy for insomnia** to go from fatigued to refreshed.

WEEK 2: THE BRAIN-BALANCING TOOLKIT

- Add **relaxation therapy, pranayama, self-hypnosis, gratitude, kindness, connection,** and **mindfulness** to supercharge your brain balancing. Go from feeling good to great.

In the following pages, I'll talk more in-depth about what each week entails; and then in the next chapter, I'll take you by the hand and walk you through each of the 14 days. One of the hardest parts for most people is just knowing exactly *what* to do each day. I wanted to make it as clear as possible because at the beginning, your brain will likely revolt and grab on to any excuse to not move forward. However, as your brain becomes less drained, the positive feedback you'll receive in the form of feeling better will make you excited about the changes you're making. This will help you adhere to the program in a strict way during the two weeks. You may wish to start this work on a weekend or a day where it will be easier for you to stick to the recommendations. This will set you up for success.

The positive feedback you'll feel will also help you continue many of these changes after the two-week program ends. After you've completed the program, I suggest you apply what I call the 80/20 rule. This means you adhere to the fundamental changes you've made 80 percent of the time, while relaxing a bit the other 20 percent of the time. So during the program, you'll eat no flour—absolutely zero flour—and you'll incorporate a probiotic superfood every single day. After you've made your way through week 2, it's okay to have an occasional slice of pizza or only eat a probiotic superfood six days a week instead of seven.

The same 80/20 rule can also be applied to the seven brain-balancing tools you'll start using in week 2 of the program. I hope that you use one or more of them regularly after you finish the daily assignments. They're wonderful to use in your day-to-day life, but they're especially helpful when you're going through difficult or stressful times. You'll learn which tools work best for you and which are most effective in specific situations. For example, you may find self-hypnosis works well for you to combat insomnia, while autogenic training is particularly helpful when you notice physical tension.

Should you ever notice your brain becoming drained, you can always come back to the program and repeat the 14 days as a brain-balancing reboot.

Please remember, these strategies are not designed to treat diseases or more serious mental illnesses that should be treated by your primary care physician, specialists, and/or other health-care professionals. Those with special conditions should consult their doctor before starting this program and modify if needed. The good news is that this program usually works synergistically with existing treatments.

Okay! Let's look more closely at what you'll be doing over the next two weeks.

WEEK 1: THE BASIC BRAIN BALANCER

During the first week, we're going to take you from drained and pessimistic to balanced and resilient by focusing on four different areas:

- **Diet:** We will remove the problematic foods that drain your brain and add foods that balance your brain and create the feel-good neurotransmitters you need.

- **Exercise:** Each day you'll do a different form of exercise to synergistically boost the effects of your healthy diet.

- **Cognition:** Each of the seven days in week 1 will focus on one of the seven pitfall thought patterns. You'll use energy-based cognitive therapy as the antidote to banish the pitfall thought patterns from mind and body, freeing you to take the necessary actions to create the life you want.

- **Cognitive Behavioral Therapy for Insomnia:** You'll use the simple techniques in CBT-I to create a personalized program with three different levels to address minor and more major sleep problems.

Let's start with the changes in diet. While they may seem intimidating at first, they also tend to get easier as they become your default lifestyle choices.

DIET OVERHAUL

To overhaul your diet, let's begin by talking about the brain-balancing foods we will *add* to your life:

- *Seven* servings of vegetables and whole fruits daily. This will ensure you're getting all the vitamin and mineral cofactors you need to produce feel-good neurotransmitters.

- One daily serving of a *probiotic*, one serving of a *prebiotic*, and one serving of a *probiotic booster* to boost levels of good gut bacteria that help you produce brain-balancing neurotransmitters.

- One daily serving of an *omega-3 superfood* to help you get adequate levels of EPA, your "stress less" omega-3, and DHA, your "sleep soundly" omega-3.

Focusing on what you're *adding* to your diet will make it easier to *take away* the following brain-draining foods:

- Sugar
- Flour
- Processed foods
- Artificial sweeteners

- Pro-inflammatory omega-6s
- Unhealthy oils like soybean oil
- Excessive caffeine
- Excessive alcohol

Our very first step is to increase brain-balancing foods while cutting out brain-draining ones (discussed in detail in Chapter 8) that shrink the brain, increase stress hormone levels, and reduce levels of feel-good neurotransmitters. Blood-sugar spikes that drain your brain disappear, and your brain shifts from an inflamed state to a calm, uninflamed one. Your gut, also known as your "second brain," gets into the brain-balancing action too, as the foods you eat help to increase good gut bacteria levels while decreasing bad ones. For most people, cutting processed, inflammation-causing foods will be the hardest step in the program since they're used to eating them.

Let's go a bit deeper—get a little more guidance on what you should and should not eat.

Say Good-bye to Sugar, Flour, and Artificial Sweeteners

As you now know, the effects of sugar and flour can be as damaging to the brain as going through a traumatic experience, and they wreak havoc with restful sleep. Even alternatives like agave have been linked to health problems, and "healthy" alternatives like whole-wheat bread often have the same glycemic index as white varieties. Artificial sweeteners can kill good gut bacteria that help balance your brain.

Eliminate:

- Agave
- All sugar
- All flour
- All bread containing flour
- Pasta
- Tortillas
- Chips

- Potatoes
- White rice
- Fruit juice or foods that say "sweetened with fruit juice"
- High-fructose corn syrup, corn syrup, corn syrup solids
- Any other kinds of syrup: carob syrup, golden syrup,

malt syrup, artificial maple syrup

- Most words ending in -*ose*, such as dextrose, fructose, galactose, glucose, maltose, sucrose

- Dextrin or maltodextrin

- Artificial sweeteners: sucralose (Splenda), aspartame (Nutrasweet), saccharin (Sweet'N Low), acesulfame potassium (acesulfame-K, Ace-K, Sunett, Sweet One, E950).

By eliminating the super sweetness from your diet, you'll start to appreciate the natural sweetness of whole fruits, which you'll be eating more of now. If you still need a little sweetener, try stevia. Favor 100 percent pure stevia extract, but other forms are acceptable as well. You may see stevia labeled with brand names like Rebiana, Truvia, or Pure Via. These are all permissible during the program.

Although real maple syrup and raw or manuka honey contain calories, the health benefit for brain-drained individuals is worth the small blood-sugar rise. But only use a maximum of 1 tablespoon of either each day. These two natural sweeteners contain antioxidants and can ease indigestion, a common symptom of stressed-out individuals, so the benefit outweighs the modest spike. They are also both prebiotics, which help your gut to manufacture brain balancers like GABA and serotonin. The other exception: sugar is acceptable if you're making one of the probiotic recipes in Appendix B from my friend Donna Schwenk. As she'll explain, sugar as an ingredient in fermented food acts as food for the bacteria—not you.

Carbs Aren't the Devil

Polarized thinking fueled the fat-free craze as Americans were told that bagels were healthy, but fat was bad. Then the no carb craze had Americans eating bacon and red meat—but no carbs. Science has proven a nuanced, gray-area approach works best; not all carbs are bad. Here are some healthy carbs you can enjoy daily. Have a maximum of 2 cups total of these foods per day:

- Brown rice

- Quinoa

- Barley

- Oatmeal

- Bulgur wheat

- Millet

- Couscous

- Spelt

You can also enjoy these carbohydrate sources, which do not count toward your 2-cup daily maximum:

- Flourless and sprouted grain bread (e.g., Ezekiel flourless bread)

- Shirataki noodles (see page 55)

- Beans

- Organic milk

- Whole fruit (or blended whole fruit, with the skin left on if edible)

Ditch Foods High in Pro-inflammatory Omega-6s

EPA is your "stress less" omega-3, and DHA is your "sleep soundly" omega-3. But remember that it's not just about the amount of omega-3s you consume each day; it's also about the ratio of omega-3s to omega-6s since they compete for space in your cells. Omega-6s are all too abundant in the modern diet. Factory-farmed animal products and soybean oils are responsible for the unbalanced omega-3 to omega-6 ratio we see in the modern world. Correcting this ratio moves the brain from a pro-inflammatory state to an anti-inflammatory one. The drained brain becomes balanced. While organic, free-roaming, and pasture-raised meat and dairy products cost more up front, they will save you money in terms of long-term health outcomes and costs.

Eliminate:

- Conventionally raised, nonorganic, or grain-fed meat, dairy, or eggs

- Margarine and trans fats

- Fried foods

- All oils except for the options listed below

Add:

- Meat, eggs, and dairy labeled with one of the following words: *organic, grass fed, pastured, free roaming,* or *free range*. Remember: omega-3 composition of animal products changes when animals eat nutritious grasses outdoors. Some deceptive food companies get away with labeling food free range, but the animals are only given access to the outdoors. Hopefully, these animals are actually outside eating nutritious plants. The best choices of all will also be labeled "Certified Humane Free Range" or "Certified Humane Pasture Raised," which guarantees the animals spend most of their waking hours outside, increasing the likelihood they're eating nutritious plants, which in turn balances your brain.

- Extra-virgin olive oil, plain olive oil, or light olive oil for cooking; flaxseed oil; cold-pressed or expeller-pressed canola oil; walnut oil; macadamia nut oil; or Malaysian palm fruit oil.

Reduce Roller-coaster Substances

Don't worry: we won't be eliminating these substances altogether. In moderation, they're quite good for the brain. But we will attempt to reduce their impact on our circadian rhythms in anticipation of the next week. So for this week, you will limit your coffee, tea, and moderate amounts of alcohol.

- A maximum of 200 mg caffeine per day (about two small cups of coffee). If you're used to sipping coffee all day long, try switching to green tea in the first week of the program. You can have four to six cups a day without going over the 200 mg limit. Or order half-caf coffee so you can have up to four small cups a day.

- A maximum of one serving of alcohol per day (preferably red wine). One serving is one 5-ounce glass of wine, one 8-ounce beer, or 1.5 ounces of liquor.

- No recreational drugs or smoking. (Note: This is not a program to treat drug or alcohol addiction.)

PRESCRIPTION DRUGS

If you are taking excess prescription medications such as sleeping pills or benzodiazepines, you may wish to talk to your prescriber about tapering off or adjusting your dose after you have completed the 14-day program. The changes in diet, exercise, sleep hygiene, and lifestyle can often make this an ideal time to cut back on overmedication as your mood and energy improve.

Add At Least One Omega-3 Superfood Per Day

During this first week, you are going to eat a serving of brain-nourishing omega-3 superfood *every single day*. Favor seafood-based superfoods since they give your brain the most concentrated doses of the two types of omega-3s, DHA and EPA. Ideally, you will have at least one serving of one of these fish per day:

- Albacore tuna, troll or pole caught, fresh or canned, U.S. or British Columbia
- Arctic char, farmed
- Barramundi, farmed, U.S.
- Black cod
- Dungeness crab, wild, California, Oregon, or Washington
- Longfin squid, wild, Atlantic
- Mussels, farmed
- Oysters, farmed
- Pacific sardines, wild
- Rainbow trout, farmed
- Spot prawns, wild, British Columbia
- Salmon, coho, farmed, U.S.
- Salmon, wild, any origin
- Shrimp

The other omega-3 superfoods are the following vegetarian options. However, these contain high levels of ALA, which your body must convert to DHA and EPA in order for you to stress less and sleep soundly, and it doesn't do this very efficiently, especially in men. There may also be variability between people of different ethnic backgrounds: African Americans may be better at converting ALA into DHA and EPA than people of European or Native American descent. Vegetarian sources of ALA include these foods:

- Walnuts (1/4 cup)
- Flaxseeds, ground (2 tablespoons) or oil (1 tablespoon)
- Chia seeds (2 tablespoons)

SHOPPING TIPS

When it comes to tuna, the "premium" whole white albacore actually has about three times *more* mercury than the very inexpensive chunk light tuna—but both still contain mercury and neither is a great source of omega-3s. You'll never regret making the switch to wild salmon or albacore that's labeled troll or pole caught!

Many people balk at this suggestion because they believe that salmon has to be expensive. But with a little creativity, you can get your daily dose of wild salmon for just over $1. I stock my pantry with vacuum-packed pouches of Chicken of the Sea Premium Wild-Caught Pink Salmon, which tastes like chunk light tuna—your kids won't be able to tell the difference—but has far more brain benefits than traditional tuna, with 500 mg of DHA and EPA per serving. If you can't find these packs at grocery stores, you can usually get them at Target or on Amazon for just over $1 per (BPA-free) pouch. Mix the salmon with some olive oil–based mayonnaise and lemon juice, toast in a toaster oven or under a broiler with a slice of organic cheese on sprouted bread, and you've got an easy, inexpensive, and brain-healthy salmon melt.

Eat at Least Seven Servings of Vegetables and Whole Fruit Per Day

The next thing you will add to your diet in week 1 is at least seven servings of vegetables and whole fruit per day. You now know just how incredibly beneficial this simple strategy can be for balancing a drained brain. Here are a few general guidelines that will help you to get the maximum benefit from these disease-fighting, brain-boosting powerhouses:

- Favor organic over conventionally grown. Refer to the list of the fruits and vegetables that are especially important to buy organic on page 62.

- Eat a variety of vegetables and fruits to ensure you're getting the different vitamins that serve as cofactors that prevent inflammation and help your body to produce brain balancers like GABA and serotonin.

- When eating fruit, ensure that it's eaten whole or blended. Don't juice it.

To get the most out of the produce you're eating, you should also drink at least *10 eight-ounce servings* of water each day.

Consume One Probiotic, One Prebiotic, and One Probiotic Booster Daily

As you know, balancing your gut—restoring the levels of healthy bacteria—is a powerful tool for fighting a drained brain. Probiotic foods are packed with healthy bacteria, and prebiotics and probiotic boosters power up the bacteria even more. So in this program, you'll eat one of each every day.

Probiotics:

- Buttermilk
- Cheese (soft varieties like Gouda, favor organic to also make sure you're getting more omega-3s)
- Fermented milk (labeled sweet acidophilus milk)
- Kefir (dairy or coconut)
- Kimchi
- Kombucha
- Kvass
- Microalgae powder, including blue-green algae, chlorella, spirulina
- Miso soup
- Natto
- Pickles
- Poi
- Sauerkraut
- Tempeh
- Yogurt (favor organic, choose varieties with no added sugar and no artificial sweeteners)
- There are also ways to ferment other foods like vegetables. Turn to Appendix B on page 263 for recipes to make your own probiotic foods.

Prebiotics:

- Asparagus
- Banana
- Chicory root
- Dandelion greens
- Garlic
- Gum arabic
- Jerusalem artichoke
- Jicama
- Leeks
- Legumes
- Maple syrup
- Oatmeal
- Onions
- Raw or manuka honey
- Wheat bran

Probiotic Boosters:

- Coffee (no sweetener except stevia; if you use milk, choose almond, coconut, or organic dairy)

- Dark chocolate that includes 50 percent or more cacao, but only a square or two

- Red grapes

- Red wine (favor pinot noir since it contains the highest levels of the antioxidant resveratrol)

- Tea (no sweetener except stevia; if you use milk, choose almond, coconut, or organic dairy)

Substitutions Are Your Friend

So now you've learned the basics of what to take out of your diet and what to put in, but I wanted to talk substitutions before we move on to the next topic. Sometimes finding alternative things to eat when you really can't imagine life without something are essential to sticking with an eating program. For example, I can't imagine living without pasta. I have always loved it. But in my quest to be healthier, I've found some things that satisfy that craving for me. They may not be one-to-one substitutions, but they hit the mark and overpower the cravings that might sabotage my success. Here are some of my favorites:

Bread Alternatives: I love flourless sprouted bread and English muffins, which provide energy-boosting carbs while cutting the glycemic index in half. My favorite is Food for Life Ezekiel 4:9, which you can get in just about any supermarket. These breads also provide brain-healthy amino acids and more protein than other types of bread. I like to toast my flourless bread, as it improves the texture.

Sweet Substitutions: You don't have to give up dessert to feed your brain! Once you give up overly sweetened processed carbs, you will be utterly amazed by the natural sweetness of foods.

- Swap fruit-flavored yogurt for plain Greek yogurt. For even more probiotics, try plain kefir mixed with your favorite whole fruit. Sprinkle a few unsweetened goji berries or flaxseeds over it for a great crunchy texture.

- For dessert, try organic, plain Greek yogurt with organic blueberries and stevia **or** a teaspoon of raw honey—preferably manuka honey.

- Make a delicious smoothie with 80 percent vegetables and 20 percent fruit.

- I also love Quest protein bars, which are made from whey protein (whereas most protein bars are made from cheap, nonorganic soy protein isolate). While some of the flavors use artificial sweeteners, many don't. Look for the flavors that say "no artificial sweeteners" on the front. I particularly like the Quest chocolate peanut butter bar. Twenty seconds in the microwave and you have my go-to dessert.

Carb Alternatives: Like I said, pasta could be my downfall. Ever since childhood, my biggest pitfall food has been bright-orange-powder macaroni and cheese. The kind in that bright-blue box. Here are some pretty simple, brain-benefiting swaps that I now eat 80 percent of the time I think about eating pasta:

- Try a pizza made with portobello mushrooms instead of dough. You can also find great recipes for a "dough" made out of cauliflower.

- Make your own fried rice at home, with only a half cup of brown rice per serving (a big difference from restaurant fried rice, which is almost all rice). Make the bulk of your home-cooked dish with organic egg or meats, onions, chopped broccoli, red pepper, and diced carrots. Use just a tablespoon or two of light olive oil to sauté, and finish with ginger, soy sauce, turmeric, and black pepper.

- Substitute shirataki noodles for pasta. These plant-based noodles have almost no carbohydrates. While once only found at health food and Asian stores, they're now available at pretty much any grocery store. Rinse them before cooking and use flavorful, healthy sauces with them.

- Instead of pasta salad, make a black bean and corn salad or organic egg salad.

- Keep large leaves of romaine to use in place of bread for sandwiches.

- Instead of pasta, try zucchini noodles. You can get these premade at many grocery stores now, or you can make your own. Buy a spiralizer to make veggies into pasta-shaped strands. I use the Veggetti Spiral Vegetable Cutter, which I bought for just $10.

- Buy cauliflower rice to use instead of regular rice. This is now available in the frozen or refrigerated section of grocery stores. Trader Joe's makes one, and major grocery stores carry the Green Giant frozen brand.

- Instead of wheat toast with peanut butter, try apples or celery with almond butter.

- Instead of mashed potatoes, try making cauliflower mashed "potatoes" or mashed garbanzo beans. Use a blender to puree a can of plain garbanzo beans with organic chicken or vegetable stock. Then heat in a saucepan with olive oil. Finish with black pepper and turmeric.

Healthier Sides and Snacks: We also get a lot of blood sugar–spiking carbs from the snack foods we munch on all day and night. Luckily, it is incredibly easy to swap out these foods with healthier alternatives. Your brain (and your waistline) will thank you!

- Instead of nachos, try celery with salsa.

- Instead of chips, eat nuts. (Find plain ones that aren't cooked in oil.)

- Instead of pita chips, try cut red peppers, baby carrots, and cherry tomatoes with your hummus.

- Instead of crackers, try organic olive oil popcorn from Trader Joe's, or make your own. Use an air popper, and then cover the popped corn with 2 tablespoons of extra-virgin olive oil. For a more decadent treat, cook your popcorn on the stove using virgin coconut oil.

Better Beverages: Since beverages are often a *huge* source of sugar in the diet, you can bring your glycemic load down a great deal simply by making smoothies and juices with an 80/20 ratio of veggies to fruit. (And since fresh lemons and limes contain just about one gram of sugar, you can count them as vegetables, too! They do wonders for adding a citrus taste to bitter vegetables.)

You may soon find that you prefer the taste of vegetables blended with fruit to those overly sweetened "smoothies" they sell at mall food courts, or even the bottled "green" ones that are marketed as vegetable juice but are made mostly of cheap fruits or apple juice. The drink will come out especially delicious if you blend the whole fruit (which keeps the skin and the fiber).

> **RECIPE:** My favorite: 1/4 cup romaine, 1/4 cup kale, 1/4 cup 'spinach, 1/4 cup broccoli, 1/4 cucumber, a squeeze of lemon, 1-inch piece of ginger, 1/2 pear with the skin on, a few pieces of cut mango, and 2 cups water. To make these as convenient as a bag of chips, I make 3 to 4 at a time and use wide-mouth Ball jars with lids to store in the fridge. Toss in your bag and go!

Vitaminwater zero is also a decent option for bringing in better beverages. It's a no-calorie, stevia-sweetened drink that's a great alternative to soda or fruit juice.

Oils, Dressings, and Sauces: A Few Condiment-Shopping Tips: My favorite marinara sauces are the $3 per bottle premium line at Trader Joe's, which are extremely affordable and use *only* olive oil.

Because some premium bottled salad dressings can cost more than $5, I recommend making your own salad dressings with extra-virgin olive oil and vinegar. They'll save you money—and they taste much better, too. And since restaurant vinaigrettes are sometimes made with soybean oil, your safest bet is to ask for vinegar and olive oil. Try different types of vinegar for variety.

Don't let food companies mislead you. Some companies will say "made with olive oil" on the front label. Turn that bottle around and read the ingredients. You'll see they often contain soybean or canola oil that's not cold or expeller pressed. I like Vegenaise since it's made with non-GMO, expeller-pressed canola oil, which is acceptable to use during the program.

EXERCISE

In addition to overhauling your diet during this first week, you'll "cross-train" your brain and body by using different types of exercise. These seven workouts will include all four basic categories of exercise you learned about since each has unique benefits in the brain. Each will have levels designed for beginners and advanced athletes alike. Choose your daily workout based on the amount of time you have, how draining your day was, and what you enjoy doing. For example, sprint interval training takes just 10 minutes. Use this form of exercise on a busy day. Meditative movement requires more time but is a perfect fit for days you may feel especially drained: Do at least one of each of the four forms of exercise during this week:

- Sustained aerobic exercise
- Interval training
- Sprint interval training
- Meditative movement

All exercise balances your brain in different ways. If you have a routine that mixes weights, cardio, intervals, and yoga on different days, great! If not, turn to pages 97–110 for some workouts that will help you add any type of exercise you may be missing to your life. These workouts will become great go-to options that are customizable based on how much time you have and what kind of mood you're in.

CHANGE YOUR THOUGHTS, CHANGE YOUR LIFE

For most people, the dietary overhaul will be the most challenging part of this program. But EBCT may help you change in profound and even spiritual ways since it can help change the way you see the world. It goes a step further than most forms of cognitive behavioral therapy, since the physical pose makes your body get into the brain-balancing process. You'll also take it a step beyond that and apply the action you see in your mind's eye to your life.

Each day, you'll tackle one of the seven pitfall thought patterns that drain your brain. In the day-by-day chapter to follow, I'll walk you through the steps to change each one. Each pitfall thought pattern will be matched with a physical pose as an antidote. You'll consider contrary evidence to help you see that thoughts aren't facts; they're information. Then you'll see the right action you'd like to take in your mind's eye and apply it to your life.

- **Paralysis-analysis:** Getting stuck in your own thoughts. ("Why couldn't I remember where I put my keys last night? What does it mean? What will I do if this keeps happening?") **Antidote:** tree pose.

- **Permanence:** Using the past or present to judge the future. ("I'm never going to get over this divorce.") **Antidote:** eye cupping.

- **Personalization**: Assuming that something is happening because of you. ("I didn't get that job because I'm not smart enough.") **Antidote:** star pose.

- **Pervasiveness**: Allowing a problem in your life to invade all parts of your life. ("I had a bad day at work. I'm going to cancel my dinner plans.") **Antidote:** shoulder shrugs or pigeon pose.

- **Pessimism**: Always believing the worst about everything. ("If I keep feeling this way, I'll probably have a panic attack when I'm driving and hit someone. How could I ever live with that guilt?") **Antidote:** the half-smile.

- **Polarization**: Seeing everything as either/or, black/white, yes/no. ("My boss didn't respond well to my presentation—I might as well just quit.") **Antidote:** spinal twist.

- **Psychic**: Feeling sure that you know what another person is thinking. ("I know she's never liked me anyway.") **Antidote:** chest thump.

SLEEP SOUNDLY

The final part of the changes you'll start in week 1 is working to improve your sleep. Basic changes to the way you live your life (e.g., diet and exercise) will make it easier for you to get the sleep you need. Higher levels of the omega-3 DHA and fewer blood-sugar spikes will improve how deeply you're sleeping. However, we'll also apply the clinically proven principles of CBT-I, which can help you fall asleep faster, stay asleep, and sleep more deeply.

This part of the program also specifically balances your 24-hour cycle of cortisol and melatonin. Changes in diet and exercise balance levels of stress hormones like cortisol while boosting feel-good neurotransmitters like serotonin and GABA that can help you fall asleep. Now CBT-I will ensure the cortisol and melatonin are following the rhythm nature intended: cortisol rises in the morning as melatonin dips; melatonin rises in the evening as cortisol dips. You'll get a natural energy boost, and this will help you get through long workdays. Stressors you may encounter will start to feel more manageable.

In the day-by-day chapter that follows, you'll use CBT-I principles and fill out a daily sleep journal that will remind you of the steps in each level. Some people will only need a few days of following the principles of level 1 to get their sleep under control. These principles include these actions:

- Setting a stable bedtime and wake time
- Establishing a 60-minute wind-down
- Reducing your exposure to light in the evening
- Using the bed only for sleep, sex, and up to 30 minutes of reading
- Ensuring your bedroom is dark and cool
- Banishing clock watching

However, if by the end of the week 1 your sleep hasn't improved using only the level 1 interventions, you can add the principles for level 2 during week 2 of the program:

- Using one of the three forms of relaxation therapy (mantra meditation, progressive muscle relaxation, autogenic training), pranayama, or self-hypnosis just before bed. You'll use these tools in the first four days of week 2, so you should be well-versed in using them by the time you need to add them.

- Identifying your sleep worries. These involve identifying the pitfall thought patterns that are sleep specific.

If you still need more, add the level 3 interventions:

- Calculating your sleep efficiency
- Setting a paradoxical intention
- Sleep compression
- Sleep expansion

- If you need it, consider adding cranial electrotherapy stimulation. Go to drmikedow.com for more information.

People with minor sleep problems who may only need level 1 will complete the CBT-I program in the first seven days. Others with more serious problems with sleep and energy will continue progressing through level 2 of CBT-I in week 2. Those who need all three levels may need longer than 14 days to complete the CBT-I program. Work your way through the CBT-I program at the pace that is beneficial for you. If you need to add level 3 interventions, turn back to page 141 to review them.

WEEK 2: THE BRAIN BALANCING TOOLKIT

Week 2 of the program is really about continuing what you started in week 1, but instead of focusing on the pitfall thought patterns, we're going to bring in some simple tools (found in Part III) to help you enhance your brain balance even more. These will become your brain-balancing toolkit. If you'd like to supercharge your balancing, you can add cranial electrotherapy stimulation to these practices. More information about this device is found on page 141 and drmikedow.com.

Each day you'll use one of the following seven tools (specified in the day-by-day program) to help take your brain balancing to the next level. Feel-good neurotransmitters go up as stress hormones go down.

- **Relaxation Therapy: Mantra Meditation:** Repeating a simple word or phrase while meditating to get your mind focused. Maintain a passive attitude to allow relaxation to unfold at its own pace.

- **Relaxation Therapy: Progressive Muscle Relaxation and Autogenic Training:** To use progressive muscle relaxation, flex each group of muscles to the count of 5 and then relax that group of muscles to the count of 10. Begin with your feet and work your way up to your head. To use autogenic training, silently tell yourself that each part of your body is warm and heavy.

- **Pranayama:** Use Diaphragmatic Breathing, 3:6 Breathing, chanting, and other breath practices. Then put them together in sequences.

- **Self-hypnosis:** Notice how your mind can easily and quickly drift into a relaxed state that feels like a pleasant sort of daydream.

- **Kindness, gratitude, and connection:** Choose a day to practice acts of kindness, reflect on specific blessings you're grateful for, and connect to others.

- **Mindfulness: Mindfulness Meditation and The Mindful Way to Worry:** Use the thought stream meditation and stimulus control to contain worry.

- **Mindfulness: The Mindful Way to Work and Mindful Coloring:** Use the "25–5" to keep your life focused on what's truly important to you, use mindful to-do lists to stay productive, and harness the power of adult coloring books to banish stress.

THE REST OF YOUR LIFE

After you finish the two-week program—sticking strictly to the rules I've laid out—you can chill out a bit. Remember the 80/20 rule I mentioned? That idea works for all areas of your life. So splurge on dessert (within reason) every once in a while. Watch TV instead of working out. Stay up late at your best friend's wedding. Just don't allow occasional indulgences to turn into your everyday behavior. That's what drains your brain. If you ever do get to the point where you're feeling overly anxious and drained again, this program will be here to jump-start you into a life of brain health.

CHAPTER 19

Day by Day

In the previous chapter, you learned about all the brain-balancing strategies you'll use over the next two weeks of the program. This chapter contains a day-by-day journal to remind you exactly what you need to do each day while also providing a place for you to track your results.

At the end of each day, I'll ask you to do a quick evaluation of where you stand after doing the work for the day. Tracking your results will help you notice how much you're improving.

Workbook for Week 1: The Basic Brain Balancer

Diet: No sugar or artificial sweeteners (page 200–201). No flour or processed snacks (page 200–201). No foods that are high in pro-inflammatory omega-6s, which include unhealthy proteins like factory-farmed meat and fats like soybean oil (page 202). Eat at least seven servings of vegetables and whole fruits daily (page 205). Consume at least one probiotic, one prebiotic, and one probiotic booster each day (page 205–207). Avoid excess caffeine or alcohol during this program. If you drink alcohol and/or caffeine, one glass of red wine, coffee, or tea can count as your daily probiotic booster. Alternatively, review the food sources of probiotic boosters (page 207). Eat at least one omega-3 superfood each day, which will help you get both your "stress less" omega-3 EPA and your "sleep soundly" omega-3 DHA (page 204). Remember, Appendix B features recipes you can use that will teach you how to incorporate many of these brain balancers into your daily diet. There are a few exceptions: a bit of honey, real maple syrup, or sugar if it's used to cook fermented foods.

Exercise: Of the different forms of exercise discussed on page 210, choose one of the four types of exercise to do each day. Throughout the program, vary the types of workouts you choose. Learn which form of exercise is right for you on certain days (e.g., sprint interval training when you're short on time, meditative movement on a day you need immediate stress relief, and so on). Remember, each form of exercise has unique brain-balancing properties, so variety is the key to balance. As a reminder, these are the four categories:

- Sustained aerobic exercise (e.g., a long brisk walk, a jog, etc.)

- Traditional interval training (e.g., alternating between high and low intensity, which consist of cardio and/or weight training)

- Sprint interval training (e.g., the 10-minute format detailed on page 107, which can be done on a bike, running, or rowing machine, etc.)

- Meditative movement (e.g., yoga, Tai Chi, etc.)

Energy-based Cognitive Therapy (EBCT): Each day you'll be on the lookout for one of the seven pitfall thought patterns. You'll use the six-step EBCT formula that includes physical poses on each day to target the pitfall thought pattern of the day. This will help you to manifest the balanced life you'd like to create for yourself.

Cognitive Behavioral Therapy for Insomnia (CBT-I): Begin the customized, three-level CBT-I program to improve your sleep and heal insomnia. Go at your own pace. Mild cases will only need to use level 1 of CBT-I during the first seven days of the program. If you struggle with moderate insomnia, you may need to progress to CBT-I level 2 during week 2 of the program. If your sleep still needs improvement, proceed to level 3 of CBT-I after you've finished the program. For a review of level 3 for those who need it, turn back to page 141.

DAY 1

LIFESTYLE TRACKING
(place a check next to each to track your progress)

Seven servings of vegetables and fruits (min.): 1____ 2____ 3____ 4____ 5____ 6____ 7____

One daily (min.): probiotic ____, prebiotic ____, probiotic booster ____

One daily omega-3 superfood (min.):_____

Type of exercise: _____

EBCT

Paralysis-analysis is the pitfall thought pattern you are targeting today. Remember, this type of thinking involves stewing and ruminating in anxious thoughts, preventing productive action from occurring.

Step 1: Notice the Pattern: Throughout the day, identify when **paralysis-analysis** shows up. Then write down how your own personal version of **paralysis-analysis** sounds to you as a thought. Also rate how true it feels for you (for a more detailed review of these steps, turn to page 114).

The paralysis-analysis pitfall thought pattern I notice:

_____

_____

How true does this worry feel from 0 to 100: _____%

Step 2: Use a Physical Pose as an Antidote: Tree pose or the discreet version of tree pose is the antidote for paralysis-analysis (see page 116).

Step 3: Find the Contrary Evidence: While in tree pose, consider the contrary evidence that proves your brain-draining worry wrong and then write it down.

My contrary evidence that I already have (e.g., What experience do you have from your own life that proves this worry could possibly be wrong?):

_____

_____

Step 4: See the Right Action You'd Like to Take: While in tree pose, see the right action you'd like to take in the future in your mind's eye.

Step 5: Revisit Your Brain-Draining Worries: Now that this antidote has worked on you physically, psychologically, and spiritually, return to the brain-draining worry you wrote in step 1. How true does this brain-draining worry feel now? Now that you have contradicted it with mind and body, does it feel less true? Rate it from 0 to 100: _____ %

Step 6: Turn Right Action into Your Reality: Make a commitment to yourself that in the future, you will choose the actions that you saw in your mind's eye.

CBT-I

Begin Level 1: Set a stable bedtime and wake time. These times should ideally be eight and a half hours apart. Your bedtime is the time you turned the lights off and went to bed—not the time you actually fell asleep. Remember: your wind-down time should be 60 minutes before your bedtime. For a review of what you need to do during level 1 (e.g., ideal sleep temperature, avoiding clock-watching, pairing your bed and sleep), turn to page 128. Since these times should ideally remain as stable as possible during CBT-I, you may wish to start the program during a period of time you won't be traveling or waking up at odd hours. Note the times you actually started to wind down, went to bed, and woke up. Journaling these times will help keep you at or near your target times. This will gradually improve the quality of your sleep.

My target wind-down time during this program (60 minutes before target bedtime): _____

My target bedtime during this program: _____

My target wake time during this program: _____

My wind-down time: _____

My bedtime: _____

END-OF-DAY EVALUATION

Rate yourself on the following on a scale from 1 to 10 (with 10 being the best):

How is my energy? _____

How well am I sleeping? _____

How well am I handling stress? _____

How am I feeling in general? _____

Today I'm most proud of myself for _____

_____

_____.

DAY 2

LIFESTYLE TRACKING
(place a check next to each to track your progress)

Seven servings of vegetables and fruits (min.): 1____ 2____ 3____ 4____ 5___ 6____ 7____

One daily (min.): probiotic ____, prebiotic ____, probiotic booster ____

One daily omega-3 superfood (min.):_____

Type of exercise: _____

EBCT

Permanence is the pitfall thought pattern you are targeting today. Remember, this type of thinking falsely assumes that just because something is a problem now, it will always be a problem.

Step 1: Notice the Pattern: Throughout the day, identify when **permanence** shows up today. Then write down how your own personal version of **permanence** sounds to you as a thought. Also rate how true it feels for you (for a more detailed review of these steps, turn to page 114).

The permanence pitfall thought pattern I notice:

_____

_____

How true does this worry feel from 0 to 100: _____%.

Step 2: Use a Physical Pose as an Antidote: Eye cupping is the antidote for permanence (see page 117 for a review).

Step 3: Find the Contrary Evidence: While cupping your eyes, consider the contrary evidence that proves your brain-draining worry wrong and then write it down.

My contrary evidence that I already have (e.g., What experience do you have from your own life that proves this worry could possibly be wrong?):

_____

_____

Step 4: See the Right Action You'd Like to Take: While eye cupping, see the right action you'd like to take in the future in your mind's eye.

Step 5: Revisit Your Brain-Draining Worries: Now that this antidote has worked on you physically, psychologically, and spiritually, return to the brain-draining worry you wrote in step 1. How true does this brain-draining worry feel now? Now that you have contradicted it with mind and body, does it feel less true? Rate it from 0 to 100: _____ %

Step 6: Turn Right Action into Your Reality: Make a commitment to yourself that in the future, you will choose the actions that you saw in your mind's eye.

CBT-I

Continue Level 1:

My wake time:_____

My wind-down time: _____

My bedtime: _____

END-OF-DAY EVALUATION

Rate yourself on the following on a scale from 1 to 10 (with 10 being the best):

How is my energy? _____

How well am I sleeping? _____

How well am I handling stress? _____

How am I feeling in general? _____

Today I'm most proud of myself for _____

_____.

DAY 3

LIFESTYLE TRACKING
(place a check next to each to track your progress)

Seven servings of vegetables and fruits (min.): 1____2____3____4____5___6____7____

One daily (min.): probiotic ____, prebiotic _____, probiotic booster _____

One daily omega-3 superfood (min.):_____

Type of exercise: _____

EBCT

Personalization is the pitfall thought pattern you are targeting today. Remember, this type of thinking places the blame entirely on yourself for something not going your way.

Step 1: Notice the Pattern: Throughout the day, identify when **personalization** shows up today. Then write down how your own personal version of **personalization** sounds to you as a thought. Also rate how true it feels for you (for a more detailed review of these steps, turn to page 114).

The personalization pitfall thought pattern I notice:

_____

_____

How true does this worry feel from 0 to 100: _____%.

Step 2: Use a Physical Pose as an Antidote: Star pose is the antidote for personalization (see page 118 for a review).

Step 3: Find the Contrary Evidence: While in star pose, consider the contrary evidence that proves your brain-draining worry wrong and then write it down.

My contrary evidence that I already have (e.g., What experience do you have from your own life that proves this worry could possibly be wrong?):

_____

_____

Step 4: See the Right Action You'd Like to Take: While in star pose, see the right action you'd like to take in the future in your mind's eye.

Step 5: Revisit Your Brain-Draining Worries: Now that this antidote has worked on you physically, psychologically, and spiritually, return to the brain-draining worry you wrote in step 1. How true does this brain-draining worry feel now? Now that you have contradicted it with mind and body, does it feel less true? Rate it from 0 to 100: _____ %

Step 6: Turn Right Action into Your Reality: Make a commitment to yourself that in the future, you will choose the actions that you saw in your mind's eye.

CBT-I

Continue Level 1:

My wake time:_____

My wind-down time: _____

My bedtime: _____

END-OF-DAY EVALUATION

Rate yourself on the following on a scale from 1 to 10 (with 10 being the best):

How is my energy? _____

How well am I sleeping? _____

How well am I handling stress? _____

How am I feeling in general? _____

Today I'm most proud of myself for _____

_____.

DAY 4

LIFESTYLE TRACKING
(place a check next to each to track your progress)

Seven servings of vegetables and fruits (min.): 1____ 2____ 3____ 4____ 5____ 6____ 7____

One daily (min.): probiotic ____, prebiotic ____, probiotic booster ____

One daily omega-3 superfood (min.):_____

Type of exercise: _____

EBCT

Pervasiveness is the pitfall thought pattern you are targeting today. Remember, this type of thinking allows something that is affecting one area of your life to spread to all areas of your life.

Step 1: Notice the Pattern: Throughout the day, identify when **pervasiveness** shows up today. Then write down how your own personal version of **pervasiveness** sounds to you as a thought. Also rate how true it feels for you (for a more detailed review of these steps, turn to page 114).

The pervasiveness pitfall thought pattern I notice:

_____

_____

How true does this worry feel from 0 to 100: ____%.

Step 2: Use a Physical Pose as an Antidote: Pigeon pose or shoulder shrugs are the antidote for pervasiveness (see pages 118–119 for a review).

Step 3: Find the Contrary Evidence: While in pigeon pose or after doing a round of shoulder shrugs, consider the contrary evidence that proves your brain-draining worry wrong and then write it down.

My contrary evidence that I already have (e.g., What experience do you have from your own life that proves this worry could possibly be wrong?):

_____

_____

Step 4: See the Right Action You'd Like to Take: While in pigeon pose or after doing a round of shoulder shrugs, see the right action you'd like to take in the future in your mind's eye.

Step 5: Revisit Your Brain-Draining Worries: Now that this antidote has worked on you physically, psychologically, and spiritually, return to the brain-draining worry you wrote in step 1. How true does this brain-draining worry feel now? Now that you have contradicted it with mind and body, does it feel less true? Rate it from 0 to 100: _____ %

Step 6: Turn Right Action into Your Reality: Make a commitment to yourself that in the future, you will choose the actions that you saw in your mind's eye.

CBT-I

Continue Level 1:

My wake time:_____

My wind-down time: _____

My bedtime: _____

END-OF-DAY EVALUATION

Rate yourself on the following on a scale from 1 to 10 (with 10 being the best):

How is my energy? _____

How well am I sleeping? _____

How well am I handling stress? _____

How am I feeling in general? _____

Today I'm most proud of myself for _____

_____.

DAY 5

LIFESTYLE TRACKING
(place a check next to each to track your progress)

Seven servings of vegetables and fruits (min.): 1____2____3____4____5___6____7____

One daily (min.): probiotic ____, prebiotic _____, probiotic booster ____

One daily omega-3 superfood (min.):_____

Type of exercise: _____

EBCT

Pessimistic thinking is the pitfall thought pattern you are targeting today. Remember, this type of thinking considers the worst-case, catastrophic scenario. It dwells in the possible—not the probable.

Step 1: Notice the Pattern: Throughout the day, identify when **pessimistic thinking** shows up today. Then write down how your own personal version of **pessimistic thinking** sounds to you as a thought. Also rate how true it feels for you (for a more detailed review of these steps, turn to page 114).

The pessimistic-thinking pitfall thought pattern I notice:

_____

_____

How true does this worry feel from 0 to 100: _____%.

Step 2: Use a Physical Pose as an Antidote: The half-smile is the antidote for pessimistic thinking (see page 119 for a review).

Step 3: Find the Contrary Evidence: While using the half-smile, consider the contrary evidence that proves your brain-draining worry wrong and then write it down.

My contrary evidence that I already have (e.g., What experience do you have from your own life that proves this worry could possibly be wrong?):

_____

_____

Step 4: See the Right Action You'd Like to Take: While using the half-smile, see the right action you'd like to take in the future in your mind's eye.

Step 5: Revisit Your Brain-Draining Worries: Now that this antidote has worked on you physically, psychologically, and spiritually, return to the brain-draining worry you wrote in step 1. How true does this brain-draining worry feel now? Now that you have contradicted it with mind and body, does it feel less true? Rate it from 0 to 100: _____ %

Step 6: Turn Right Action into Your Reality: Make a commitment to yourself that in the future, you will choose the actions that you saw in your mind's eye.

CBT-I

Continue Level 1:

My wake time:_____

My wind-down time: _____

My bedtime: _____

END-OF-DAY EVALUATION

Rate yourself on the following on a scale from 1 to 10 (with 10 being the best):

How is my energy? _____

How well am I sleeping? _____

How well am I handling stress? _____

How am I feeling in general? _____

Today I'm most proud of myself for _____

_____.

DAY 6

LIFESTYLE TRACKING
(place a check next to each to track your progress)

Seven servings of vegetables and fruits (min.): 1____ 2____ 3____ 4____ 5____ 6____ 7____

One daily (min.): probiotic ____, prebiotic ____, probiotic booster ____

One daily omega-3 superfood (min.):_____

Type of exercise: _____

EBCT

Polarized thinking is the pitfall thought pattern you are targeting today. Remember, this type of thinking has a binary, black-or-white pattern. The words *always* or *never* are frequently found in this type of thought pattern.

Step 1: Notice the Pattern: Throughout the day, identify when **polarized thinking** shows up today. Then write down how your own personal version of **polarized thinking** sounds to you as a thought. Also rate how true it feels for you (for a more detailed review of these steps, turn to page 114).

The polarized thinking pitfall thought pattern I notice:

_____

_____

How true does this worry feel from 0 to 100: _____%.

Step 2: Use a Physical Pose as an Antidote: The spinal twist is the antidote for polarized thinking (see pages 119–120 for a review).

Step 3: Find the Contrary Evidence: While using the spinal twist, consider the contrary evidence that proves your brain-draining worry wrong and then write it down.

My contrary evidence that I already have (e.g., What experience do you have from your own life that proves this worry could possibly be wrong?):

_____

_____

Step 4: See the Right Action You'd Like to Take: While using the spinal twist, see the right action you'd like to take in the future in your mind's eye.

Step 5: Revisit Your Brain-Draining Worries: Now that this antidote has worked on you physically, psychologically, and spiritually, return to the brain-draining worry you wrote in step 1. How true does this brain-draining worry feel now? Now that you have contradicted it with mind and body, does it feel less true? Rate it from 0 to 100: _____ %

Step 6: Turn Right Action into Your Reality: Make a commitment to yourself that in the future, you will choose the actions that you saw in your mind's eye.

CBT-I

Continue Level 1:

My wake time:_____

My wind-down time: _____

My bedtime: _____

END-OF-DAY EVALUATION

Rate yourself on the following on a scale from 1 to 10 (with 10 being the best):

How is my energy? _____

How well am I sleeping? _____

How well am I handling stress? _____

How am I feeling in general? _____

Today I'm most proud of myself for _____

_____.

DAY 7

LIFESTYLE TRACKING
(place a check next to each to track your progress)

Seven servings of vegetables and fruits (min.): 1____ 2____ 3____ 4____ 5___ 6____ 7____

One daily (min.): probiotic ____, prebiotic _____, probiotic booster _____

One daily omega-3 superfood (min.):_____

Type of exercise: _____

EBCT

Psychic thinking is the pitfall thought pattern you are targeting today. Remember, this type of thinking expects people around us to read our minds without us verbalizing what we need. Or, it assumes we know what others are thinking without them verbalizing it to us.

Step 1: Notice the Pattern: Throughout the day, identify when **psychic thinking** shows up today. Then write down how your own personal version of **psychic thinking** sounds to you as a thought. Also rate how true it feels for you (for a more detailed review of these steps, turn to page 114).

The psychic-thinking pitfall thought pattern I notice:

_____

_____

How true does this worry feel from 0 to 100: _____%.

Step 2: Use a Physical Pose as an Antidote: The chest thump or Lion's Breath is the antidote for psychic thinking (see page 120 for a review).

Step 3: Find the Contrary Evidence: While using the chest thump or Lion's Breath, consider the contrary evidence that proves your brain-draining worry wrong and then write it down.

My contrary evidence that I already have (e.g., What experience do you have from your own life that proves this worry could possibly be wrong?):

_____

_____

Step 4: See the Right Action You'd Like to Take: While using the chest thump or Lion's Breath, see the right action you'd like to take in the future in your mind's eye.

Step 5: Revisit Your Brain-Draining Worries: Now that this antidote has worked on you physically, psychologically, and spiritually, return to the brain-draining worry you wrote in step 1. How true does this brain-draining worry feel now? Now that you have contradicted it with mind and body, does it feel less true? Rate it from 0 to 100: _____ %

Step 6: Turn Right Action into Your Reality: Make a commitment to yourself that in the future, you will choose the actions that you saw in your mind's eye.

CBT-I

Continue Level 1:

My wake time:_____

My wind-down time: _____

My bedtime: _____

END-OF-DAY EVALUATION

Rate yourself on the following on a scale from 1 to 10 (with 10 being the best):

How is my energy? _____

How well am I sleeping? _____

How well am I handling stress? _____

How am I feeling in general? _____

Today I'm most proud of myself for _____

_____.

Workbook for Week 2: The Brain-Balancing Toolkit

Diet: Continue with the changes you've made in week 1. You'll continue to track this each day.

Energy-Based Cognitive Therapy: Now that you know what the seven pitfall thought patterns sound like, feel free to use the antidotes whenever you notice one of the pitfall thought patterns showing up in your daily life.

Exercise: Continue to choose one of the four types of exercise each day for week 2. You'll continue to track this each day.

Cognitive Behavioral Therapy for Insomnia (CBT-I): Continue level 1 of CBT-I by keeping your wind-down, bedtime, and wake times stable while also tracking them each day. If your sleep still needs improvement, then you'll also add on level 2 of CBT-I by following the instructions below. Level 2 includes using a form of EBCT to *reframe* your sleep worry. It also includes adding an additional tool to *relax* when you go to bed.

Your toolkit: Each day you'll use a different brain-balancing tool at some point during the day. If you are implementing CBT-I level 2, you'll also use one of these tools while you're in bed.

DAY 8

LIFESTYLE TRACKING
(place a check next to each to track your progress)

Seven servings of vegetables and fruits (min.): 1____ 2____ 3____ 4____ 5___ 6____ 7____

One daily (min.): probiotic ____, prebiotic _____, probiotic booster _____

One daily omega-3 superfood (min.):_____

Type of exercise: _____

TOOL OF THE DAY: Relaxation therapy: mantra meditation. You can find a guided video of this at www.facebook.com/drmikedow. Do this at least once today.

- Find a comfortable seated position and close your eyes.
- Relax your muscles, starting with your feet, and allow the relaxation to spread all the way up to your head.
- Breathe easily and comfortably through your nose, and mindfully become aware of the breath.
- Attach a mantra like the word *one* to your breath. Say this word to yourself on each inhale and exhale. You can also choose another soothing word if you'd like.
- Maintain a passive attitude so that relaxation unfolds at its own pace.
- Continue for 10 to 20 minutes.

CBT-I

Continue Level 1:

My wake time:_____

My wind-down time: _____

My bedtime: _____

If You Need It, Also Add on CBT-I Level 2:

Relax: In addition to practicing relaxation therapy (mantra meditation) during the day, add another practice of this tool to your nighttime routine. Do another round while you're in bed to help lull you to sleep.

Reframe: Using the information that starts on page 138, work to identify your biggest sleep worry and write it down here:

The pitfall thought pattern that disrupts my sleep the most is _____.

It leads to a sleep worry that sounds something like . . .

SLEEP WORRY: _____ (HOW TRUE DOES THIS FEEL: ___%).

Change Your Thoughts, See Your Success: Once you have identified your sleep worry, overcome and change it using the strategies you learned from EBCT. First, use a physical pose. Second, find the *contrary evidence* from knowledge and experience you already have in your life. Third, see your success in your mind's eye.

After using a physical pose (listed on page 140), reflecting on this contrary evidence, and seeing your future in your mind's eye, how true does it feel now?

SLEEP WORRY FROM ABOVE: HOW TRUE DOES IT FEEL NOW: _____%

For many people, this process significantly reduces how true this worry feels. This reframing is the *cognitive* part of cognitive behavioral therapy. Sleep worries become less powerful, and they may bother you a little less. This helps to ease sleep worries that prevent restful sleep.

END-OF-DAY EVALUATION

Rate yourself on the following on a scale from 1 to 10 (with 10 being the best):

How is my energy? _____

How well am I sleeping? _____

How well am I handling stress? _____

How am I feeling in general? _____

Today I'm most proud of myself for _____

_____.

DAY 9

LIFESTYLE TRACKING
(place a check next to each to track your progress)

Seven servings of vegetables and fruits (min.): 1____ 2____ 3____ 4____ 5___ 6____ 7____

One daily (min.): probiotic ____, prebiotic _____, probiotic booster _____

One daily omega-3 superfood (min.):_____

Type of exercise: _____

TOOL OF THE DAY: Relaxation therapy: progressive muscle relaxation and autogenic training. Practice each one at least once today.

Progressive Muscle Relaxation: You can memorize it easily. Or you can see and hear me guiding you through it on my Facebook page (www.facebook.com/drmikedow).

- Begin by finding a comfortable seated or lying down position and closing your eyes.

- Inhale through your nose for a count of 5. At the same time, flex your feet and tense your calf muscles. Notice the feeling of tension in this part of the body.

- Exhale through your nose for a count of 10 while releasing and feeling all the tension dissolve. Notice the difference between tension and total relaxation.

- While inhaling through your nose for a count of 5, squeeze your leg muscles as you straighten your knees. Notice the feeling of tension in this part of the body.

- While exhaling through your nose for a count of 10, release and feel all the tension dissolve. Notice the difference between tension and total relaxation.

- Inhale through your nose for a count of 5. At the same time, squeeze your buttocks together. Notice the feeling of tension in this part of the body.

- Exhale through your nose for a count of 10 while releasing and feeling all the tension dissolve. Notice the difference between tension and total relaxation.

- While inhaling through your nose for a count of 5, squeeze your abs as if you're doing crunches. Notice the feeling of tension in this part of the body.

- While exhaling through your nose for a count of 10, release and feel all the tension dissolve. Notice the difference between tension and total relaxation.

- Inhale through your nose for a count of 5. At the same time, squeeze your back muscles by squeezing your shoulder blades toward each other. Notice the feeling of tension in this part of the body.

- Exhale through your nose for a count of 10 while releasing and feeling all the tension dissolve. Notice the difference between tension and total relaxation.

- While inhaling through your nose for a count of 5, make fists with both your hands, straighten your elbows, and contract your biceps and triceps. Notice the feeling of tension in this part of the body.

- While exhaling through your nose for a count of 10, release and feel all the tension dissolve. Notice the difference between tension and total relaxation.

- Inhale through your nose for a count of 5. At the same time, raise your shoulders and tense your neck as you bring your chin to your chest. Notice the feeling of tension in this part of the body.

- Exhale through your nose for a count of 10 while releasing and feeling all the tension dissolve. Notice the difference between tension and total relaxation.

- While inhaling through your nose for a count of 5, tense your jaw, wrinkle your nose, and squeeze your eyes even more closed. Notice the feeling of tension in this part of the body.

- While exhaling through your nose for a count of 10, release and feel all the tension dissolve. Notice the difference between tension and total relaxation.

- Inhale through your nose for a count of 5. At the same time, raise your eyebrows as you feel tension in your forehead and across your scalp. Notice the feeling of tension in this part of the body.

- Exhale through your nose for a count of 10 while releasing and feeling all the tension dissolve. Notice the difference between tension and total relaxation.

Autogenic Training: Say these phrases silently to yourself in a comfortable seated or lying position. You can also see and hear me reading this script on my Facebook page (www.facebook.com/drmikedow).

- I am completely calm.
- My arms are heavy. (six times)
- I am completely calm.
- My arms are warm. (six times)
- I am completely calm.
- My legs are heavy. (six times)
- I am completely calm.
- My legs are warm. (six times)
- I am completely calm.
- My heart beats calmly and regularly. (six times)
- I am completely calm.
- My breathing is calm and regular. (six times)
- I am completely calm.
- My abdomen is warm. (six times)
- I am completely calm.
- My forehead is pleasantly cool. (six times)
- I am completely calm.

    If you use this practice to fall asleep, stop the practice here and allow yourself to drift to sleep whenever you're ready as you take whatever time you need to do so. If not, continue.
- Arms firm, breathe deeply, open eyes.

CBT-I

Continue Level 1:

My wake time:_____

My wind-down time: _____

My bedtime: _____

If You Need It, Also Add on CBT-I Level 2:

Relax: In addition to practicing both forms of relaxation therapy during the day, add an additional practice of one of them before you go to bed.

END-OF-DAY EVALUATION

Rate yourself on the following on a scale from 1 to 10 (with 10 being the best):

How is my energy? _____

How well am I sleeping? _____

How well am I handling stress? _____

How am I feeling in general? _____

Today I'm most proud of myself for _____

_____.

DAY 10

LIFESTYLE TRACKING
(place a check next to each to track your progress)

Seven servings of vegetables and fruits (min.): 1____ 2____ 3____ 4____ 5____ 6____ 7____

One daily (min.): probiotic ____, prebiotic _____, probiotic booster _____

One daily omega-3 superfood (min.):_____

Type of exercise: _____

TOOL OF THE DAY: Practice pranayama today. You can use the breathing exercises and the sequences listed beginning on page 161. You can memorize the exercises, or you can also see and hear me guiding you through them on my Facebook page (www.facebook.com/drmikedow).

CBT-I

Continue Level 1:

My wake time:_____

My wind-down time: _____

My bedtime: _____

If You Need It, Also Add on CBT-I Level 2:

Relax: In addition to pranayama during the day, add another practice of one of the breathing exercises to your nighttime routine. Choose any of the pranayama practices that are calming or a calming sequence.

END-OF-DAY EVALUATION

Rate yourself on the following on a scale from 1 to 10 (with 10 being the best):

How is my energy? _____

How well am I sleeping? _____

How well am I handling stress? _____

How am I feeling in general? _____

Today I'm most proud of myself for _____

_____.

DAY 11

LIFESTYLE TRACKING
(place a check next to each to track your progress)

Seven servings of vegetables and fruits (min.): 1____ 2____ 3____ 4____ 5___ 6____ 7____

One daily (min.): probiotic ____, prebiotic _____, probiotic booster _____

One daily omega-3 superfood (min.):_____

Type of exercise: _____

TOOL OF THE DAY: Practice self-hypnosis today. You can memorize this script, or you can also see and hear me guiding you through this on my Facebook page (www.facebook.com/drmikedow).

Begin by settling into a comfortable seated or lying down position in a place that's safe, comfortable, and quiet. Place one of your hands in front of you with your palm facing away from you. Begin with your fingers pressed gently together. Your elbow is bent so that your hand is at eye level.

Now fix your gaze on your middle finger with your eyes still open. You may notice that after some time, the finger will go in and out of focus or perhaps the eyes become tired. Notice any interesting sensations in your hand. I wonder if you've already begun to notice any changes associated with your intention to relax. You may notice tension has dissolved in the shoulders or neck, or perhaps your body begins to feel lighter. You may even feel a slight tingling or warming sensation throughout the body. I don't know what exactly you'll experience, but that's not important. All that really matters is you enjoy this time, because you deserve to rest.

As you become more and more comfortable and relaxed, the fingers will begin to spread. I don't know which finger will move first. Maybe it will be the index finger. Maybe it will be the pinky, or maybe they'll move at the same time. As soon as the mind is ready to deeply relax, then the hand will begin to move closer and closer to your face. That's right. Good.

You feel the eyelids becoming heavier as your hand moves toward you. Heavier and heavier. Closer and closer. As soon as you're ready to relax even more deeply, the hand will make its way to your face, the eyes will close fully, and the hand finds its way to a comfortable position.

The next five breaths will take you down into an even deeper state of relaxation. As you're descending into this peaceful and calm state, you may notice the body feel like it's floating in the air like a feather. I wonder if the body will even begin to feel like a rag doll as a wonderful ease spreads. Every sensation you notice and feel in this moment takes you to a deeper state of rest and relaxation.

Breathing easily in a wonderful and relaxed way, you may even wish to imagine that every breath is spreading a calming energy through every cell and organ in your body and brain. You may wish to see a color of your choosing in your mind's eye. Your mind, your body, and your spirit are all becoming so calm and so comfortable. Spread this peace throughout the body from the toes to the top of the head. That's right. Perfect.

This calming energy may even feel like a pleasant type of daydream. I wonder what easy, relaxed, and comfortable sensations you will feel. Linger here.

(If you use this practice to fall asleep, stop the meditation here and allow yourself to drift to sleep whenever you're ready as you take whatever time you need to do so. If not, continue.)

Really notice the quality of this sensation. In the future, you'll be surprised by this calm energy returning to you whenever you need it.

Now allow the next five inhales and exhales you take to be refreshing, invigorating ones, bringing a balanced energy to every cell in your body. Each breath is bringing you back up to a fully awake state. As soon as you're feeling fully alert, then the eyes will open. When that happens, you'll feel an urge to move and stretch your limbs. You'll go about the rest of your day with a relaxed confidence you need to move through it with grace and ease.

CBT-I

Continue Level 1:

My wake time:_____

My wind-down time: _____

My bedtime: _____

If You Need It, Also Add on CBT-I Level 2:

Relax: Add one of the breathing practices to your nighttime routine. Choose any of the pranayama practices that are calming to you.

END-OF-DAY EVALUATION

Rate yourself on the following on a scale from 1 to 10 (with 10 being the best):

How is my energy? _____

How well am I sleeping? _____

How well am I handling stress? _____

How am I feeling in general? _____

Today I'm most proud of myself for _____

_____.

DAY 12

LIFESTYLE TRACKING
(place a check next to each to track your progress)

Seven servings of vegetables and fruits (min.): 1____ 2____ 3____ 4____ 5____ 6____ 7____

One daily (min.): probiotic ____, prebiotic _____, probiotic booster _____

One daily omega-3 superfood (min.):_____

Type of exercise: _____

TOOL OF THE DAY: Kindness, gratitude, and connection.

Kindness: Do five acts of kindness today. Remember, these can be big and/or small acts. Write them down here:

1. _____

2. _____

3. _____

4. _____

5. _____

Gratitude: Be grateful today. Remember to be specific. Also be reflective by finishing your gratitude journal with the word *because*. As you do this, you may even wish to take a moment to consider what your life would be like without these blessings.

I am grateful for _____

_____

because _____

_____.

Connection: Make a conscious effort to connect to someone today. It could be having a dinner with someone you love, a phone conversation with a friend, or a day at the dog park.

Today, I chose to connect by _____

_____.

CBT-I

Continue Level 1:

My wake time:_____

My wind-down time: _____

My bedtime: _____

If You Need It, Also Add on CBT-I Level 2:

Relax: Add one of the calming practices (e.g., mantra meditation, progressive muscle relaxation, autogenic training, self-hypnosis) to your nighttime routine.

END-OF-DAY EVALUATION

Rate yourself on the following on a scale from 1 to 10 (with 10 being the best):

How is my energy? _____

How well am I sleeping? _____

How well am I handling stress? _____

How am I feeling in general? _____

Today I'm most proud of myself for _____

_____.

DAY 13

LIFESTYLE TRACKING
(place a check next to each to track your progress)

Seven servings of vegetables and fruits (min.): 1____ 2____ 3____ 4____ 5___ 6____ 7____

One daily (min.): probiotic ____, prebiotic _____, probiotic booster _____

One daily omega-3 superfood (min.):_____

Type of exercise: _____

TOOL OF THE DAY: Thought stream meditation and stimulus control.

Thought Stream Meditation: Set aside 12 minutes today to do the thought stream meditation (for a review, turn to page 188). Walk yourself through the below meditation in your mind. You can also listen to me guide you through this on my Facebook page (www.facebook.com/drmikedow).

Imagine yourself sitting by the side of a peaceful river. The river represents the thoughts and feelings in your mind. For the next 12 minutes, spend some time just watching what's in your river at this moment. Without any judgment . . . without trying to slow the river down or speed it up . . . just watch your river.

And while you're at it, notice the difference between *you* sitting next to the river and the *river* itself. Most of the time, we have a tendency to overidentify with our thoughts and feelings. We believe that we are our thoughts and feelings, and we forget who we really are. But we're so much *more* than our thoughts. Feelings come and feelings go. They're useful information to help guide our lives. But we also must remember who we are and not feel imprisoned by them.

This happens when we proverbially *jump into* our river. When you notice you've "jumped in," simply find your way out of the river and feel yourself back on the side of the bank.

You'll be left with the feeling of peace when you sense that part of you that is you. It's the part of you that always has been and always will be. It's the part of you that is connected to all living beings.

Stimulus Control: Also use *stimulus control*, which I call "the mindful way to worry." The first step in this process is to *pick your worry time and place*. Do this at the beginning of your day. Remember, your "worry time" will be 5 to 30 minutes where you will concentrate solely on worrying. You'll also choose a neutral place to worry, avoiding places like your bedroom or office. This will prevent you associating worry with places you'd like to be sleeping or working. (For a full review of this process, turn to page 189.)

My worry time will be _____.

My worry place will be _____.

Now that you have your prescribed time and place for later today, be mindful of worry when it surfaces throughout the day. Catch yourself as soon as you discover you're worrying.

When you have reached your prescribed "worry time" and "worry place," write in a worry journal or just use a piece of paper. Alternatively, you can use a computer to type your worries. You can also speak them out loud. Worry in a free-flowing format while staying immersed in the worry. Also consider a few questions as you worry. What am I going to *do* about this worry? What are *solutions* to this problem?

CBT-I

Continue Level 1:

My wake time:_____

My wind-down time: _____

My bedtime: _____

If You Need It, Also Add on CBT-I Level 2:

Relax: Add one of the calming practices (e.g., mantra meditation, progressive muscle relaxation, autogenic training, self-hypnosis) to your nighttime routine.

END-OF-DAY EVALUATION

Rate yourself on the following on a scale from 1 to 10 (with 10 being the best):

How is my energy? _____

How well am I sleeping? _____

How well am I handling stress? _____

How am I feeling in general? _____

Today I'm most proud of myself for _____

_____.

DAY 14

LIFESTYLE TRACKING
(place a check next to each to track your progress)

Seven servings of vegetables and fruits (min.): 1_____ 2_____ 3_____ 4_____ 5_____ 6_____ 7_____

One daily (min.): probiotic _____, prebiotic _____, probiotic booster _____

One daily omega-3 superfood (min.):_____

Type of exercise: _____

TOOL OF THE DAY: The 25–5, mindful to-do lists, and coloring.

The 25–5: The first step is to list your top 25 goals in your life. They can professional and personal. Write your top 25 goals here in no particular order:

1. _____

2. _____

3. _____

4. _____

5. _____

6. _____

7. _____

8. _____

9. _____

10. _____

11. _____

12. _____

13. _____

14. _____

15. _____

16. _____

17. _____

18. _____

19. _____

20. _____

21. _____

22. _____

23. _____

24. _____

25. _____

After you've written your top 25 goals, go back and circle the 5 most important ones. This is your mindful "big picture" focus of your life. In general, keep the focus of your life on these five most important goals. Keep your life's focus on these goals until you have achieved them. When you have reached a life goal at some point a few weeks, months, or years from now, you can come back to this list and circle a new goal to add to your top five. Or you may wish to return to this exercise and do a new 25–5. It's a great exercise to use when you're opening a new chapter in your life. It reminds us to work diligently and to spend time on tasks that are most important to us.

Mindful To-Do Lists: Now that you know what to keep your focus on in your life, create a mindful to-do list of 5 to 10 things you'd like to get done today. Remember, these consist of household tasks like cleaning out a closet, work-related ones like finishing your quarterly expenses on a spreadsheet, or personal ones like sending a thank-you note.

These tasks should be small enough so that you could potentially get all 10 done in one day. Remember, you may need to break larger tasks into smaller ones (e.g., if you would need a week to clean out the whole garage, perhaps you'd write: take the charity boxes in the garage to Salvation Army for your list today).

Today's Mindful To-Do List:

1. _____

2. _____

3. _____

4. _____

5. _____

6. _____

7. _____

8. _____

9. _____

10. _____

At the end of your day, write a list of 5–10 tasks you'd like to get done *tomorrow*. If you didn't finish all your tasks today, simply move them onto tomorrow's list. Prioritize the tasks so that anything that *needs* to get done tomorrow will be the first or second task on the list.

Tomorrow's Mindful To-Do List:

1. _____

2. _____

3. _____

4. _____

5. _____

6. _____

7. _____

8. _____

9. _____

10. _____

Color: Go online and download free mandala coloring pages. (There are a ton out there!) And then get out some colored pencils or crayons. When you feel stressed, spend a few minutes coloring today.

CBT-I

Continue Level 1:

My wake time:_____

My wind-down time: _____

My bedtime: _____

If You Need It, Also Add on CBT-I Level 2:

Relax: Add one of the calming practices (e.g., mantra meditation, progressive muscle relaxation, autogenic training, self-hypnosis) to your nighttime routine.

END-OF-DAY EVALUATION

Rate yourself on the following on a scale from 1 to 10 (with 10 being the best):

How is my energy? _____

How well am I sleeping? _____

How well am I handling stress? _____

How am I feeling in general? _____

Today I'm most proud of myself for _____

_____.

END-OF-PROGRAM EVALUATION

What I've learned about myself through this journey is _____

_____

_____.

Overall I'm most proud of myself for _____

_____

_____.

Of the changes I've made and the tools I've learned, the ones I'm going to make part of

my everyday life are:_____

_____

_____.

Conclusion

Congratulations! You have made it through the Drained Brain program. By now you probably feel an overall sense of calm along with more lasting supplies of energy. Brain-balancing neurotransmitters have already begun to rise as draining stress hormones have fallen. Of course, these initial improvements are just the beginning, since the daily choices you have made have set off a chain reaction in both brain and body. The improvements in energy, mood, and sleep will actually make it easier to make heathier choices in the future. Positive feedback in the way you feel will keep the momentum going. You can ensure a lifetime of balance and health benefits by making the changes you've made in this program a way of life.

From now on, follow the 80/20 rule. This means that 80 percent of the time, you are consuming a probiotic daily, choosing yoga with friends over a night on the couch, and avoiding draining foods like sugar and flour. But since a lifetime of perfection is unrealistic and can be draining in and of itself, it's okay to miss a day of interval training or have a piece of pizza now and again.

There's also something different about you that will come in handy the next time life throws you a curveball. You are now armed with an entire toolkit of stress-relieving practices you can call on whenever you feel overwhelmed. You now know which ones work best for you.

I know that no matter who you are, where you may live, or how old you may be, healing your drained brain will help you to live the life you were born to live.

Natural Herbs, Adaptogens, and Supplements

Throughout this book, you've heard about some of the natural ways to fight stress, anxiety, and insomnia, but I didn't include everything. Herbs and adaptogens are kinds of supplements that some people love; however, there is some controversy surrounding their safety and effectiveness—especially in the UK and U.S. where they are not regulated.

Herbs

Even with the controversy, some herbs have been proven to be both safe and effective. And when specifically talking about anxiety, stress, and insomnia, many of the pharmaceutical treatments like benzodiazepines and sleeping pills have proven to be anything but "safe" and are associated with addiction and an increasing number of fatal overdoses.

If you are going to use any of the herbs listed below, consult your doctor to make sure you don't have any conditions or are not taking any drugs or supplements that could have dangerous interactions. Always take these under the guidance of a licensed healthcare professional who is aware of your health history, including the medications or supplements you take. This person can help you determine if an herb is safe for you. Even commonly used and widely accepted as "safe" herbs could have interactions (e.g., too much chamomile can interfere with the effectiveness of birth control pills).

Also, it's a good idea to find reputable companies with reputable track records when purchasing herbs or supplements so you're more likely to get the amount of the herb listed on the label. Remember: herbs and supplements are not regulated like prescription medications. I like New Chapter, Gaia Herbs, Natrol, herbal Yogi teas, and Traditional Medicinals since they're all well-established, trusted companies.

With a bit of precaution and diligence, the herbs listed below can be a natural and effective part of helping you manage stress and insomnia. And they tend to be safer than pharmaceuticals like Ambien and benzodiazepines, which have become increasingly problematic in recent years. So while there is some controversy and needed diligence when it comes to some natural remedies, they can help. I recommend, however, that you try the energy-based cognitive behavioral therapy, nutrition, exercise, and clinically proven forms of meditation that you learned in this book before adding additional supplements. Basic lifestyle changes are safe and risk-free ways to treat anxiety and insomnia.

- **Chamomile, catnip, and lemon balm:** These herbs are often made into calming teas. Chamomile can help insomnia and has even been shown to modestly reduce anxiety in people with generalized anxiety disorder. It has also been shown to have a positive effect on blood pressure, inflammation, and digestive problems like gas and diarrhea. It may even have anticancer effects in the body. Chamomile may, however, have dangerous interactions for people taking birth control pills, estrogens, warfarin, and cancer drugs. Catnip can help anxiety, insomnia, and GI upset but can interact with lithium. Lemon balm is a calming herb from the mint family that can be helpful with restlessness, anxiety, insomnia, and GI upset. One small study found it lowered anxiety by 18 percent and insomnia by 42 percent.[1] Since all three of these herbs are sedatives, they shouldn't be mixed with other sedatives like alcohol, sleeping pills, or benzodiazepines.

- **Licorice:** Extracts of this plant can increase low cortisol levels, which can potentially be helpful for people with atypical presentations of drained brains where low cortisol is present (e.g., Drop Drain, X-treme Drain).[2] However, there are some major precautions when using licorice. Look for deglycyrrhizinated licorice (DGL), which may reduce one of the major dangers of this herb: high blood pressure. Since drained-brained individuals are at increased risk for developing this dangerous condition, be sure to use it under a doctor's supervision. It should not be taken by pregnant or nursing women and should only be used for very short amounts of time.

- **Passionflower and kava:** These herbs are often taken in teas or in supplements. Both of these herbs can boost levels of GABA and help promote a sense of calm. Passionflower is used to relieve anxiety, calm muscle spasms, reduce pain, help with symptoms of fibromyalgia, and induce sleep. It shouldn't be used with other prescription sedatives. Kava is used to reduce anxiety but has a long list of interactions and safety concerns, including liver damage. It is banned from the market in Canada and Europe but is still available in the U.S. market, but likely has too many concerns to make it a viable and safe choice for most people.

- **Valerian:** This herb is often made into a tea or supplement, or even added to a bath to promote sleep. It is often used to treat insomnia and can help people wean themselves off prescription sleep aids, especially when combined with the cognitive behavioral strategies that are now the primary recommended treatment for insomnia. Valerian works primarily by increasing GABA in the brain. The usual dose is 150 mg, two to three times per day. It has been shown to help people fall asleep more quickly and also have more slow-wave sleep.[3] It has also been shown to treat anxiety without causing sedation and chronic fatigue syndrome.[4] It should not be taken with other depressants like alcohol, sleep aids, or benzodiazepines and also may interact with other prescription drugs. It should not be taken by pregnant or nursing women.

ADAPTOGENS & OTHER SUPPLEMENTS

Adaptogens are a class of herb originally defined as substances that enhance the "state of nonspecific resistance" in stress. Now, however, an adaptogen is defined as a substance that "increases your ability to adapt to environmental factors and to avoid damage from these factors." The ultimate goal is to condition your body to stress. By regulating cortisol production, they can help promote a healthier stress response in people. In fact, they were initially studied and developed for soldiers in World War II facing extreme conditions. Some adaptogens can be simultaneously stimulating while also calming, but they are different from stimulants in that the goal is decreased sensitivity to stress in the future. In many ways, they're like a stress vaccine.

Adaptogens may be helpful for people who experience extreme stress, fatigue, chronic fatigue syndrome, or adrenal fatigue. While drained brains tend to have high levels of cortisol in general, this may not always be the case. For example, adrenal fatigue may result when someone has been under prolonged, intense stress with sky-high levels of cortisol.

This can lead to the stress response no longer functioning as it should and *low* levels of cortisol, like in people with PTSD. Adaptogens can help balance cortisol levels. In many cases, they bring cortisol levels up initially, which later helps your body to be "used to" that level of response, which eventually means a decreased sensitivity to stress and lower levels of cortisol in the long run. On a cellular level, certain adaptogens can even create stress proteins that are linked to increased survival rate. Again, take these under the guidance of a licensed health-care professional and advise them of any other medications or supplements you may be taking.

- **Ginseng:** There are many forms of ginseng, and each has slightly different effects. *Panax ginseng* which is also known as Korean, Chinese, or Asian ginseng, is the most popular. Ginseng helps the body cope with fatigue and psychological and physical stress and acts primarily on the adrenal glands. It can cause contradictory effects where it can be both stimulating and calming. People who are sensitive to stimulants may want to avoid ginseng. If you are pregnant, have diabetes, or are on blood-thinning medication, do not take ginseng. It can be too activating when mixed with caffeine.

- **Rhodiola (*Rhodiola rosea*, golden root, arctic root):** This adaptogenic herb can improve physical endurance and cognitive performance and reduce fatigue associated with stress. One large study of people with stress-related fatigue taking rhodiola showed fewer cortisol spikes in the face of a stressor, which improved performance and decreased burnout.[5] Unlike most adaptogens, which act primarily on the adrenal glands, rhodiola appears to act directly on the central nervous system and may affect levels of cortisol, serotonin, and norepinephrine. Pregnant women should avoid it.

- **Ashwagandha (*Withania somnifera*, Indian ginseng):** This Ayurvedic herb is used to treat stress and fatigue. One study of chronically stressed individuals taking 500 mg of ashwagandha daily for 60 days found they had 30 percent less cortisol compared with those taking a placebo.[6] In a head-to-head study, patients taking ashwagandha reduced anxiety more than those assigned to traditional psychotherapy.[7] It can even help men with sterility problems improve semen quality due to a reduction in oxidative stress.[8] Immunosuppressants and sedatives like sleeping pills, benzodiazepines, and alcohol should not be taken with ashwagandha.

- **Holy basil (*Ocimum tenuiflorum*, tulsi):** This herb is known for its ability to reduce blood sugar, help people manage stress, decrease pain and inflammation, and improve immune function. One study involving people with generalized anxiety disorder treated with holy basil for 60 days showed an improvement in their anxiety symptoms.[9] It has been shown to decrease

cortisol levels in the bloodstream.[10] Anticoagulants may interact v
holy basil.

- **Bacopa:** This herb has been shown to be as potent on anxiety as the
  benzodiazepine lorazepam (Ativan) while also enhancing cognitive
  function.[11] It may help to stabilize serotonin levels and reduce adrenaline
  when facing a stressor.[12] A study with elderly people experiencing anxiety
  demonstrated a daily dose of bacopa over 12 weeks helped decrease
  anxiety while improving cognitive performance.[13] Pregnant or nursing
  women, people with thyroid conditions, or those with a slow heart rate
  should avoid it.

- **DHEA:** This supplement is a hormone produced by the adrenal glands.
  There is an inverse relationship between DHEA and cortisol. When stress
  in encountered, cortisol will rise and DHEA levels go down. Healthy
  levels of DHEA have even been shown to prevent the pitfall thought
  pattern paralysis-analysis and anticipatory anxiety.[14] Production of this
  hormone typically declines with age. It tends to improve mood but can also
  affect levels of testosterone and estrogen. Many of the natural strategies
  recommended in this program can naturally increase DHEA levels without
  needing to take it as a supplement. If you do supplement, Natrol makes an
  affordable option.

- **5-HTP:** This supplement is a serotonin precursor and has been shown
  to relieve symptoms of both anxiety and insomnia.[15, 16] With this and
  all supplements, check with your prescriber before taking it. If 5-HTP is
  taken with medications that also boost serotonin such as antidepressants
  or triptans, it could lead to a condition called serotonin syndrome. Natrol
  makes an affordable option.

- **CBD Oil:** While more research is needed, there is good evidence to
  suggest that CBD oil which is derived from hemp may be an effective
  and nonaddictive treatment for drained brains. Unlike THC, CBD is not
  psychoactive. One recent study found CBD oil to be an effective treatment
  for social anxiety.[17] It has also been shown to reduce cortisol levels, and may
  be a proven add-on treatment to psychotherapy for patients with PTSD and
  phobias.[18] Laws surrounding CBD are changing rapidly, so check the most
  up-to-date state laws regarding this product. One other problem: a 2016
  analysis from the FDA found only a few of the products they tested had
  anywhere near the dose claimed on the label.[19] More research, legislation
  changes, and monitoring of products may make therapeutic dosing of CBD
  oil a viable treatment alternative in the near future.

Brain-Healthy Recipes

In this appendix, I've included 42 recipes—20 from Liana Werner-Gray, the author of *The Earth Diet* and *10-Minute Recipes*, and 22 from Donna Schwenk, the author of *Cultured Food for Life, Cultured Food for Health,* and her latest book, *Cultured Food in a Jar.* Liana's recipes all go along with the rules I've laid out in my program, as do Donna's—plus hers are all probiotic. About half of these recipes are pulled directly from their books—but the other half are only to be found here! This should give you plenty of material as you work your way through the program.

RECIPES FROM LIANA WERNER-GRAY

Zucchini Spaghetti with Tomato Sauce and Walnut "Meatballs"

This is a completely raw, plant-based vegan dish, no cooking required. It is extremely nutrient rich, leaving you fulfilled yet light so you can continue on with your day without feeling sluggish! The Walnut Meatballs are a great alternative to meat and excellent nourishment for the brain.

Serves 4

2 large zucchini
1 batch Raw Tomato Sauce (page 265)
1 batch Walnut "Meatballs" (page 266)
Nutritional yeast, to taste (optional)

Use a spiralizer or vegetable peeler to make spaghetti strips with the zucchini. Place in bowls. Evenly divide the Raw Tomato Sauce and "meatballs" between the bowls, and sprinkle nutritional yeast, if desired, on top.

Tips:

- To save some time, you can make this recipe without the Walnut "Meatballs," and just have the Zucchini Spaghetti and Tomato Sauce.

- Top with cashew cheese.

Raw Tomato Sauce

Serves 4

2 large tomatoes
1 cup sundried tomatoes
1 clove garlic
¼ red or yellow onion
1 tablespoon extra-virgin olive oil
¼ teaspoon black pepper
¼ teaspoon chili flakes or cayenne pepper
1 tablespoon fresh basil or ½ tablespoon dried basil
½ teaspoon dried thyme
½ teaspoon dried parsley
½ teaspoon dried oregano

Add all ingredients to your blender and mix for 1 minute or until well combined.

Tip:

Soak the sundried tomatoes for 1 hour to make the blender process easier and the sauce smoother.

Walnut "Meatballs"

You can make raw tacos by wrapping up a few of these "meatballs" in lettuce with the toppings of your choice. They also go well on a bed of brown-rice pasta, bean pasta, or zucchini pasta. Serve with dipping sauce and organic corn chips for a great party snack.

Serves 4 to 6

1½ cups walnuts
1 cup sundried tomatoes
2 tablespoons extra-virgin olive oil
1 teaspoon dried sage
1 teaspoon fennel seeds
1 teaspoon dried thyme
1 teaspoon dried rosemary
1 teaspoon dried oregano
1 pinch black pepper
1 pinch cayenne pepper
1 pinch salt

Add all ingredients to your blender and mix for 5 minutes or until well combined. The mixture should be moist and stick together. Roll mixture with your hands to make "meatballs."

Tips:

- If you do not have a blender, you can use a mortar and pestle to crush the walnuts. Then dice the sundried tomatoes, and mix everything together in a bowl.

- For a nut-free version, use pumpkin seeds or sunflower seeds instead of walnuts.

- If you use essential oils instead of dried herbs, be sparing. Start with just the amount of oil you get when you dip a clean toothpick in the bottle, then increase to taste.

Grass-Fed Beef Tacos

I love tacos and grew up eating them once per week. Thanks, Mum! I love to top mine with avocado, grated carrot, and lettuce. It's very important the beef is high quality grass fed so it is good brain food; if it's not, the beef is often contaminated with hormones, antibiotics, and GMOs.

Serves 3 (2 tacos each)

FILLING:

1 tablespoon extra-virgin coconut oil, for cooking

1 pound ground beef

1 teaspoon salt

1 teaspoon cumin

1 teaspoon turmeric

1 teaspoon garlic powder or 1 tablespoon garlic, minced

1 teaspoon onion powder

½ teaspoon paprika

¼ teaspoon black pepper

Dash of cayenne pepper

CHOOSE YOUR SHELL:

6 organic taco shells

6 tortilla wraps

6 lettuce leaves

CHOOSE YOUR TOPPINGS:

Nutritional yeast

Organic cheese, grated

Carrots, grated

Lettuce, shredded

Avocado, cubed

Peppers, diced

Taco sauce

Fresh cilantro

Black beans, cooked

Vegan sour cream

Mango salsa

Ketchup

If you are choosing taco shells, bake them in the oven at 350°F for 5 minutes. While they are baking, heat a large frying pan with oil and add the beef. Use a wooden spoon to break up the beef.

Add all of the spices to the beef and stir.

Cook for 8 minutes or until done.

Wrap the meat in tortilla wraps, taco shells, or lettuce leaves. Add the toppings of your choice.

Tips:

- To make things even faster, use 2 tablespoons of taco seasoning instead of the listed spices.
- Stretch out the filling and serve more people by adding 1/4 cup ketchup and 1/2 cup beans.
- Use large, soft, organic tortillas to make burritos.
- Use this filling for beef nachos.

Super Green Juice

You can get all your essential greens in one drink with this recipe.

Serves 1

1 cucumber
1 green apple or ¾ cup pineapple
3 celery stalks
½ cup kale
½ cup spinach
¼ cup parsley
¼ cup cilantro

Juice all the ingredients in your juicer. Drink.

Tips:

- Add dandelion greens for more intense flavor.
- If you want a sugar-free juice, make this without the apple, which is something I often do.

Simple Ginger Tea

This is a simple recipe but has powerful health benefits. Ginger is a natural pain reliever and also anti-inflammatory, helping to cleanse any brain fog and create clarity in mood and thinking. You can add a dash of turmeric and cayenne pepper too for added health benefits. Drink this one every night before bed, and it will assist you in having a great night's sleep as well as wake up feeling fresh.

Serves 2

2-inch piece of ginger, diced
A dash of turmeric and cayenne pepper after boiling, optional

Add 4 cups water and ginger to a pot and bring to a boil for 5 minutes.

Strain the liquid as you pour it into a mug, then serve.

Cauliflower Popcorn

I enjoy this recipe whenever I am craving popcorn! It has a similar smell and taste. You can eat this one raw once you mix everything together in the bowl, where it then becomes a 10-minute recipe, or you can roast it for 20 minutes. I usually do half and half; I will eat half of it raw because it tastes so delicious, and we get a lot of nutrition from raw vegetables; we should all strive to eat more raw vegetables. Plus I sometimes can't wait for it to be roasted—ha ha! And then I will roast the other half and enjoy that nice and hot.

Serves 4

2½ tablespoons extra-virgin olive oil
½ cup nutritional yeast
¾ teaspoon salt
1 head cauliflower, chopped into bite-sized pieces

Preheat the oven to 325°F.

In a large bowl, mix the oil, nutritional yeast, and salt until combined.

Add the cauliflower pieces to the bowl and toss until the pieces are well coated.

Bake for 20 minutes until golden brown.

Tip:

Add 1 tablespoon sesame seeds for extra flavor.

Basic French Fries (Sweet Potato or Jicama!)

Did you know that potatoes are high in vitamin C? This makes them immune boosting. As root vegetables they have grounding properties. If you are experiencing anxiety, depression, and stress, potatoes can help provide relief for the mind. Fry the potatoes in coconut oil because it has a higher smoke point than olive oil and creates buttery French fries.

But you don't have to be depressed to love French fries. They're a classic, mouthwatering, salty and savory comfort food with excellent mouthfeel. Crunchy on the outside and soft in the middle! No need to beat yourself up when you eat them.

Serves 2

2 tablespoons extra-virgin coconut oil, for cooking
2 sweet potatoes (or jicama)
Salt, to taste

Add the coconut oil to a pan and heat on high.

As the oil is heating, wash the potatoes and then cut them into thin to medium strips. (If you cut them too big, they will take longer to cook.)

Add the potatoes to the oil and let cook for 4 1/2 minutes, and then flip them over. They should have a golden-brown side. Cook for another 4 1/2 minutes, and then turn off the heat.

Season with salt.

Tips:

- Use a spiralizer to make fun "Curly Wurly Fries."

- You can cook these in tigernut oil, which has a higher smoke point than olive oil, plus is a natural prebiotic!

Variations:

- Chipotle Fries: Add a dash of cayenne and 1 teaspoon chipotle powder to the fries before cooking.

- Garlic Fries: Add 2 teaspoons garlic powder to the fries before cooking.

- Cheese Fries: Add 2 tablespoons nutritional yeast to the fries before cooking.

- Lemon Herb French Fries: Sprinkle 2 tablespoons tigernut flour or almond flour and 1 to 2 teaspoons thyme over the fries before cooking. Squeeze juice of 1 lemon over finished fries.

Four-Ingredient Green Salad

This salad is quite surprising as it is built on a foundation of herbs, and it is so easy yet really flavorful and refreshing. It seems so simple, but there are a lot of flavors, and it's a powerful detox salad that will surprisingly fill you up!

Serves 1

1 avocado, cubed
1 cup fresh parsley leaves
1 cup fresh cilantro leaves
1 lemon
Salt and pepper, to taste

Place the avocado, parsley, and cilantro in a bowl.

Squeeze lemon juice over the salad. Season with salt and pepper, to taste.

Tip:

Include the stems from the parsley and cilantro for added nutrients.

Variation:

Five-Ingredient Green Salad: Add 1 chopped cucumber.

Bean Burgers

This is a great vegan meal and can fulfill a burger craving! It's nice and light, yet high in protein and brain fueling. This burger is a prebiotic superfood!

Serves 4 (1 burger each)

2 tablespoons extra-virgin coconut oil, for cooking

One 15-ounce can organic beans, drained (butter, kidney, or black beans work best)

½ cup almond meal (blended almond)

1 small yellow onion, chopped

¼ cup nutritional yeast

½ teaspoon cumin

¼ teaspoon garlic powder

¼ teaspoon fennel

¼ teaspoon thyme

¼ teaspoon sage

¼ teaspoon salt

¼ teaspoon black pepper

Pinch of cayenne pepper

1 Flax Egg Alternative (page 274)

Heat the oil in a large pan over medium heat. Mash beans with the rest of the ingredients. Taste and add more spices or salt to your liking. Divide into 4 equal parts and shape into patties.

Fry the patties until golden, about 4 minutes on each side.

Tips:

- Top these burgers with fresh parsley, cilantro, and basil.

- Serve on gluten-free rolls, kale, collard greens, lettuce, Turmeric Saffron Coconut Meat Wraps (page 277), or gluten-free tortillas.

- Nonvegans can use one egg in this recipe instead of Flax Egg Alternative (page 274).

- Replace the nutritional yeast with more almond meal for a less cheesy flavor.

Variations:

- Bean Balls: Roll the mixture into 10 balls and serve on brown rice pasta or zucchini pasta.

- Nut-Free Bean Burgers: Replace the almond meal with pumpkin-seed, sunflower-seed, or hemp-seed meal.

- Spicy Bean Burgers: Add extra cayenne pepper.

- Lentil Burgers: Use lentils instead of beans.

- Tigernut Bean Burgers: Replace the brown rice flour and flax meal with 1/2 cup tigernut flour.

Flax Egg Alternative

For every egg in an original recipe, use one serving of this flax mix. This is a great vegan alternative to egg.

Makes 1 serving

3 teaspoons ground flaxseed

In a bowl, whisk the flaxseed and 4 teaspoons water together.

Let it sit for 7 minutes. During this resting period, it will become gummy, just like eggs.

Seafood Sticks

These make a great entertaining platter and party food. And it's important to use a good quality salt like Himalayan salt, sea salt, or Real Salt so it is pure minerals, not a salt that has an anticaking agent, which is not good for the brain at all.

Serves 4

1 pound white fish
1 pound shrimp, peeled and deveined
Real Salt and pepper, to taste
8 skewers
1 tablespoon coconut oil, for cooking
1 lemon

Cut the fish into cubes and sprinkle with salt and pepper. Alternate shrimp and fish cubes on each skewer.

Place skewers on a hot grill or lightly oiled frying pan. Cook for about 3 minutes on each side, or until done. Squeeze lemon juice over the cooked skewers.

Tip:

You can also use crabmeat for these Seafood Sticks.

Cauliflower Rice

This recipe goes great with spicy food, curries, soups, and salads. This is an epic recipe that fulfills rice cravings without the heavy carbs; it's incredible and will leave you feeling light afterward. A great way to incorporate more vegetables in your diet.

Serves 4

1 head cauliflower
1 tablespoon coconut oil
Salt and pepper, to taste

Use a food processor or vegetable chopper to chop the cauliflower into tiny rice-sized pieces.

Sauté in a hot pan with oil for 9 minutes. Season with salt and pepper.

Tips:

- Add one small diced yellow onion, for extra flavor.
- You may chop the cauliflower by hand, but it will take longer.

Sweet Potato Toast

Instead of using bread, just pop a slice of sweet potato in the toaster!

Serves 2

1 sweet potato
1 tablespoon coconut oil
1 avocado, mashed or sliced
1 teaspoon lemon juice
½ teaspoon garlic salt
Dash of turmeric
Dash of paprika
Dash of black pepper
Dash of saffron (optional)

Slice the sweet potato lengthwise into 1/4-inch thick slices, so it resembles a piece of bread.

Put the slices in a toaster and toast. You may need to toast it twice until it is soft enough and enjoyable to eat.

Spread buttery coconut oil on each slice and let melt.

Top toast with avocado and remaining ingredients.

Tip:

Serve with a dash of saffron.

Turmeric Saffron Coconut Meat Wraps

Use these instead of flour tortillas. These are a delicious alternative and gluten free. They do take some patience since they'll need to sit in the dehydrator for 12 hours, but they're absolutely worth it. Make a huge batch at once so you can store them in the fridge for up to a month.

Makes 2 wraps

2 cups raw coconut meat (only from young coconuts)
1½ tablespoons raw coconut water
½ teaspoon Real Salt
¼ teaspoon turmeric
Small pinch of saffron

Put the coconut meat in a food processor or blender and mix until it becomes smooth. Add the coconut water, salt, turmeric, and saffron, and blend until completely smooth.

Spread the coconut batter on a dehydrator sheet (or you can use parchment paper) about 1/4 inch thick, not too thin or it will end up with holes.

Place this in the dehydrator at 110 degrees for 12 hours. It is ready when it is dry and solid, but not so dry that it cracks when you bend it.

Baked Salmon with a Saffron Walnut Crust

This dish features two powerhouse brain-health foods, salmon and walnuts, so it'll help power up your brain while satisfying your taste buds.

Serves 4

1½ pounds skinless wild salmon, cut into 4 pieces
1 egg
¼ cup walnuts, blended into a nut meal (some small chunks okay)
2 pinches of saffron
½ teaspoon salt

Preheat oven to 380°F. Prepare a baking sheet with parchment paper or a thin coating of coconut oil.

Place the salmon on the baking sheet. Beat the egg in a separate bowl, and pour it over the salmon until well coated on all sides. Press it with your hands to make the egg soak into the fish more.

Mix the walnut meal, saffron, and salt together on a plate. Press each fillet into the walnut mixture to coat. Place the salmon back in the baking sheet.

Bake for 7 minutes, turn the salmon over, and bake for another 7 minutes, or to your desired doneness.

Flax Oil Salad Dressing

This dressing is made with two simple ingredients: flax oil, which is packed with brain-healthy ALA, and lemon juice. It's super simple, and you can add so many different things to spice it up. I've added some of my favorite variations below the basic recipe. You can keep this for up to two months in an airtight container in the refrigerator.

Makes 1/4 cup dressing (serves 4, or for one large salad)

Juice of 1 lemon
¼ cup flax oil

Add the ingredients to a bowl and mix until well combined.

Variations:

- Add 1 tablespoon honey or maple syrup for Sweet Flax Salad Dressing.
- Add ½ teaspoon cayenne pepper for Spicy Salad Dressing.
- Add 1 avocado to the mixing bowl for Creamy Dressing.
- Add 1 tablespoon nutritional yeast to the dressing and mix for Cheesy Dressing.
- Add 2 tablespoons hummus for Hummus Salad Dressing.
- Add 2 tablespoons tahini for Tahini Salad Dressing.
- Add 2 cloves garlic with a squeeze of lemon for Flax Garlic Salad Dressing.
- Add 1-inch piece ginger with a squeeze of lemon for Flax Ginger Salad Dressing.
- Add ½ teaspoon turmeric powder to any of the above for added health benefits, especially the Hummus and Flax Ginger Dressing.

Saffron Turmeric Quinoa with Raw Green Toppings

This delicious dish is created around the complex carb quinoa and includes healthy toppings like avocado and Swiss chard.

Serves 3

1 cup uncooked quinoa
1 teaspoon cumin
2 pinches of saffron
1 teaspoon turmeric powder
1 teaspoon real salt
1 teaspoon extra-virgin coconut oil or flax oil
1 teaspoon black pepper
½ teaspoon cayenne pepper, if you like a little kick

Toppings:

1 avocado, cut into cubes
Handful fresh parsley, chopped
Juice of 1 lemon
½ cup Swiss chard, chopped

In a pot, combine 21/2 cups water and the quinoa. Bring this to a boil over high heat.

Reduce the heat to low, cover, and simmer for 15 minutes. The quinoa will absorb the water during the process.

Add the remaining ingredients and continue to cook, stirring occasionally, for another 5 minutes, or until the quinoa is moist and soft.

Add toppings and serve.

Blueberry Ice Cream

You can't get any simpler than this ice cream made with just two ingredients: frozen blueberries and bananas! No added sugar, no added anything! Also just straight up frozen blueberries make a great frozen treat. Whenever you have that craving, just go to the freezer and grab a handful of blueberries.

Serves 1–2

1 frozen banana
1 cup frozen or fresh blueberries

Add the bananas and blueberries to a blender and mix until the blended fruit is smooth and fluffy exactly like ice cream. At first it will appear chunky, and then it will become juicy and smooth like soft serve ice cream.

Tips:

- The banana must be frozen in this recipe to make the instant ice cream. To freeze bananas, peel them and then wrap them in plastic and put in the freezer. Grab however many you need whenever you want to make a smoothie or ice cream.

- Serve with toppings like fresh berries and or nuts.

Green Juice with Swiss Chard, Kale, and Asparagus

The apple in this recipe makes it slightly sweet and more enjoyable to drink. If you want it to be pure vegetable, just make it without the apple.

Serves 2–3

2 cucumbers
2 green apples
6 celery stalks
½ bunch kale
6 asparagus stalks
4 cups Swiss chard
1 lemon, peeled
1 thumb-sized piece of ginger

Put all the ingredients in the juicer and juice.

Turmeric Hummus

Hummus is a great healthy snack. Chickpeas contain a lot of zinc and vitamin B6, which can help calm the mind. It's also a good way to get in those servings of vegetables— I love to eat this with raw veggies.

Serves 4–6

One 14-ounce can chickpeas
¼ cup aquafaba (water from the chickpeas can)
2 tablespoons garlic salt
1½ tablespoons lemon juice
1½ tablespoons sesame seeds
1½ tablespoons turmeric powder
1 tablespoon sesame seed oil
1 tablespoon flax oil, extra-virgin olive oil, or tigernut oil
½ teaspoon Real Salt

In a food processor, combine all ingredients and process until smooth.

Tips:

- As an alternative to chickpeas, try almonds, pumpkin seeds, sunflower seeds, or hemp seeds.

- Add more lemon juice and massage mixture into kale or lettuce leaves for a Hummus Salad Dressing.

Carrot Winter Squash Turmeric Ginger Soup

The idea of a soup is that it's meant to be super simple, yet also delicious and immune boosting. Soups started when people began throwing a bunch of vegetables in some water and boiling it until the desired consistency. It was a way to stretch vegetables out further, by adding more water. Soups can be so rewarding when you add your favorite flavors and toppings at the end, too. This one is hearty and beautiful for winter; it's a vibrant orange color that uplifts the spirit while you're eating it.

Serves 4

3 cups butternut squash soup (use an organic carton)*
4 large carrots, peeled and cut into bite-sized pieces
2 teaspoons flax oil
1½ teaspoons garlic salt
1 tablespoon turmeric powder (or 2 thumb-sized fresh turmeric root pieces)
1½ tablespoons ginger powder (or 3 thumb-sized fresh ginger root pieces)
6 cups water

TOPPINGS

Sprinkle of sesame seeds and flaxseeds
1 cup bean sprouts or pea shoots
Dash of cayenne pepper or ¼ teaspoon red pepper flakes
Handful of chopped Swiss chard and fresh parsley

Place all the soup ingredients in large, clean pot and bring to a boil. Reduce heat to medium and boil for 10 to 15 minutes until carrots are soft. Let it cool for a few minutes before serving. If you want a smooth soup, put the soup in a blender and blend for a few minutes until completely smooth.

* If you want to use fresh butternut squash, get 1 large butternut squash, scoop out the insides, and discard the seeds (or roast them later with some olive oil and Real Salt for a delicious snack). Chop the butternut squash into small bite-sized pieces and boil for 15 minutes until soft, and then proceed with recipe.

Roast Turmeric Lemon Chicken with Gluten-Free Gravy, Sweet Potatoes, and Peas

In just over two hours total, you can have a delicious, healthy meal—and you can impress anyone you may be entertaining. This meal has a wow factor to it!

Serves 6

1 whole organic chicken (about 3 pounds)
2 teaspoons onion powder
2 teaspoons garlic powder
2 teaspoons turmeric powder
1 teaspoon sage
½ teaspoon salt
½ teaspoon pepper
½ cup extra-virgin olive oil
2 lemons
6 medium sweet potatoes

½ cup juices from the chicken (or coconut oil)
5 tablespoons chicken fat or olive oil
4 tablespoons tapioca flour
1 tablespoon brown rice flour
2 cups chicken stock
Dash Real Salt
Dash black pepper
Dash each of thyme, rosemary, and sage
1½ cups peas

1. Preheat the oven to 375°F.

2. Place the chicken in a roasting pan.

3. In a bowl mix the onion powder, garlic powder, turmeric, sage, salt, and pepper.

4. Coat the chicken in the olive oil, and sprinkle the spice mixture over the chicken. Then squeeze one lemon over the entire chicken.

5. Place the sweet potatoes around the chicken to bake with it.

6. Cut the other lemon into quarters and place them inside the chicken for baking.

7. Bake uncovered for 1 hour and 15 minutes, then take the chicken out of the oven and baste the chicken with the pan drippings.

8. Bake for another 30 minutes, or until the chicken is completely cooked through.

9. After you've finished baking the chicken, make the gravy. Heat juices from the chicken and the chicken fat over medium-low in a small saucepan until shimmering. Sprinkle in the flours. Whisk well; it should be a thick paste.

10. Add the stock gradually, whisking in 1 cup and then slowly adding the remaining cup stock in a steady stream. For a thinner gravy, add up to another 2 cups of stock.

11. Cook the gravy until it gently bubbles and thickens, about 5 minutes. This step improves both the flavor and texture. Add the salt, pepper, and herbs to the gravy and season as desired.

12. Add the peas to boiling water and let sit for 3 minutes or until soft and cooked to your desire.

13. Serve the chicken, sweet potatoes, and peas and drizzle gravy over plates.

RECIPES FROM DONNA SCHWENK

KEFIR RECIPES

Easy Kefir

There are two ways to make kefir: using kefir starter culture packets and using live grains. The live grains will last forever as long as you care for them. I've had mine for more than 14 years. The starter culture packets don't last forever, but they're really easy and you don't have to care for any grains. The packets are how I started. There are a number of brands available, but I recommend Easy Kefir from Cutting Edge Cultures. I have to be honest, I work with this company, but their cultures truly are the best. The Easy Kefir packets are actually made from kefir grains ground into a powder, so you get all the varied strains of bacteria possible. Other brands aren't made in this way, so they have fewer strains in them, which means that they aren't as gut balancing.

You can use nearly any type of milk that's available. Whole milk, reduced fat, nonfat, goat's milk, cow's milk, pasteurized, or homogenized—whatever you choose. However, I think fresh, raw, whole cow's milk makes the most delicious kefir. The only thing I recommend you avoid is ultra-pasteurized or lactose-free milk. These don't provide enough food to keep the bacteria happy. And never use a jar still hot from the dishwasher. Heat and lack of food are the two things that will kill the probiotics in your kefir.

Makes 1 quart, 8 servings

4 cups milk
1 packet Easy Kefir

Place the milk in a glass jar that can be securely sealed, and stir in the Easy Kefir. Or you can simply seal the jar and shake it to mix everything together.

Leave the jar on your kitchen counter, out of direct sunlight, or in a cabinet at room temperature (between 68°F and 72°F), for 18 to 24 hours. If your home is cooler than 72°F, you may have to let it ferment for a bit longer. If your home is cooler than 65°F, your kefir may not ferment properly.

When the milk has thickened and has a distinctive, sour fragrance, your kefir is ready. The final consistency is like drinkable yogurt.

Place the kefir in the refrigerator. The fermentation process will continue, but the cold temperature will slow it down. You can keep the kefir perfectly preserved in your fridge in a sealed container for many months, but the longer it's in the refrigerator, the more sour it will become, and the fewer probiotics it will have.

Save 1/4 cup of this kefir to culture a new batch. Simply add 3 3/4 cups milk to this kefir, seal the jar, and let it ferment again. You can do this anywhere from two to seven times, with the exact number depending on the freshness of your kefir. I recommend reculturing within seven days of making each batch.

Red Velvet Kefir Smoothie

Homemade kefir has 50-plus beneficial bacteria, while yogurt only has 3–10 strains. This smoothie can give you not only billions of probiotics, but also the yummy flavor of a red velvet cake without all the sugar. Healthy food made fun!

Makes 2 servings

1 cup kefir
¾ cup coconut or almond milk
1 cup frozen strawberries
1 cup raspberries
2 cups fresh spinach
1 tablespoon cocoa or cacao powder
1 teaspoon vanilla
1 tablespoon liquid stevia

Add all ingredients into a high-speed blender and blend until smooth and well combined.

Serve immediately.

Second-Fermented Citrus Kefir

This is one of my favorite ways to flavor my kefir. It can mellow out the tart taste of unflavored kefir. Adding a small amount of lemon peel is a prebiotic, which is food for bacteria. It will allow the microbes to grow and multiply, giving you more probiotics in each spoonful and changing the taste to a milder, more delightful flavor.

Makes 1/2 gallon, 4 servings

2 cups kefir
1 organic lemon

Place the kefir in a glass jar that can be securely sealed.

Using a vegetable peeler, peel one strip of zest from the lemon—the equivalent of one time around the fruit. Avoid the white pith, which is bitter.

Place the zest in the jar with the kefir and close securely.

Leave the jar on your kitchen counter, out of direct sunlight, for 1 to 3 hours to ferment a second time.

Transfer the jar to the refrigerator, leaving in the zest. This kefir can be stored in the fridge in its jar for one year.

Kefir Cheese

This probiotic cheese has the texture of cream cheese or sour cream. If you like it firmer, let it strain a little longer. What's exciting about this cheese is how versatile it is while being loaded with probiotics. I use it for everything that calls for yogurt, cream cheese, or sour cream. It's little substitutions like this that can make a big difference in helping your body achieve wellness, and you get to have yummy cheese!

Makes 1 cup kefir cheese

2 cups kefir

Place a basket-style coffee filter in a strainer and set the strainer over a bowl.

Pour the kefir into the coffee filter. Cover the bowl with plastic wrap and place it in the refrigerator overnight. The bowl will catch the liquid whey. The next day you'll have a beautiful chunk of kefir cheese. If you would like firmer cheese, you can let the whey continue to drain for a full day or longer.

Almond Milk Kefir

When making nondairy kefir, you just need to be sure the nondairy milk has at least 8 grams of carbohydrates to give the bacteria something to eat. It uses the sugars and creates probiotics for you. You don't get the sugar, but instead you get lots of healthy bacteria. We add a small teaspoon of date paste or raw sugar so the bacteria will have something to eat. Remember the sugar is not for you; it's for the bacteria.

Makes 8 servings

1 cup almonds sliced or whole (raw if possible)
4 cups water
1 packet Easy Kefir
1 teaspoon date paste or raw sugar

Cover almonds in water and soak for at least 4 hours or overnight.

Strain almonds and discard water.

Place almonds and 4 cups of fresh water in a blender. Blend on high speed until almonds are incorporated and blended into a smooth consistency.

If you want a thinner consistency, strain this mixture through a nut bag to remove the small pieces. For a thicker consistency, leave the pulp in.

Place mixture into a glass jar and mix in 1 packet Easy Kefir and date paste with a spoon or whisk until all ingredients are thoroughly combined.

Place a lid on the jar and let it sit at room temperature for 16 to 24 hours or until tart or sour tasting. It might separate into whey and curds. This is normal for nondairy milks.

Place almond kefir in the refrigerator or enjoy immediately. It should keep for at least a month, although it will continue to get more sour and tart.

If you would like to make more almond milk kefir, take 1/4 cup of this almond milk kefir, add to 3 - 3/4 cups of fresh almond milk, and culture again for 16 to 24 hours or until tart. You can do this many, many times over or until it stops working and making the milk tart. Then you will need a new Easy Kefir packet.

Cranberry Walnut Chickpea Salad

You can make this wonderful salad in a snap. You'll get two cultured foods and millions of probiotics. Each cultured food is unique and contains different strains of probiotics, which are doing hundreds of processes in your body all day long without your awareness. This salad has a mixture of flavors, and so each bite can be unique. This is a living salad with enzymes and probiotics that quite literally change you from the inside out.

Makes 6 servings

¼ cup kefir
1 teaspoon Dijon mustard
1 tablespoon honey or 1 packet stevia powder
3 cups canned garbanzo beans (chickpeas)
½ cup chopped red grapes
¼ cup Curried Cauliflower chopped into bite-sized pieces (page 308)
½ cup organic dried cranberries, raisins, or chopped dates
½ cup roughly chopped walnuts or pecans
½ cup thinly sliced green onions
Celtic Sea Salt and pepper to taste

Mix together the kefir, mustard, and honey in a small bowl. Set aside.

In a medium bowl, combine the garbanzo beans, grapes, cauliflower, cranberries, nuts, and green onions, and season with salt and pepper.

Pour the kefir mixture into the garbanzo bean mixture and stir until well combined. Serve over a bed of lettuce.

Clementine Kefir Smoothie

Many think of clementines as baby oranges, but they deserve their own recognition. Clementines are loaded with minerals such as calcium, magnesium, potassium, and phosphorous. They also add essential vitamins such as vitamin C (ascorbic acid) and folate to the body. I love how they make this smoothie taste like you've just picked something fresh from the tree. You'll also never know there's a cup of greens in there, too.

Makes 1 serving

4 clementines
½ cup kefir
1 banana previously chopped and frozen
1 cup greens, spinach or kale
2 teaspoons of stevia

Place all ingredients into a blender and blend until smooth.

Serve immediately.

Breakfast Kefir Bowl

Breakfast bowls are all the rage these days, and for good reason—they're incredibly healthy and easy to make. I have often made these types of bowls for dinner when I'm tired and want something easy and comforting. Kefir can have a calming effect on the body, and with the addition of all the greens, you get an anti-inflammatory meal. It's a great option to have any time of day.

Makes 1 serving

½ ripe avocado
1 medium banana previously sliced and frozen
1 cup frozen mixed berries (strawberries, raspberries, blueberries)
1 handful of kale, large stems removed
1 cup spinach
1 cup kefir
1 tablespoon almond butter
1 tablespoon chia seeds
stevia to taste
Toppings, as desired: sunflower seeds, flaxseeds, poppy seeds, granola, raw or roasted nuts (almonds, pecans, walnuts, etc.), shredded unsweetened coconut, or fresh berries

Add all smoothie ingredients to a blender and blend until creamy and smooth.

Add stevia if more sweetness is needed.

Place in a bowl and add desired toppings.

Serve immediately.

Minty Cucumber Kefir Salad

I love cucumbers and kefir. They go very well together, and adding fresh mint and toasted pine nuts makes for a wonderful side dish you can serve with any meal. You can add a little fresh dill too, if you'd like, or extra garlic. Taste it and experiment to suit your taste. It's simple to make, creamy, savory, and loaded with flavor.

Makes 4 servings

½ cup pine nuts
¼ cup golden raisins
1 cup plain kefir
1 cup Kefir Cheese (page 290)
2 cloves of garlic, minced or finely grated
1 tablespoon fresh mint, minced
2 teaspoon Celtic Sea Salt to taste
1 teaspoon freshly ground black pepper
1 Persian or English cucumber

Preheat oven to 350°F. Place nuts in a single layer in a shallow baking pan. Bake 5 to 10 minutes or until they are golden brown. Set aside to cool.

Place the raisins in a bowl and add enough water to cover. Cover and let plump for 20 minutes. Drain.

In a large bowl, whisk the kefir, Kefir Cheese, garlic, mint, salt, and pepper.

Add the raisins, cucumbers, and nuts to the kefir mixture. Taste and add more salt if needed.

Serve immediately and garnish with more chopped mint and nuts if desired.

Instant Kefir Ice Cream

Fast, easy, and probiotic ice cream that doesn't need an ice-cream maker. Fresh summer peaches are my favorite flavor—at least for today they are! You can't ask for a better and faster way to get probiotics in your kids, too.

Makes 3 servings

2 heaping cups fruit (peaches, strawberries, blueberries) cut into 1-inch pieces
1/3 cup Easy Kefir
2 tablespoons honey or stevia

Place the fruit in the freezer on parchment paper or a cookie sheet and freeze for at least 4 hours.

Place the frozen fruit in a food processor and pulse until it starts to get creamy.

Add the kefir and honey, and process until creamy like ice cream.

Serve immediately or place it in a bowl in the freezer for 30 minutes to firm up.

KOMBUCHA RECIPES

Basic Kombucha

Making your own kombucha can make you feel very artisanal—I know it made me feel like that. It gives you a sense of accomplishment unlike any of the other cultured foods, because how many people do you know who make their own carbonated beverages? It may seem a little daunting at first, but it's quite easy. One of the things I recommend to most people before they try making kombucha at home is to buy a bottle of kombucha at the store to get a feel for how it is supposed to look and taste.

One of the supplies I've listed for making your own kombucha is a SCOBY (symbiotic culture of bacteria and yeast). To get one, you can go one of a number of ways. If you have a friend who makes kombucha, he or she probably has a SCOBY to spare. There is also a worldwide sharing group where you can find people who are willing to share their cultures (www.kefirhood.com). Otherwise, you can buy a starter kit online. I offer them in my store (www.culturedfoodlife.com/store) or you can get them from Wise Choice Market (www.wisechoicemarket.com). Whatever kit you get should come with one SCOBY and one cup of fermented tea. I don't recommend getting a dehydrated SCOBY as these don't work as well.

I'd like to make a comment here about sugar. You'll see in the recipe below that I list three types of sugar: Sucanat, white sugar, and coconut sugar. Sucanat is a brand of pure, dried sugarcane juice. Because it is minimally processed, it retains the nutrients that are removed from white sugar in the refining process. It also contains less sucrose than refined sugar. However, it does have a slight maple or barley taste, so it's not for everyone. Most of the time, I use regular white sugar when I make kombucha because I like the way it makes my kombucha taste. Also, the sugar gets eaten as the good bacteria proliferate, so I don't have to worry that I will consume too much sugar.

One last thing to discuss: the type of tea to use. I've noted in the recipe that you should use black or green tea, but honestly, almost any type of tea (or combination of teas) will work. You just have to figure out which one you like best. Do, however, avoid herbal teas or fruit-flavored teas with oils, as they have antibacterial qualities that could affect the outcome of your kombucha.

A note before you begin: At the end of this process, you will have created your very own SCOBY. Make sure to keep this—plus one cup of the kombucha you've made—to use as the starter for your next batch.

Makes 3 quarts

3 quarts filtered water (not distilled)
1 cup Sucanat, white sugar, or coconut sugar
4 or 5 tea bags (organic green tea is preferred, but black tea is good, too)
1 SCOBY
1 cup fermented kombucha tea

Wash all utensils with hot, soapy water and rinse well.

Bring the water to a rolling boil in a large pot over medium-high heat. Add the sugar and continue to boil for 5 minutes.

Turn off the heat and add the tea bags. Steep for 10 to 15 minutes, then remove the tea bags and let the tea cool to room temperature.

Pour the cool tea into a 1-gallon glass jar.

Add the SCOBY, placing it so that the smooth, shiny surface faces up.

Add the fermented kombucha tea.

Place a linen cloth or napkin completely over the opening of the glass jar and secure it with a rubber band. This keeps dust, mold, spores, and vinegar flies out of the fermenting tea.

Let the covered container sit undisturbed in a well-ventilated and dark place at a temperature between 65°F and 90°F for 6 to 15 days. To keep the temperature stable, using a seedling mat is highly recommended. You can get these from a local brew store or online. The store on my website—www.culturedfoodlife.com/store—has a link to products on Amazon that I really like.

To determine whether the tea is ready, do a taste test every couple of days, starting on the fourth day. The tea should be tart, not sweet. However, it should not be overly sour or vinegary. If the tea is sweet, the sugar hasn't been fully converted. If it tastes like sparkling apple cider, it is ready to drink, unless you want it more tart. If the vinegar taste is too prominent, it's probably fermented a bit too long. It won't hurt you to drink at this point, but you won't receive as many health benefits because the healthy bacteria die off over time as the food supply is gradually reduced. Your tea should also be a little bubbly if it has not been cultured too long. The good yeast makes naturally occurring carbonation, which dissipates over time. If this happens, the kombucha still has health benefits, but it has more probiotics when it is bubbly.

When the tea is brewed to your taste, pour it into sturdy glass bottles with clamp-down lids. You can repurpose beer bottles with these lids, such as those from Grolsch, or you can buy new bottles that are specifically designed for brewing. Bottles bought at craft stores aren't as sturdy and may explode. Once the bottles are filled, clamp the lids down, and place the bottles in the refrigerator. The tea can be stored there for one year or longer. It will eventually turn to vinegar, which you can use as you would any vinegar. The finished kombucha can be second-fermented with various juices, but it's also delicious as is.

Save your SCOBY and 1 cup of tea from each batch of kombucha to use as a starter for your next batch. Simply make another pot of tea with sugar and add this to your starter and culture to start the process again.

Berry Kombucha Spritzer

I love to add frozen berries to my kombucha. It's a great after-dinner treat or midday snack. Kombucha will give you a boost when you're struggling with low energy. It assists the liver in detoxification and also gives you a special probiotic yeast called *Saccharomyces boulardii*. This probiotic is a good yeast and will help you bring balance to your microbiome. It also cannot be killed by antibiotics.

Makes 2 servings

1 cup frozen berries (strawberry, blackberries, raspberries, blueberries)
2 cups Ginger Blueberry Kombucha (page 302—you can also substitute a different flavor)

Place frozen berries in chilled glasses.
Pour kombucha over berries and serve.

Sunny Kombucha

This has two special juices in it, and remember the sugar in the juice is not for you, but rather for the microbes to consume and to make into probiotics for you! Add the anti-inflammatory—turmeric—and you have an amazing bubbly beverage. It tastes like sunshine!

Makes 16 ounces

1 tablespoon turmeric root, grated or juice
2 tablespoons carrot juice
2 tablespoons orange juice
13 ounces Basic Kombucha (page 297)

You can either juice the turmeric root in a juicer or you can use a garlic press to "grate" some of it.

Add all ingredients to a 16-ounce thick glass bottle made for brewing.

Let sit 5–14 days. (If you're using freshly pressed orange or carrot juice, the fermenting time will be shorter—closer to 5–7 days, depending on the warmth of your house.)

Remember: Always use thick glass bottles made for brewing.

Pink Lemonade Kombucha

Pomegranates are an antioxidant-rich superfood and also a good source of vitamin C. In addition to these two wonderful components, you'll get probiotics and a wonderful replacement for soda pop in your diet.

Makes 16 ounces

Juice of ½ lemon
2 tablespoons pomegranate juice
14 ounces of Basic Kombucha (page 297)

Add lemon and pomegranate juices to a 16-ounce thick glass bottle made for brewing.

Fill with plain kombucha, leaving at least 1/2 inch of space at the top.

Cap your bottle and let the kombucha sit on your counter for anywhere from a few days to several weeks. It depends on how strong your kombucha is and how warm your house is. Check it every day by opening the bottle. When you find it bubbly, it is ready.

Store bottle in the refrigerator. It will keep for several months refrigerated.

Ginger Blueberry Kombucha

I can't say enough about ginger. I have it almost every day and have found it can work like food medicine in the body. There are numerous studies on the health benefits of ginger, and it gives this drink a spicy kick you can't beat.

Makes 16 ounces

2-inch slice of ginger root
1 tablespoon lemon juice
2 ounces blueberry juice
13 ounces of Basic Kombucha (page 297)

Using a clean garlic press, squeeze the ginger root through the garlic press. You can also use a juicer to extract the juice. Fresh-squeezed ginger works much better than placing a piece of ginger root in the bottle to ferment with the kombucha.

Place lemon juice, ginger juice, and blueberry juice in a thick glass bottle made for brewing.

Fill with kombucha, leaving a little headspace at the top of the bottle.

Clamp the bottle closed and date the bottle so you'll know how long it has fermented.

Let the kombucha sit on your counter for anywhere from a few days to several weeks. It depends on how strong your kombucha is and how warm your house is. Check it every day by opening the bottle.

Once it's bubbly and suits your taste, transfer to the refrigerator.

CULTURED VEGGIES RECIPES

Cultured Sweet Potato

This cultured sweet potato has endless possibilities. I love to experiment with different cultured toppings, and so I included different ones for you to try. Curried cauliflower can give it a wonderful blend of spicy flavors, and mixing in some kefir cheese will make it creamy. Or change it up and add fermented salsa with just a dollop of kefir cheese, and you'll have one of my favorite and unique combos.

Makes 1 serving

1 large sweet potato
1 heaping spoonful Curried Cauliflower (page 308) or Fermented Salsa (page 305)
1 large spoonful Kefir Cheese (page 290)
Black pepper and Celtic Sea Salt to taste

Preheat the oven to 350°F.

Wash the potato thoroughly and use a fork to pierce it eight to ten times. Then place the potato directly on a baking rack in the oven. Bake until you can easily push a fork into the potato, about an hour.

After the potato is baked, split it open lengthwise and let it cool slightly, about 5 minutes. Then top with cultured veggies, kefir cheese, and pepper and salt.

Serve immediately and enjoy.

Cultured Avocado Boat

I could eat guacamole every day. This recipe is one I serve to my friends when they come over to visit. I know they will be receiving billions of probiotics with each bite, and it thrills me when they all ask for the recipe. It's really a complete meal and oh so good for you.

Makes 2 servings

1 avocado
1 hard-boiled egg, chopped into bite-sized pieces
1 tablespoon Fermented Salsa (page 305)
2 tablespoons chopped cilantro
1 tablespoon Kefir Cheese (page 290)
½ teaspoon coriander
1/8 teaspoon Celtic Sea Salt
1/8 teaspoon pepper
¼ lime

Cut the avocado in half, remove the pit, and scoop out the flesh, making sure to leave the shells intact. Place the avocado flesh in a small bowl.

Add the hard-boiled egg to the avocado.

Add the Fermented Salsa, cilantro, Kefir Cheese, coriander, salt, and pepper to the bowl and mix thoroughly.

Scoop the mixture back into the avocado shells and squeeze the lime on top.

Fermented Salsa

If you're hesitant about making cultured foods, you should make this dish. It will prove to you how easy and delicious probiotic foods are. It will last for a month in your fridge, and you can serve this with so many things. I made a dip with this recipe that I included in this book, and you won't want to miss making that one either. It's three ingredients and crazy good!

Makes 1/2 gallon

¼ teaspoon Cutting Edge Cultures plus ½ cup water
4 large tomatoes, chopped
1 large yellow onion, chopped
2 cups packed cilantro leaves, chopped
Juice of 1 large lime (about 2 tablespoons)
1 small jalapeño, chopped
2 teaspoons Celtic Sea Salt

Stir together the culture and water. Let the mixture sit while you prepare the other ingredients—around 10 minutes.

Place tomatoes, onions, cilantro, and lime juice in a bowl and toss until incorporated. Add the jalapeño and salt to the vegetable mixture and stir gently to combine. Spoon the salsa into 2 large mason jars (or any other glass jar you prefer).

Gently press the mixture so the juices cover the salsa.

Add the starter culture and fill the jar with filtered water, leaving 2 to 3 inches of headspace to let the mixture bubble and expand as it ferments.

Seal the container and let it sit on your kitchen counter, out of direct sunlight, for 2 days.

After two days of fermenting, place it in the refrigerator.

This can be kept in an airtight jar in the refrigerator for up to one month.

Fermented Salsa Dip

Three ingredients, stir, and serve! That's it, and you've got a probiotic food that will deliver huge amounts of probiotics to your body. Forget the supplements, eat the probiotic foods instead! They work better and are less expensive and taste great!

Makes 6 servings

½ cup Kefir Cheese (page 290)
½ cup Fermented Salsa (page 305), drained
½ cup salsa (store bought or homemade)

In a small bowl, mix together the Kefir Cheese and salsas until well combined.

Serve with cut-up vegetables, if desired.

Spicy Kale Kimchi

I can't say enough about kimchi. It's a pretty incredible food, and the country of Korea has made this their national food. I've been making different versions of kimchi since we eat so much of it, and this one has the addition of kale. I think you'll love the flavor, and if you want to turn down the heat, just add less Korean chili powder.

Makes 1/2 gallon, 32 servings

¼ teaspoon Cutting Edge Starter Culture plus ½ cup water
1 head Napa cabbage
3 cups shredded kale
2 carrots shredded
1 bunch green onions, chopped
1 clove garlic chopped
1-inch piece ginger root, peeled and chopped
1/8 cup fish sauce
¼ cup Korean chili powder or Aleppo pepper (you can add less if you like less spice)
1 tablespoon Celtic Sea Salt

Stir together the culture and water. Let the mixture sit while you prepare the other ingredients—around 10 minutes.

Remove and discard the end core from the cabbage.

Shred or chop the cabbage using a food processor or hand grater.

Combine the cabbage, kale, carrots, and green onions in a large bowl.

Add the garlic, ginger, fish sauce, Korean chili powder, and salt to the vegetable mixture and toss gently but thoroughly to combine. You can also mix it with your hands, but if you do, wear rubber gloves to avoid chili burn.

Transfer the vegetable mixture to two 1-quart glass or ceramic containers that can be securely sealed.

Divide the culture between the containers. Then fill the containers with filtered water, leaving 2 inches of headspace to let the vegetables bubble and expand as they ferment.

Seal the containers and let them sit on your kitchen counter, out of direct sunlight, for 3 days.

Check the vegetables every day to make sure they stay fully submerged in water. If they have risen above the water, simply push them down so they are fully covered by the water. If any white yeast formed because the veggies rose above the water, do not worry. Remember, this isn't harmful. Just scoop out the vegetables it's on and push the rest under the water.

When the veggies are done fermenting, place them in the refrigerator.

These veggies can be stored in airtight containers in the refrigerator for up to 9 months.

Curried Cauliflower

This Indian curried vegetable is a little addictive. I've been not only eating it straight from the jar but adding it to multiple dishes. I love using it as a topping for some rice and stir fry. It's a wonderful addition to any curry meal, and the health benefits of turmeric and curry are something you'll want to make sure you don't miss out on.

Makes 1/2 gallon, 32 servings

¼ teaspoon Cutting Edge Starter Culture plus ½ cup water
1 small head of cauliflower, cut into bite-sized pieces
1 tablespoon curry powder
1 tablespoon chili powder
1 teaspoon cayenne
1 teaspoon turmeric
3 cloves garlic
1 tablespoon Celtic Sea Salt
6 golden raisins

Stir together the culture and water. Let the mixture sit while you prepare the other ingredients—around 10 minutes.

In a large bowl, combine cauliflower, curry, chili, cayenne, turmeric, garlic, salt, and raisins until well combined.

Transfer the vegetable mixture to two 1-quart glass or ceramic containers that can be securely sealed.

Divide the culture between the containers. Then fill the containers with filtered water, leaving 2 inches of headspace to let the vegetables bubble and expand as they ferment.

Seal the containers and let them sit on your kitchen counter, out of direct sunlight, for 3 days.

Check the vegetables every day to make sure they stay fully submerged in water. If they have risen above the water, simply push them down so they are fully covered by the water. If any white yeast formed because the veggies rose above the water, do not worry. Remember, this isn't harmful. Just scoop out the vegetables it's on and push the rest under the water.

When the veggies are done fermenting, place them in the refrigerator.

These veggies can be stored in airtight containers in the refrigerator for up to 9 months.

Sweet and Spicy Kimchi Pinwheels

This is a recipe from my book *Cultured Food in a Jar*. The flavors are so unique that half the time this mixture never makes it to the tortilla; I wind up eating it by the spoonful. It's crazy good, and you can also use this on vegetables as a topping.

Makes 3 servings

1 small zucchini, chopped
1 cup walnuts
1-inch piece of ginger
1 clove garlic
1 to 2 dates, pitted
Pinch of Celtic Sea Salt
3 gluten-free tortillas
½ cup Spicy Kale Kimchi (page 306)
3 romaine lettuce leaves, shredded

Put the zucchini, walnuts, ginger, garlic, dates, and salt into your food processor and pulse until well combined.

Spread the zucchini mixture on the tortillas and top it with kimchi and shredded lettuce.

Roll these up and cut them crosswise into pinwheels.

Endnotes

Chapter 1: An Epidemic of Drained Brains

1. *Stress in America: Coping with Change*, American Psychological Association (2017): www.apa.org/news/press/releases/stress/2016/coping-with-change.PDF.

2. R. Kessler et al., "Prevalence, Severity, and Comorbidity of Twelve-Month DSM-IV Disorders in the National Comorbidity Survey Replication (NCS-R)," *Archives of General Psychiatry* 62, no. 6 (June 2005): 617–27; R. Kessler et al., "Lifetime Prevalence and Age-of-Onset Distributions of Mental Disorders in the World Health Organization's World Mental Health Survey Initiative," *World Psychiatry* 6, no. 3 (October 2007): 168–76.

3. S. Bacon et al., "The Impact of Mood and Anxiety Disorders on Incident Hypertension at One Year," *International Journal of Hypertension* 2014 (2014).

4. J. W. Smoller et al, "Panic Attacks and Risk of Incident Cardiovascular Events Among Postmenopausal Women in the Women's Health Initiative Observational Study," *Archives of General Psychiatry* 64, no. 10 (October 2007): 1153–60.

5. W. A. Shibeshi, Y. Young-Xu, and C. M. Blatt, "Anxiety Worsens Prognosis in Patients with Coronary Artery Disease," *Journal of the American College of Cardiology* 49, no. 20 (May 2007), 2021–7.

6. L. A. Chilcott and C. M. Shaprio, "The Socioeconomic Impact of Insomnia. An Overview," *Pharmacoeconomics*, 10, Suppl. 1 (1996): 1–14.

7. R. Kessler et al., "Insomnia and the Performance of US Workers: Results from the America Insomnia Survey," *Sleep* 34, no. 9 (September 2011): 1161–71.

8. D. M. Bush, *Emergency Department Visits for Adverse Reactions Involving the Insomnia Medication Zolpidem*. (2013). Substance Abuse and Mental Health Services Administration, Center for Behavioral Health Statistics and Quality. Rockville, MD.

9.   M. A. Bachhuber et al, "Increasing Benzodiazepine Prescriptions and Overdose Mortality in the United States, 1996–2013," *American Journal of Public Health* 106, no. 4 (April 2016): 686–8.

10. Centers for Disease Control, "Opioids Drive Continued Increase in Drug Overdose Deaths" (February 20, 2013): www.cdc.gov/media/releases/2013/p0220_drug_overdose_deaths.html.

Chapter 2: A Symphony of Draining Chemicals

1.   P. E. Barnett and D. T. Benedetti, "A Study in 'Vicarious Conditioning,'" presented at the meeting of the Rocky Mountain Psychological Association, Glenwood Springs, Colorado (May 1960); S. M. Berber, "Conditioning through Vicarious Instigation," *Psychological Review* 69 (September 1962): 450–66.

2.   M. A. Schuster et al, "A National Survey of Stress Reactions after the September 11, 2001, Terrorist Attacks," *New England Journal of Medicine* 345, no. 20 (November 2001): 1507–12.

3.   M. Slone, "Responses to Media Coverage of Terrorism," *Journal of Conflict Resolution* 44, no. 4 (August 2000): 508–22.

4.   A. Bandura, *Social Learning Theory* (Englewood Cliffs, NJ: Prentice Hall, 1977).

5.   S. Fiske, "Attention and Weight in Person Perception: The Impact of Negative and Extreme Behavior," *Journal of Personality and Social Psychology* 38, no. 6 (June 1980): 889–906; O. Hideki, W. M. Winton, and M. Oyama, "Effects of Stimulus Valence on Recognition Memory and Endogenous Eyeblinks: Further Evidence for Positive-Negative Asymmetry," *Personality and Social Psychology Bulletin* 24, no. 9 (September 1998): 986–93.

6.   S. E. Taylor, "Asymmetrical Effects of Positive and Negative Events: The Mobilization-Minimization Hypothesis," *Psychological Bulletin* 110, no. 1 (July 1991): 67–85.

7.   J. B. Watson and R. Rayner, "Conditioned Emotional Reactions," *Journal of Experimental Psychology* 3 (1920): 1–14.

8.   R. G. Tedeschi and L. G. Calhoun, *Trauma and Transformation: Growing in the Aftermath of Suffering* (Thousand Oaks, CA: Sage Publications, Inc., 1995).

9.   R. G. Tedeschi and L. G. Calhoun, "Posttraumatic Growth: Conceptual Foundations and Empirical Evidence," *Psychological Inquiry* 15 (2004): 1–18.

10. J. A. Bellingtier, S. D. Neupert, and D. Kotter-Grühn, "The Combined Effects of Daily Stressors and Major Life Events on Daily Subjective Ages," *The Journals of Gerontology Series B: Psychological Sciences and Social* Sciences 72, no. 4 (2015): 613-621.

Chapter 3: The Mind-Body Connection

1. M. Irwin et al., "Reduction of Immune Function in Life Stress and Depression," *Biological Psychiatry* 27, no. 1 (January 1990): 22–30.

2. N. N. Liźko, V. M. Silov, and G. D. Syrych, [Events in the Development of Dysbacteriosis of the Intestines in Man under Extreme Conditions], *Die Nahrung* 28, nos. 6–7 (1984): 599–605.

3. R. J. Gilken, Jr., "The Spectrum of Irritable Bowel Syndrome: A Clinical Review," *Clinical Therapeutics* 27, no. 11 (November 2005): 1696–1709.

4. M. J. Spence and R. Moss-Morris, "The Cognitive Behavioural Model of Irritable Bowel Syndrome: A Prospective Investigation of Patients with Gastroenteritis," *Gut* 56, no. 8 (August 2007): 1006–71.

5. G. Ranjith, "Epidemiology of Chronic Fatigue Syndrome," *Occupational Medicine* 55, no. 1 (January 2005): 13–9.

6. R. K. Naviaux et al., "Metabolic Features of Chronic Fatigue Syndrome," *Proceedings of the National Academy of Sciences* 113, no. 37 (September 2016): E5472–80.

7. C. Heim et al., "Childhood Trauma and Risk for Chronic Fatigue Syndrome: Association with Neuroendocrine Dysfunction," *Archives of General Psychiatry* 66, no. 1 (January 2009): 72–80.

8. H. K. Kang et al., "Post-Traumatic Stress Disorder and Chronic Fatigue-like Illness among Gulf War Veterans: A Population-Based Survey of 30,000 Veterans," *American Journal of Epidemiology* 157, no. 2 (January 2003): 141–8.

9. S. M. Collin et al., "Chronic Fatigue Syndrome at Age 16 Years," *Pediatrics* 137, no. 2 (February 2016): doi:10.1542/peds.2015-3434.

10. L. A. Aaron, M. M. Burke, and D. Buchwald, "Overlapping Conditions among Patients with Chronic Fatigue Syndrome, Fibromyalgia, and Temporomandibular Disorder," *Archives of Internal Medicine* 160, no. 2 (January 2000): 221–227; D. J. Clauw, "Fibromyalgia: A Clinical Review," *Journal of the American Medical Association* 311, no. 15 (April 2014): 1547–55.

11. J. S. Seng et al., "Posttraumatic Stress Disorder and Physical Comorbidity among Female Children and Adolescents: Results from Service-Use Data," *Pediatrics* 116, no. 6 (December 2005), e767–76.

12. D. S. Ciccone et al., "Sexual and Physical Abuse in Women with Fibromyalgia Syndrome: A Test of the Trauma Hypothesis," *Clinical Journal of Pain* 21, no. 5 (September–October 2005): 378–86.

13. H. Cohen et al., "Confirmation of an Association between Fibromyalgia and Serotonin Transporter Promoter Region (5-HTTLPR) Polymorphism, and Relationship to Anxiety-Related Personality Traits," *Arthritis & Rheumatism* 46, no. 3 (March 2002): 845–7.

14. J. W. Smoller et al, "Panic Attacks and Risk of Incident Cardiovascular Events Among Postmenopausal Women in the Women's Health Initiative Observational Study," *Archives of General Psychiatry* 64, no. 10 (October 2007): 1153–60.

15. C. M. Albert et al., "Phobic Anxiety and Risk of Coronary Heart Disease and Sudden Cardiac Death among Women," *Circulation* 111, no. 4 (February 2005): 480–7.

16. W. A. Shibeshi, Y. Young-Xu, and C. M. Blatt, "Anxiety Worsens Prognosis in Patients with Coronary Artery Disease," *Journal of the American College of Cardiology* 49, no. 20 (May 2007), 2021–27.

17. M. S. Player and L. E. Peterson, "Anxiety Disorders, Hypertension, and Cardiovascular Risk: A Review," *International Journal of Psychiatry in Medicine* 41, no. 4 (2011): 365–77.

18. A. E. Moyer et al., "Stress-Induced Cortisol Response and Fat Distribution in Women," *Obesity Research* 2, no. 3 (May 1994): 255–62.

19. K. R. Sahakyan et al., "Normal-Weight Central Obesity: Implications for Total and Cardiovascular Mortality," *Annals of Internal Medicine* 163, no. 11 (December 2015): 827–35.

20. Y. Chida et al., "Do Stress-Related Psychosocial Factors Contribute to Cancer Incidence and Survival?" *Nature Clinical Practice Oncology* 5, no. 8 (August 2008): 466–75.

21. A. K. Sood and S. K. Lutgendorf, "Stress Influences on Anoikis," *Cancer Prevention Research* 4, no. 4 (April 2011): 481–85.

22. C. P. Le et al., "Chronic Stress in Mice Remodels Lymph Vasculature to Promote Tumour Cell Dissemination," *Nature Communications* 7 (March 2016): doi:10.1038/ncomms10634.

23. M. Vythilingam et al., "Childhood Trauma Associated with Smaller Hippocampal Volume in Women with Major Depression," *American Journal of Psychiatry* 159, no. 12 (December 2002): 2072–80.

24. A. S. Hill, A. Sahay, and R. Hen, "Increasing Adult Hippocampal Neurogenesis Is Sufficient to Reduce Anxiety and Depression-Like Behaviors," *Neuropsychopharmacology* 40, no. 10 (September 2015): 2368–78.

25. E. B. Ansell et al., "Cumulative Adversity and Smaller Gray Matter Volume in Medial Prefrontal, Anterior Cingulate, and Insula Regions," *Biological Psychiatry* 72, no. 1 (July 2012): 57–64.

Chapter 4: Wired for Brain Drain

1. A. Kline et al., "Effects of Repeated Deployment to Iraq and Afghanistan on the Health of New Jersey Army National Guard Troops: Implications for Military Readiness," *American Journal of Public Health* 100, no. 2 (February 2010): 276–83.

2. F. S. Goes et al., "Co-Morbid Anxiety Disorders in Bipolar Disorder and Major Depression: Familial Aggregation and Clinical Characteristics of Co-Morbid Panic Disorder, Social Phobia, Specific Phobia and Obsessive-Compulsive Disorder," *Psychological Medicine* 42, no. 7 (July 2012): 1449–59.

3. D. R. Miles et al., "A Twin Study on Sensation Seeking, Risk Taking Behavior and Marijuana Use," *Drug and Alcohol Dependence* 62, no. 1 (March 2001): 57–68.

4. Y. Neria et al., "Sensation Seeking, Wartime Performance, and Long-Term Adjustment among Israeli War Veterans," *Personality and Individual Differences* 29, no. 5 (November 2000): 921–32.

5. Z. Zaleski, "Sensation-Seeking and Preference for Emotional Visual Stimuli," *Personality and Individual Differences* 5, no. 5 (1984): 609–11.

6. J. R. Koopmans et al., "A Multivariate Genetic Analysis of Sensation Seeking," *Behavior Genetics* 25, no. 4 (July 1995): 349–56.

7. S. M. Clinton, S. J. Watson, and H. Akil, "High Novelty-Seeking Rats Are Resilient to Negative Physiological Effects of the Early Life Stress," *Stress* 17, no. 1 (January 2014): 97–107.

8. C. Blair, D. Granger, and R. Peters Razza, "Cortisol Reactivity Is Positively Related to Executive Function in Preschool Children Attending Head Start," *Child Development* 76, no. 3 (May–June 2005): 554–67.

9. C. Blair and C. C. Raver, "Child Development in the Context of Adversity: Experiential Canalization of Brain and Behavior," *American Psychologist* 67, no. 4 (May–June 2012): 309–18.

10. A. M. Penney, V. C. Miedema, and D. Mazmanian, "Intelligence and Emotional Disorders: Is the Worrying and Ruminating Mind a More Intelligent Mind?" *Personality and Individual Differences* 74 (February 2015): 90–3.

11. J. D. Coplan et al., "The Relationship between Intelligence and Anxiety: An Association with Subcortical White Matter Metabolism," *Frontiers in Evolutionary Neuroscience* 3 (2011): 8.

12. Ibid.

13. M. El Zein, V. Wyart, and J. Grèzes, "Anxiety Dissociates the Adaptive Functions of Sensory and Motor Response Enhancements to Social Threats," *eLife* 4 (2015): e10274.

14. R. J. Valentino, D. Bangasser, and E. J. Van Bockstaele, "Sex-Biased Stress Signaling: The Corticotropin-Releasing Factor Receptor as a Model," *Molecular Pharmacology* 83, no. 4 (April 2013): 737–45.

15. J. M. Hettema et al., "The Structure of Genetic and Environmental Risk Factors for Anxiety Disorders in Men and Women," *Archives of General Psychiatry* 62, no. 2 (February 2005): 182–9.

16. I. M. Goldenberg et al., "The Infrequency of 'Pure Culture' Diagnoses among the Anxiety Disorders," *Journal of Clinical Psychiatry* 57, no. 11 (November 1996): 528–33.

17. I. Dincheva et al., "FAAH Genetic Variation Enhances Fronto-Amygdala Function in Mouse and Human," *Nature Communications* 6 (March 2015): 6395.

18. H. M. Haughey et al., "Marijuana Withdrawal and Craving: Influence of the Cannabinoid Receptor 1 (CNR1) and Fatty Acid Amide Hydrolase (FAAH) Genes," *Addiction* 103, no. 10 (October 2008): 1678–86.

19. I. Dincheva et al., "FAAH Genetic Variation Enhances Fronto-Amygdala Function in Mouse and Human," *Nature Communications* 6 (March 2015): 6395.

20. S. Lyubomirsky, *The How of Happiness: A Scientific Approach to Getting the Life You Want* (New York: Penguin Press, 2007).

21. I. Ben-Ami Bartal et al., "Anxiolytic Treatment Impairs Helping Behavior in Rats," *Frontiers in Psychology* 8, no. 7 (June 2016): 850.

Chapter 6: Balance Your Blood Sugar

1. J. Maniam et al., "Sugar Consumption Produces Effects Similar to Early Life Stress Exposure on Hippocampal Markers of Neurogenesis and Stress Response," *Frontiers in Molecular Neuroscience* 19, no. 8 (January 2016): 86.

2. F. N. Jacka et al., "Western Diet Is Associated with a Smaller Hippocampus: A Longitudinal Investigation," *BMC Medicine* 13, no. 1 (September 2015): doi:10.1186/s12916-015-0461-x.

3. S. I. Martire et al., "Extended Exposure to a Palatable Cafeteria Diet Alters Gene Expression in Brain Regions Implicated in Reward, and Withdrawal from this Diet Alters Gene Expression in Brain Regions Associated with Stress," *Behavioural Brain Research* 265 (May 2015): 132–41.

4. S. M. Schmid et al., "A Single Night of Sleep Deprivation Increased Ghrelin Levels and Feelings of Hunger in Normal-Weight Healthy Men," *Journal of Sleep Research* 17, no. 3 (September 2008): 331–34.

5. C. S. Harrell et al., "High-Fructose Diet During Periadolescent Development Increases Depressive-like Behavior and Remodels the Hypothalamic Transcriptome in Male Rats," *Psychoneuroendocrinology* 62 (December 2015): 252–64.

6. Y. Kwon, E. Apostolidis, and K. Shetty, "Inhibitory Potential of Wine and Tea Against A-Amylase and A-Glucosidase for Management of Hyperglycemia Linked to Type 2 Diabetes," *Journal of Food Biochemistry* 32, no. 1 (February 2008): 15–31.

7. Ibid.

Chapter 7: Calm Your Brain

1. M. P. St-Onge et al., "Fiber and Saturated Fat Are Associated with Sleep Arousals and Slow Wave Sleep," *Journal of Clinical Sleep Medicine* 12, no. 1 (January 2016): 19–24.

2. C. Bell, J. Abrams, and D. Nutt, "Tryptophan Depletion and Its Implications for Psychiatry," *The British Journal of Psychiatry* 178, no. 5 (May 2001): 399–405.

3. L. Wang, T. J. Maher, and R. J. Wurtman, "Oral L-glutamine Increases GABA Levels in Striatal Tissue and Extracellular Fluid," *FASEB Journal* 21, no. 4 (April 2007): 1227–32.

4. D. G. Blanchflower et al., "Is Psychological Well-Being Linked to the Consumption of Fruit and Vegetables?" *Social Indicators Research* 114, no. 3 (December 2013): 785–801.

5. G. Zhang et al., "Thiamine Nutritional Status and Depressive Symptoms Are Inversely Associated among Older Chinese Adults," *Journal of Nutrition* 143, no. 1 (January 2013): 53–8; D. Benton, J. Haller, and J. Fordy, "Vitamin Supplementation for 1 Year Improves Mood," *Neuropsychobiology* 32, no. 2 (1995): 98–105.

6. A. Rosanoff, C. M. Weaver, and R. K. Rude, "Suboptimal Magnesium Status in the United States: Are the Health Consequences Underestimated?" *Nutrition Reviews* 70, no. 3 (March 2012): 153–64.

7.   S. W. Golf et al., "Plasma Aldosterone, Cortisol, and Electrolyte Concentrations in Physical Exercise after Magnesium Supplementation," *Journal of Clinical Chemistry and Clinical Biochemistry* 22, no. 11 (November 1984): 717–21.

8.   S. Brody et al., "A Randomized Controlled Trial of High Dose Ascorbic Acid for Reduction of Blood Pressure, Cortisol, and Subjective Responses to Psychological Stress," *Psychopharmacology* 159, no. 3 (January 2002): 319–24.

9.   American Chemical Society, "Scientists Say Vitamin C May Alleviate the Body's Response to Stress," *ScienceDaily* (August 23, 1999): www.sciencedaily.com/releases/1999/08/990823072615.htm.

10. E. M. Peters et al., "Vitamin C Supplementation Attenuates the Increases in Circulating Cortisol, Adrenaline and Anti-Inflammatory Polypeptides Following Ultramarathon Running," *International Journal of Sports Medicine* 22, no. 07 (October 2001): 537–43.

11. I. Bjelland et al., "Choline in Anxiety and Depression: The Hordaland Health Study," *American Journal of Clinical Nutrition* 90, no. 4 (October 2009): 1056–60.

12. P. Appleby et al., "Comparative Fracture Risk in Vegetarians and Nonvegetarians in EPIC-Oxford," *European Journal Clinical Nutrition* 61, no. 12 (December 2007): 1400–6.

13. L. E. Williams and J. A. Bargh, "Experiencing Physical Warmth Promotes Interpersonal Warmth," *Science* 322, no. 5901 (October 2008): 606–7.

Chapter 8: Eat Peaceful Proteins and Feel-Good Fats

1.   R. E. Morgan et al., "Plasma Cholesterol and Depressive Symptoms in Older Men," *Lancet* 341, no. 8837 (January 1993): 75–9.

2.   J. Delarue et al., "Fish Oil Prevents the Adrenal Activation Elicited by Mental Stress in Healthy Men," *Diabetes & Metabolism* 29, no. 3 (June 2003): 289–95.

3.   K. Hamazaki et al., "Effect of W-3 Fatty Acid-Containing Phospholipids on Blood Catecholamine Concentrations in Healthy Volunteers: A Randomized, Placebo-Controlled, Double-Blind Trial," *Nutrition* 21, no. 6 (June 2005): 705–10.

4.   J. K. Kiecolt-Glaser et al., "Omega-3 Supplementation Lowers Inflammation and Anxiety in Medical Students: A Randomized Controlled Trial," *Brain, Behavior, and Immunity* 25, no. 8 (November 2011): 1725–34.

5.   C. B. Gesch et al., "Influence of Supplementary Vitamins, Minerals and Essential Fatty Acids on the Antisocial Behaviour of Young Adult Prisoners. Randomised, Placebo-Controlled Trial," *British Journal of Psychiatry* 181, no. 1 (July 2002): 22–8.

6.   L. Buydens-Branchey and M. Branchey, "Long-Chain N-3 Polyunsaturated Fatty Acids Decrease Feelings of Anger in Substance Abusers," *Psychiatry Research* 157, nos. 1–3 (January 2008): 95–104.

7. P. Montgomery et al., "Fatty Acids and Sleep in UK Children: Subjective and Pilot Objective Sleep Results from the DOLAB Study–A Randomized Controlled Trial," *Journal of Sleep Research* 23, no. 4 (August 2014): 364–88.

8. J. B. Ladesich et al., "Membrane Level of Omega-3 Docosahexaenoic Acid Is Associated with Severity of Obstructive Sleep Apnea," *Journal of Clinical Sleep Medicine* 7, no. 4 (August 2011): 391–6.

9. C. A. Daley et al., "A Review of Fatty Acid Profiles and Antioxidant Content in Grass-Fed and Grain-Fed Beef," *Nutrition Journal* (March 2010): www.nutritionj.com/content/9/1/10.

10. P. I. Ponte et al., "Restricting the Intake of a Cereal-Based Feed in Free-Range-Pastured Poultry: Effects on Performance and Meat Quality," *Poultry Science* 87, no. 10 (October 2008): 2032–42; P. I. Ponte et al., "Influence of Pasture Intake on the Fatty Acid Composition, and Cholesterol, Tocopherols, and Tocotrienols Content in Meat from Free-Range Broilers," *Poultry Science* 87, no. 1 (January 2008): 80–8; A. G. D'Alessandro et al., "How the Nutritional Value and Consumer Acceptability of Suckling Lambs Meat Is Affected by the Maternal Feeding System," *Small Ruminant Research* 106, no. 2–3 (August 2012) 83–91.

11. "Research Shows Eggs from Pastured Chickens May Be More Nutritious," *Penn State News* (July 20, 2010): news.psu.edu/story/166143/2010/07/20/research-shows-eggs-pastured-chickens-may-be-more-nutritious.

12. K. L. Weaver et al., "The Content of Favorable and Unfavorable Polyunsaturated Fatty Acids Found in Commonly Eaten Fish," *Journal of the American Dietetic Association* 108, no. 7 (July 2008): 1178–85.

13. F. Visioli et al., "Dietary Intake of Fish vs. Formulations Leads to Higher Plasma Concentrations of N-3 Fatty Acids," *Lipids* 38, no. 4 (April 2003): 415–18.

14. D. Mozaffarian and E. B. Rimm, "Fish Intake, Contaminants, and Human Health: Evaluating the Risks and the Benefits," *Journal of the American Medical Association* 297, no. 6 (February 2007): 590.

15. O. Ouédraogo and M. Amyot, "Effects of Various Cooking Methods and Food Components on Bioaccessibility of Mercury from Fish," *Environmental Research* 111, no. 8 (November 2011): 1064–69.

16. Y. Yokoyama et al., "Vegetarian Diets and Blood Pressure: A Meta-Analysis," *JAMA Internal Medicine* 174, no. 4 (April 2014): 577–87.

17. D. Mozaffarian and E. B. Rimm, "Fish Intake, Contaminants, and Human Health: Evaluating the Risks and the Benefits," *Journal of the American Medical Association* 297, no. 6 (February 2007): 590.

18. *IARC Monographs on the Evaluation of the Carcinogenic Risk of Chemicals to Humans: Polynuclear Aromatic Compounds. Chemical, Environmental and Experimental Data, Volume 32* (Lyons, France: International Agency for Research on Cancer, 1983); M. G. de Verdier et al., "Meat, Cooking Methods and Colorectal Cancer: A Case-Referent Study in Stockholm," *International Journal of Cancer* 49, no. 4 (October 1991): 520–5.

19. T. R. Dhiman et al. "Conjugated Linoleic Acid Content of Milk from Cows Fed Different Diets," *Journal of Dairy Science* 82, no. 10 (1999): 2146–2156.

20. L. A. Smit et al., "Conjugated Linoleic Acid in Adipose Tissue and Risk of Myocardial Infarction," *American Journal of Clinical Nutrition* 92, no. 1 (July 2010): 34–40.

21. L. Schaefer et al., "Role of Nutrition in Reducing Antemortem Stress and Meat Quality Aberrations," *Journal of Animal Science* 79, Suppl. (2001): E91–E101.

22. J. Hellhammer et al., "Effects of Soy Lecithin Phosphatidic Acid and Phosphatidylserine Complex (PAS) on the Endocrine and Psychological Responses to Mental Stress," *Stress* 7, no. 2 (June 2004): 119–26.

23. W. N. Jefferson, E. Padilla-Banks, and R. R. Newbold, "Adverse Effects on Female Development and Reproduction in CD-1 Mice Following Neonatal Exposure to the Phytoestrogen Genistein at Environmentally Relevant Doses," *Biology of Reproduction* 73, no. 4 (October 2005): 798–806.

24. F. N. Jacka et al., "Western Diet Is Associated with a Smaller Hippocampus: A Longitudinal Investigation," *BMC Medicine* 13, no. 1 (September 2015): doi:10.1186/s12916-015-0461-x.

25. L. Pimpin et al., "Is Butter Back? A Systematic Review and Meta-Analysis of Butter Consumption and Risk of Cardiovascular Disease, Diabetes, and Total Mortality," *PloS ONE* 11, no. 6 (June 2016): doi:10.1371/journal.pone.0158118.

Chapter 9: Embrace the Power of Probiotics

1. W. Gomm et al., "Association of Proton Pump Inhibitors with Risk of Dementia: A Pharmacoepidemiological Claims Data Analysis," *JAMA Neurology* 73, no. 4 (April 2016): 410–6.

2. G. Hoarau et al. "Bacteriome and Mycobiome Interactions Underscore Microbial Dysbiosis in Familial Crohn's Disease," *mBio* 7, no. 5 (September 2016): doi:10.1128/mBio.01250-16.

3. S. Bacon et al., "The Impact of Mood and Anxiety Disorders on Incident Hypertension at One Year," *International Journal of Hypertension* 2014 (2014).

4. T. G. Dinan and J. F. Cryan, "Melancholic Microbes: A Link Between Gut Microbiota and Depression?" *Neurogastroenterology and Motility* 25, no. 9 (September 2014): 713–9.

5. Shoskes et al., "Longitudinal Effects of Chronic Stress on the Murine Gut Microbiota," presented at the Society for Neuroscience Conference (2015).

6. T. Vanuytsel et al., "Psychological Stress and Corticotropin-Releasing Hormone Increase Intestinal Permeability in Humans by a Mast Cell-Dependent Mechanism," *Gut* 63, no. 8 (August 2014): 1293–9.

7. T. G. Dinan and J. F. Cryan, "Melancholic Microbes: A Link Between Gut Microbiota and Depression?" *Neurogastroenterology and Motility* 25, no. 9 (September 2014): 713–9.

8. S. M. Collins, M. Surette, and P. Bercik, "The Interplay Between the Intestinal Microbiota and the Brain," *Nature Reviews Microbiology* 10, no. 11 (November 2012): 735–42.

9. K. M. Neufeld et al., "Reduced Anxiety-like Behavior and Central Neurochemical Change in Germ-Free Mice," *Neurogastroenterology and Motility* 23, no. 3 (March 2011): 255–64.

10. J. C. Clemente et al., "The Microbiome of Uncontacted Amerindians," *Science Advances* 1, no. 3 (April 2015): doi:10.1126/sciadv.1500183.

11. C. De Filippo et al., "Impact of Diet in Shaping Gut Microbiota Revealed by a Comparative Study in Children from Europe and Rural Africa," *Proceedings of the National Academy of Sciences* 107, no. 33 (August 2010): 14,691–6.

12. J. M. Krueger and J. A. Majde, "Microbial Products and Cytokines in Sleep and Fever Regulation," *Critical Reviews in Immunology* 14, no. 3–4 (1994): 355–79.

13. R. M. Voigt et al., "Circadian Disorganization Alters Intestinal Microbiota," *PloS ONE* 9, no. 5 (May 2014): doi.org/10.1371/journal.pone.0097500.

14. A. Wallis et al., "Support for the Microgenderome: Associations in a Human Clinical Population," *Scientific Reports* 6 (2016): doi:10.1038/srep19171.

15. K. Tillisch et al., "Consumption of Fermented Milk Product with Probiotic Modulates Brain Activity," *Gastroenterology* 144, no. 7 (June 2013): 1394–1401.

16. T. G. Dinan and J. F. Cryan, "Melancholic Microbes: A Link Between Gut Microbiota and Depression?" *Neurogastroenterology and Motility* 25, no. 9 (September 2013): 713–9.

17. P. Allen et al., "Probiotic May Help Alleviate Stress-Related Conditions: The Bacteria Strain *Bifidobacterium longum 1714* Reduces Stress, Improves Memory in Study of Healthy Men," presented at the Society for Neuroscience Conference (2015).

18. Q. Zhang, Y. Wu, and X. Fei, "Effect of Probiotics on Body Weight and Body-Mass Index: A Systematic Review and Meta-Analysis of Randomized, Controlled Trials," *International Journal of Food Sciences and Nutrition* 67, no. 5 (August 2015): 571–80.

19. C. Dominianni et al., "Sex, Body Mass Index, and Dietary Fiber Intake Influence the Human Gut Microbiome," *PloS ONE* 10, no. 4 (April 2015): doi.org/10.1371/journal.pone.0124599.

20. Ibid.

21. T. Stefka et al., "Commensal Bacteria Protect Against Food Allergen Sensitization," *Proceedings of the National Academy of Sciences* 111, no. 36 (September 2014): 13145–50.

22. R. A. Kemperman et al., "Impact of Polyphenols from Black Tea and Red Wine/Grape Juice on a Gut Model Microbiome," *Food Research International* 53, no. 2 (October 2013): 659–69.

23. D. C. Vodnar and C. Socaciu, "Green Tea increases the Survival Yield of Bifidobacteria in Simulated Gastrointestinal Environment and During Refrigerated Conditions," *Chemistry Central Journal* 6, no. 1 (June 2012): 61.

24. M. Jacquet et al., "Impact of Coffee Consumption on the Gut Microbiota: A Human Volunteer Study," *International Journal of Food Microbiology* 130, no. 2 (March 2009): 117–21.

25. S. F. Clarke et al., "Exercise and Associated Dietary Extremes Impact on Gut Microbial Diversity," *Gut* 63, no. 12 (December 2014): 1913–20.

Chapter 10: Jog for Joy

1. H. Boecker et al., "The Runner's High: Opioidergic Mechanisms in the Human Brain," *Cerebral Cortex*, 18, no. 11 (November 2008): 2523–31.

2. J. Fuss et al., "A Runner's High Depends on Cannabinoid Receptors in Mice," *Proceedings of the National Academy of Sciences* 112, no. 42 (October 2015): 13105–8.

3. R. J. Maddock et al., "Acute Modulation of Cortical Glutamate and GABA Content by Physical Activity," *Journal of Neuroscience* 36, no. 8 (February 2016): 2449–57.

4. F. Lucertini et al., "High Cardiorespiratory Fitness Is Negatively Associated with Daily Cortisol Output in Healthy Aging Men," *PloS ONE* 10, no. 11 (November 2015): doi.org/10.1371/journal.pone.0141970.

5. N. Cherbuin et al., "Being Overweight Is Associated with Hippocampal Atrophy: The PATH Through Life Study," *International Journal of Obesity* 39, no. 10 (October 2015): 1509–14.

6. P. D. Loprinzi and B. J. Cardinal, "Association between Objectively-Measured Physical Activity and Sleep, NHANES 2005–2006," *Mental Health and Physical Activity* 4, no. 2 (December 2011): 65–9.

7. J. Chedda et al., "Physical Activity and Habitual Sleep Duration: Does the Specific Type of Activity Matter?" *Sleep* 38, Abstract Supplement (June 2015): A89–90.

8. K. Jayakody, S. Gunadasa, and C. Hosker, "Exercise for Anxiety Disorders: Systematic Review," *British Journal of Sports Medicine* 48, no. 3 (February 2014): 187–96.

9. I. Marks, "Treatment of Panic Disorder," *American Journal of Psychiatry* 156, no. 7 (July 1999): 1129–30.

10. T. A. Manger and R. W. Motta, "The Impact of an Exercise Program on Posttraumatic Stress Disorder, Anxiety, and Depression," *International Journal of Emergency Mental Health* 7, no. 1 (Winter 2005): 49–57.

11. H. H. Kyu et al., "Physical Activity and Risk of Breast Cancer, Colon Cancer, Diabetes, Ischemic Heart Disease, and Ischemic Stroke Events: Systematic Review and Dose-Response Meta-Analysis for the Global Burden of Disease Study 2013," *BMJ 354* (August 2016): doi.org/10.1136/bmj.i3857.

12. S. Nokia "Physical Exercise Increases Adult Hippocampal Neurogenesis in Male Rats Provided It Is Aerobic and Sustained," *Journal of Physiology* 594, no. 7 (April 2016): 1855–73.

13. Ibid.

14. Heenan and N. F. Troje, "Both Physical Exercise and Progressive Muscle Relaxation Reduce the Facing-the-Viewer Bias in Biological Motion Perception," *PloS ONE* 9, no. 7 (July 2014): doi.org/10.1371/journal.pone.0099902.

15. Centers for Disease Control and Prevention, "Adult Participation in Aerobic and Muscle-Strengthening Physical Activities—United States, 2011," *Morbidity and Mortality Weekly Report* 62, no. 17 (May 2013): 326–30.

16. E. G. Ciolac, "High-Intensity Interval Training and Hypertension: Maximizing the Benefits of Exercise," *American Journal of Cardiovascular Disease* 2, no. 2 (2012): 102–10.

17. A. H. Boal et al., "Monotherapy with Major Antihypertensive Drug Classes and Risk of Hospital Admissions for Mood Disorders," *Hypertension* 68, no. 5 (November 2016): 1132–8.

18. A. Smyth et al., "Physical Activity and Anger or Emotional Upset as Triggers of Acute Myocardial Infarction: The INTERHEART Study," *Circulation* 134, no. 15 (October 2016): 1059–67.

19. J. L. Talanian et al., "Two Weeks of High-Intensity Aerobic Interval Training Increases the Capacity for Fat Oxidation during Exercise in Women," *Journal of Applied Physiology* 102, no. 4 (April 2007): 1439–47.

20. S. H. Boutcher, "High-Intensity Intermittent Exercise and Fat Loss," *Journal of Obesity* 2011 (2010): doi:10.1155/2011/868305.

21. J. B. Gillen et al., "Twelve Weeks of Sprint Interval Training Improves Indices of Cardiometabolic Health Similar to Traditional Endurance Training Despite a Five-Fold Lower Exercise Volume and Time Commitment," *PloS ONE* 11, no. 4 (April 2016): doi:10.1371/journal.pone.0154075.

22. K. N. Harkess et al., "Brief Report on the Psychophysiological Effects of a Yoga Intervention for Chronic Stress," *Journal of Psychophysiology* 31 (2017): 38–48.

23. B. G. Berger and D. R. Owen, "Stress Reduction and Mood Enhancement in Four Exercise Modes: Swimming, Body Conditioning, Hatha Yoga, and Fencing," *Research Quarterly for Exercise and Sport* 59, no. 2 (June 1988): 148–59.

24. D. S. Shannahoff-Khalsa et al., "Randomized Controlled Trial of Yogic Meditation Techniques for Patients with Obsessive-Compulsive Disorder," *CNS Spectrums* 4, no. 12 (December 1999): 34–47; G. R. Norton and W. E. Johnson, "A Comparison of Two Relaxation Procedures for Reducing Cognitive and Somatic Anxiety," *Journal of Behavior Therapy and Experimental Psychiatry* 14, no. 3 (September 1983): 209–14; A. Broota and C. Sanghvi, "Efficacy of Two Relaxation Techniques in Examination Anxiety," *Journal of Personality and Clinical Studies* 10, no. 1–2 (March–September 1994): 29–35.

25. G. Sahasi, D. Mohan, and C. Kacker, "Effectiveness of Yogic Techniques in the Management of Anxiety," *Journal of Personality and Clinical Studies* 5 (1989): 51–5.

26. N. S. Vahia et al., "Psychophysiologic Therapy Based on the Concepts of Patanjali: A New Approach to the Treatment of Neurotic and Psychosomatic Disorders," *American Journal of Psychotherapy* 27, no. 4 (October 1973): 557–65.

27. C. C. Streeter et al., "Yoga Asana Sessions Increase Brain GABA Levels: A Pilot Study," *Journal of Alternative and Complementary Medicine* 13, no. 4 (May 2007): 419–26.

28. M. S. Lee et al., "Qigong Reduced Blood Pressure and Catecholamine Levels of Patients with Essential Hypertension," *International Journal of Neuroscience* 113, no. 12 (December 2003): 1691–701.

29. M. Nedeljkovic et al., "Getting Started with Taiji: Investigating Students Expectations and Teachers Appraisals of Taiji Beginners Courses," *Evidence-Based Complementary and Alternative Medicine* 2012 (2012): doi:10.1155/2012/595710.

30. P. Jin, "Efficacy of Tai Chi, Brisk Walking, Meditation, and Reading in Reducing Mental and Emotional Stress," *Journal of Psychosomatic Research* 36, no. 4 (May 1992): 361–70.

31. J. G. Zhang et al., "The Effects of Tai Chi Chuan on Physiological Function and Fear of Falling in the Less Robust Elderly: An Intervention Study for Preventing Falls," *Archives of Gerontology and Geriatrics* 42, no. 2 (March–April 2006): 107–16.

Chapter 11: Shift Your Thoughts with Energy-Based Cognitive Therapy

1. T. L. Kraft and S. D. Pressman. "Grin and Bear It: The Influence of Manipulated Facial Expression on the Stress Response." *Psychological Science* 23, no. 11 (2012): 1372–1378.

Chapter 12: Sleep Better with Cognitive Behavioral Therapy for Insomnia

1. Yong Liu et al., "Prevalence of Healthy Sleep Duration among Adults—United States, 2014," *Morbidity and Mortality Weekly Report* 65, no. 6 (February 2016): 137–41.

2. F. C. Baker, A. R. Wolfson, and K. A. Lee, "Association of Sociodemographic, Lifestyle, and Health Factors with Sleep Quality and Daytime Sleepiness in Women: Findings from the 2007 National Sleep Foundation 'Sleep in America Poll,'" *Journal of Women's Health* 18, no. 6 (June 2009): 841–49.

3. C. de Weerth, R. H. Zijl, and J. K. Buitelaar, "Development of Cortisol Circadian Rhythm in Infancy," *Early Human Development* 73, no. 1–2 (August 2003): 39–52.

4. A. Scher et al., "Sleep Quality, Cortisol Levels, and Behavioral Regulation in Toddlers," *Developmental Psychobiology* 52, no. 1 (January 2010): 44–53.

5. C. S. Möller-Levet et al., "Effects of Insufficient Sleep on Circadian Rhythmicity and Expression Amplitude of the Human Blood Transcriptome," *Proceedings of the National Academy of Sciences* 110, no. 12 (March 2013): E1132–41.

6. T. C. Erren, R. J. Reiter, and C. Piekarski, "Light, Timing of Biological Rhythms, and Chronodisruption in Man," *Naturwissenschaften* 90, no. 11 (November 2003): 485–94.

7. F. P. Cappuccio et al., "Sleep Duration and All-Cause Mortality: A Systematic Review and Meta-Analysis of Prospective Studies," *Sleep* 33, no. 5 (May 2010): 585–92.

8. K. Opstad, "Circadian Rhythm of Hormones Is Extinguished During Prolonged Physical Stress, Sleep and Energy Deficiency in Young Men," *European Journal of Endocrinology* 131, no. 1 (July 1994): 56–66.

9. D. Neckelmann, A. Mykletun, and A. A. Dahl, "Chronic Insomnia as a Risk Factor for Developing Anxiety and Depression," *Sleep* 30, no. 7 (July 2007): 873–80.

10. C. E. Sexton et al., "Poor Sleep Quality Is Associated with Increased Cortical Atrophy in Community-Dwelling Adults," *Neurology* 83, no. 11 (September 2014): 967–73.

11. L. Xie et al, "Sleep Drives Metabolite Clearance from the Adult Brain," *Science* 342, no. 6156 (October 2013): 373–7.

12. R. H. Pietrzak et al., "Plasma Cortisol, Brain Amyloid-β, and Cognitive Decline in Preclinical Alzheimer's Disease: A 6-Year Prospective Cohort Study," *Biological Psychiatry: Cognitive Neuroscience and Neuroimaging* 2, no. 1 (January 2017): 45–52.

13. M. Bellesi et al., "Effects of Sleep and Wake on Oligodendrocytes and Their Precursors," *Journal of Neuroscience* 33, no. 36 (September 2013): 14,288–300.

14. H. P. Van Dongen et al., "The Cumulative Cost of Additional Wakefulness: Dose-Response Effects on Neurobehavioral Functions and Sleep Physiology from Chronic Sleep Restriction and Total Sleep Deprivation," *Sleep* 26, no. 2 (March 2003): 117–26.

15. C. M. Morin, *Insomnia: Psychological Assessment and Management* (New York: Guilford Press, 1993).

16. A. Qaseem et al., "Management of Chronic Insomnia Disorder in Adults: A Clinical Practice Guideline from the American College of Physicians," *Annals of Internal Medicine* 165, no. 2 (July 2016): 125–33.

17. C. M. Morin et al., "Psychological Management of Insomnia: A Clinical Replication Series with 100 Patients," *Behavior Therapy* 25, no. 2 (Spring 1994): 291–309.

18. C. M. Morin et al. "Efficacy of Cognitive-Behavioral Treatments for Insomnia: A Meta-Analytic Review," *Sleep Research* 18 (1989): 272.

19. M. T. Smith et al., "Comparative Meta-Analysis of Pharmacotherapy and Behavior Therapy for Persistent Insomnia," *American Journal of Psychiatry* 159, no. 1 (January 2002): 5–11.

20. "FDA Drug Safety Communication: Risk of Next-Morning Impairment after Use of Insomnia Drugs; FDA Requires Lower Recommended Doses for Certain Drugs Containing Zolpidem (Ambien, Ambien CR, Edluar, and Zolpimist)" (2013): www.fda.gov/Drugs/DrugSafety/ucm334033.htm.

21. J. Glass et al., "Sedative Hypnotics in Older People with Insomnia: Meta-Analysis of Risks and Benefits," *BMJ* 331, no. 7526 (November 2005): 1169.

22. Substance Abuse and Mental Health Services Administration, Center for Behavioral Health Statistics and Quality. (May 1, 2013). *Emergency Department Visits for Adverse Reactions Involving the Insomnia Medication Zolpidem*. Rockville, MD.

23. D. F. Kripke, R. D. Langer, and L. E. Kline, "Hypnotics' Association with Mortality or Cancer: A Matched Cohort Study," *BMJ Open* 2, no. 1 (January 2012): doi:10.1136/bmjopen-2012-000850.

24. L. H. Jacobson, G. E. Callander, and D. Hoyer, "Suvorexant for the Treatment of Insomnia." *Expert Review of Clinical Pharmacology* 7, no. 6 (November 2014): 711–30.

25. L. B. Goldstein et al., "Guidelines for the Prim vention of Stroke: A Guideline for Healthcare Professionals from the American Heart Association/American Stroke Association," *Stroke* 42, no. 2 (January 2011): 517–84.

26. K. J. Reid et al., "Timing and Intensity of Light Correlate with Body Weight in Adults," *PloS ONE* 9, no. 4 (April 2014): doi.org/10.1371/journal.pone.0092251.

27. E. Morita et al., "A Before and After Comparison of the Effects of Forest Walking on the Sleep of a Community-Based Sample of People with Sleep Complaints," *BioPsychoSocial Medicine* 5 (October 2011): 13.

28. S. S. Tworoger et al., "Effects of a Yearlong Moderate-Intensity Exercise and a Stretching Intervention on Sleep Quality in Postmenopausal Women," *Sleep* 26, no. 7 (November 2003): 830–6.

29. D. L. Kirsch and F. Nichols, "Cranial Electrotherapy Stimulation for Treatment of Anxiety, Depression, and Insomnia," *Psychiatric Clinics of North America* 36, no. 1 (March 2013): 169–76.

30. R. G. Lande and C. Gragnani. "Efficacy of Cranial Electric Stimulation for the Treatment of Insomnia: A Randomized Pilot Study," *Complementary Therapies in Medicine* 21, no. 1 (February 2013): 8–13; S. Klawansky et al., "Meta-Analysis of Randomized Controlled Trials of Cranial Electrostimulation: Efficacy in Treating Selected Psychological and Physiological Conditions," *Journal of Nervous and Mental Disease* 183, no. 7 (July 1995): 478–84.

31. J. Varughese and R. P. Allen, "Fatal Accidents Following Changes in Daylight Savings Time: The American Experience," *Sleep Medicine* 2, no. 1 (January 2001): 31–6.

Chapter 13: Relaxation Therapy

1. J. A. Dusek et al., "Genomic Counter-Stress Changes Induced by the Relaxation Response," *PloS ONE* 3, no. 7 (July 2008): doi.org/10.1371/journal.pone.0002576.

2. H. Benson and M. Z. Klipper, *The Relaxation Response* (New York: Avon, 1975).

3. F. Stetter and S. Kupper, "Autogenic Training: A Meta-Analysis of Clinical Outcome Studies," *Applied Psychophysiology and Biofeedback* 27, no. 1 (March 2002): 45–98.

Chapter 14: Pranayama

1. Y. F. Chen et al., "The Effectiveness of Diaphragmatic Breathing Relaxation Training for Reducing Anxiety," *Perspectives in Psychiatric Care* (August 2016): doi:10.1111/ppc.12184.

2. A. Vedamurthachar et al., "Antidepressant Efficacy and Hormonal Effects of Sudarshana Kriya Yoga (SKY) in Alcohol Dependent Individuals," *Journal of Affective Disorders* 94, no. 1–3 (August 2006): 249–53.

3. N. Janakiramaiah et al., "Therapeutic Efficacy of Sudarshan Kriya Yoga (SKY) in Dysthymic Disorder," *NIMHANS* 17 (January 1998): 21–8; V. V. Agte and S. A. Chiplonkar, "Sudarshan Kriya Yoga for Improving Antioxidant Status and Reducing Anxiety in Adults," *Alternative and Complementary Therapies* 14, no. 2 (April 2008): 96–100.

4. J. Eyerman, "A Clinical Report of Holotropic Breathwork in 11,000 Psychiatric Inpatients in a Community Hospital Setting," *MAPS Bulletin Special Edition* (Spring 2013): 24–7; S. W. Holmes et al., "Holotropic Breathwork: An Experiential Approach to Psychotherapy," *Psychotherapy* 33, no. 1 (March 1996): 114–20.

5. N. Janakiramaiah, "Antidepressant Efficacy of Sudarshan Kriya Yoga (SKY) in Melancholia: A Randomized Comparison with Electroconvulsive Therapy (ECT) and Imipramine," *Journal of Affective Disorders* 57, no. 1–3 (January–March 2000): 255–9.

6. T. Descilo et al., "Effects of a Yoga Breath Intervention Alone and in Combination with an Exposure Therapy for Post-Traumatic Stress Disorder and Depression in Survivors of the 2004 South-East Asia Tsunami," *Acta Psychiatrica Scandinavica* 121, no. 4 (April 2010): 289–300.

7. S. Kumar et al., "Meditation on OM: Relevance from Ancient Texts and Contemporary Science," *International Journal of Yoga* 3, no. 1 (January 2010): 2–5.

Chapter 15: Self-Hypnosis

1. H. Spiegel and D. Spiegel, *Trance and Treatment: Clinical Uses of Hypnosis* (Arlington, VA: American Psychiatric Publishing, Inc., 2008).

2. A. Raz, J. Fan, and M. I. Posner, "Hypnotic Suggestion Reduces Conflict in the Human Brain," *Proceedings of the National Academy of Sciences* 102, no. 28 (July 2005): 9978–83.

3. M. C. Gay, "Effectiveness of Hypnosis in Reducing Mild Essential Hypertension: A One-Year Follow-Up," *International Journal of Clinical and Experimental Hypnosis* 55, no. 1 (January 2007): 67–83.

4. P. J. Whorwell, A. Prior, and E. B. Faragher, "Controlled Trial of Hypnotherapy in the Treatment of Severe Refractory Irritable-Bowel Syndrome," *Lancet* 324, no. 8414 (December 1984): 1232–4.

5. A. Alladin and A. Alibhai, "Cognitive Hypnotherapy for Depression: An Empirical Investigation," *International Journal of Clinical and Experimental Hypnosis* 55, no. 2 (April 2007): 147–66.

6. C. Liossi and P. White, "Efficacy of Clinical Hypnosis in the Enhancement of Quality of Life of Terminally Ill Cancer Patients," *Contemporary Hypnosis* 18, no. 3 (September 2001): 145–60.

7. J. K. Kiecolt-Glaser et al., "Hypnosis as a Modulator of Cellular Immune Dysregulation During Acute Stress," *Journal of Consulting and Clinical Psychology* 69, no. 4 (August 2001): 674–82.

Chapter 16: Kindness, Gratitude, and Connection

1. E. B. Raposa, H. B. Laws, and E. B. Ansell, "Prosocial Behavior Mitigates the Negative Effects of Stress in Everyday Life," *Clinical Psychological Science* 4, no. 4 (July 2016): 691–8.

2. S. Lyubomirsky, C. Tkach, and K. M. Sheldon, "Pursuing Sustained Happiness through Random Acts of Kindness and Counting One's Blessings: Tests of Two Six-Week Interventions," Department of Psychology, University of California, Riverside, unpublished raw data, 2004.

3. Ibid.

4. S. E. Taylor et al., "Biobehavioral Responses to Stress in Females: Tend-and-Befriend, Not Fight-or-Flight," *Psychological Review* 107, no. 3 (July 2000): 411–29.

5. K. C. Light et al., "Oxytocin Responsivity in Mothers of Infants: A Preliminary Study of Relationships with Blood Pressure During Laboratory Stress and Normal Ambulatory Activity," *Health Psychology* 19, no. 6 (November 2000): 560–7.

6. K. Uvnäs-Moberg, "Antistress Pattern Induced by Oxytocin," *News in Physiological Sciences* 13 (February 1998): 22–5.

7. P. Kirsch et al., "Oxytocin Modulates Neural Circuitry for Social Cognition and Fear in Humans," *Journal of Neuroscience* 25, no. 49 (December 2005): 11,489–93.

8. M. van Zuiden et al., "Intranasal Oxytocin to Prevent Posttraumatic Stress Disorder Symptoms: A Randomized Controlled Trial in Emergency Department Patients," *Biological Psychiatry* 81, no. 12 (June 2017): 1030–40.

9. M. Niwa et al., "Adolescent Stress-Induced Epigenetic Control of Dopaminergic Neurons Via Glucocorticoids," *Science* 339, no. 6117 (January 2013): 335–9.

10. E. Friedmann and S. A. Thomas, "Pet Ownership, Social Support, and One-Year Survival after Acute Myocardial Infarction in the Cardiac Arrhythmia Suppression Trial (CAST)," *American Journal of Cardiology* 76, no. 17 (December 1995): 1213–7; E. Friedmann et al., "Relation between Pet Ownership and Heart Rate Variability in Patients with Healed Myocardial Infarcts," *American Journal of Cardiology* 91, no. 6 (March 2003): 718–21.

11. R. A. Johnson, J. S. Odendaal, and R. L. Meadows, "Animal-Assisted Interventions Research: Issues and Answers," *Western Journal of Nursing Research* 24, no. 4 (June 2002): 422–40.

12. K. M. Cole et al., "Animal-Assisted Therapy in Patients Hospitalized with Heart Failure," *American Journal of Critical Care* 16, no. 6 (November 2007): 575–85.

Chapter 17: Mindfulness

1. P. E. Dux et al., "Training Improves Multitasking Performance by Increasing the Speed of Information Processing in Human Prefrontal Cortex," *Neuron* 63, no. 1 (July 2009): 127–38.

2. J. S. Rubinstein, D. E. Meyer, and J. E. Evans, "Executive Control of Cognitive Processes in Task Switching," *Journal of Experimental Psychology: Human Perception and Performance* 27, no. 4 (August 2001): 763–97.

3. T. D. Borkovec et al., "Stimulus Control Applications to the Treatment of Worry," *Behaviour Research and Therapy* 21, no. 3 (1983): 247–51.

4. B. Verkuil et al., "Pretreatment of Worry Enhances the Effects of Stress Management Therapy: A Randomized Clinical Trial." *Psychotherapy and Psychosomatics* 80, no. 3 (2011): 189–190.

5. E. J. Masicampo and R. F. Baumeister, "Consider It Done! Plan Making Can Eliminate the Cognitive Effects of Unfulfilled Goals," *Journal of Personality and Social Psychology* 101, no. 4 (October 2011): 667–83.

6. N. A. Curry and T. Kasser, "Can Coloring Mandalas Reduce Anxiety?" *Art Therapy* 22, no. 2 (January 2005): 81–5.

7. R. van der Vennet and S. Serice, "Can Coloring Mandalas Reduce Anxiety? A Replication Study," *Art Therapy* 29, no. 2 (2012): 87–92.

Appendix A: Natural Herbs, Adaptogens, and Supplements

1. J. Cases et al., "Pilot Trial of *Melissa officinalis* L. Leaf Extract in the Treatment of Volunteers Suffering from Mild-to-Moderate Anxiety Disorders and Sleep Disturbances," *Mediterranean Journal of Nutrition and Metabolism* 4, no. 3 (December 2011): 211–8.

2. M. T. Epstein et al., "Licorice Raises Urinary Cortisol in Man," *Journal of Clinical Endocrinology and Metabolism* 47, no. 2 (August 1978): 397–400.

3. F. Donath et al., "Critical Evaluation of the Effect of Valerian Extract on Sleep Structure and Sleep Quality," *Pharmacopsychiatry* 33, no. 2 (March 2000): 47–53.

4. R. Kohnen and W. D. Oswald, "The Effects of Valerian, Propranolol, and Their Combination on Activation, Performance, and Mood of Healthy Volunteers under Social Stress Conditions," *Pharmacopsychiatry* 21, no. 6 (November 1988): 447–8.

5. E. M. Olsson, B. von Schéele, and A. G. Panossian, "A Randomised, Double-Blind, Placebo-Controlled, Parallel-Group Study of the Standardised Extract shr-5 of the Roots of *Rhodiola rosea* in the Treatment of Subjects with Stress-Related Fatigue," *Planta Medica* 75, no. 2 (February 2009): 105–12.

6. B. Auddy et al., "A Standardized *Withania somnifera* Extract Significantly Reduces Stress-Related Parameters in Chronically Stressed Humans: A Double-Blind, Randomized, Placebo-Controlled Study," *Journal of the American Nutraceutical Association* 11, no. 1 (2008): 50–6.

7. K. Cooley et al., "Naturopathic Care for Anxiety: A Randomized Controlled Trial ISRCTN78958974," *PLoS ONE* 4, no. 8 (August 2009): doi.org/10.1371/journal.pone.0006628.

8. M. K. Ahmad et al., "*Withania somnifera* Improves Semen Quality by Regulating Reproductive Hormone Levels and Oxidative Stress in Seminal Plasma of Infertile Males," *Fertility and Sterility* 94, no. 3 (August 2010): 989–96.

9. D. Bhattacharyya et al., "Controlled Programmed Trial of *Ocimum sanctum* Leaf on Generalized Anxiety Disorders," *Nepal Medical College Journal* 10, no. 3 (September 2008): 176–9.

10. S. Gholap and A. Kar, "Hypoglycaemic Effects of Some Plant Extracts Are Possibly Mediated through Inhibition in Corticosteroid Concentration," *Die Pharmazie* 59, no. 11 (November 2004): 876–8.

11. S. K. Bhattacharya and S. Ghosal, "Anxiolytic Activity of a Standardized Extract of *Bacopa monniera:* An Experimental Study," *Phytomedicine* 5, no. 2 (April 1998): 77–82.

12. N. Sheikh et al., "Effect of *Bacopa monniera* on Stress Induced Changes in Plasma Corticosterone and Brain Monoamines in Rats," *Journal of Ethnopharmacology* 111, no. 3 (May 2007): 671–6.

13. C. Calabrese et al, "Effects of a Standardized *Bacopa monnieri* Extract on Cognitive Performance, Anxiety, and Depression in the Elderly: A Randomized, Double-Blind, Placebo-Controlled Trial," *Journal of Alternative and Complementary Medicine* 14, no. 6 (July 2008): 707–13.

14. M. Boudarene, J. J. Legros, and M. Timsit-Berthier, "[Study of the Stress Response: Role of Anxiety, Cortisol and DHEAs]," *L'Encephale* 28, no. 2 (March–April 2002): 139–46.

15. R. S. Kahn et al, "Effect of a Serotonin Precursor and Uptake Inhibitor in Anxiety Disorders; A Double-blind Comparison of 5-hydroxytryptophan, Clomipramine and Placebo." *International Clinical Psychopharmacology* 2, no. 1 (January 1987): 33-45.

16. A. Soulairac and H. Lambinet. "The Effects of 5-hydroxy-tryptophan, a Precursor of Serotonin, on Sleep Disorder." *Annales Medico-Psychologiques 1*, no 5. (May 1977): 792–797.

17. M. M. Bergamaschi et al., "Cannabidiol Reduces the Anxiety Induced by Simulated Public Speaking in Treatment-Naïve Social Phobia Patients," *Neuropsychopharmacology* 36, no. 6 (May 2011): 1219–26.

18. A. W. Zuardi, F. S. Guimarães, and A. C. Moreira, "Effect of Cannabidiol on Plasma Prolactin, Growth Hormone and Cortisol in Human Volunteers," *Brazilian Journal of Medical and Biological Research* 26, no. 2 (1993): 213–7; R. K. Das et al., "Cannabidiol Enhances Consolidation of Explicit Fear Extinction in Humans," *Psychopharmacology* 226, no. 4 (April 2013): 781–92.

19. "2016 Warning Letters and Test Results for Cannabidiol-Related Products," U. S. Food and Drug Administration (2016): www.fda.gov/NewsEvents/PublicHealthFocus/ucm484109.htm.

Index

E

F

M

Macadamia oil, 85
Magnesium, 66
Malaysian palm fruit oil, 85
Mantra, relaxation through, 152–153
Mantra Breathing
  in Drained Brain program, 213
  Lifestyle Tracking exercise, 233
  overview, 165
Manuka honey, 54, 201
Maple syrup, 54, 201
Margarine spreads, 85
Marpac Dohm, 136
M Café, 83
McGill University, 174–175
Meat
  in modified Mediterranean diet, 80–81
  omega-3s from, 75–76
Meat substitute products, 82–83
Meditation. *See also* Mantra Breathing; Mindfulness
  meditative movement, 108–110, 113
  thought stream meditation, Lifestyle Tracking exercise, 246
  thought stream meditation, overview, 188–189
  Transcendental Meditation, 151, 152
Mediterranean diet, modified. *See* Modified Mediterranean diet
Melatonin
  blood sugar and, 52
  evening levels of, 17, 163
  overview, 16–17
  stress-sleep cycle and, 126
  supplements, 64, 134
Memory problems, 7–8
Mercury, in fish, 78
Mesmer, Franz, 173–174
Metabolic equivalent (MET) minutes, for exercise, 101
Microbiome, 88–92
Mind-body connection, 23–32
  brain structure and stress, 30
  overview, 23–26
  physical effects from stress, 26–30
  pitfall thought patterns and, 31–32
Mindfulness, 187–194
  coloring for, 194
  Lifestyle Tracking exercises, 249–252
  mindfulness-based cognitive therapy (MBCT), 187
  multitasking *versus* single-tasking, 188

overview, 187
thought stream meditation, 188–189
using in Drained Brain program, 214
for work, 192–193
for worry (stimulus control), Lifestyle Tracking Exercise, 247
for worry (stimulus control), overview, 189–191
Mindful to-do lists
  Lifestyle Tracking exercise, 251–252
  overview, 192–193
Minerals. *See* Vitamins and minerals; *individual minerals*
Minor insomnia, cognitive behavioral therapy for insomnia for, 131–137
Minty Cucumber Kefir Salad, 295
Moderate insomnia, cognitive behavioral therapy for insomnia for, 138–141
Modified Mediterranean diet
  beans and soybeans in, 82–84
  fish and alternatives in, 76–79
  meat, dairy, and eggs in, 80–81
  oils and fats in, 84–86
Monounsaturated fats, 84
Monsanto, 85
Monterey Bay Aquarium, 78
Mood. *See also* Anxiety; Stress
  danger of exercising while upset, 106
  genetics and, 38 (*See also* Genetic tendency for stress)
Moon Channel (breathing exercise), 166–167
Multitasking, 188
Muscles
  muscle-strengthening exercise, 105
  progressive muscle technique, 153–155, 213, 235–236
Myalgic encephalomyelitis, 27–28
Mycobiome, 89
Myelin, 127

N

Nancy (France) School, 174
Napping, 132
National Institute of Mental Health, 4
National Institutes of Health (NIH), 174
Natrol, 134
Natural killer (NK) cell activity, 26
Negative bias, 10–11
Nervous system. *See also* Hormones
  breath control for, 159–160
  overview, 12–14

identifying, 114–115
Lifestyle Tracking exercise, 224–225
overview, 31, 112–113
pigeon pose and shoulder shrugs for,
 118–119
sleep issues from, 139
using in Drained Brain program, 211
Pessimistic thought patterns. *See also* Energy-
 based cognitive therapy
half-smile exercise for, 119
identifying, 114–115
Lifestyle Tracking exercise, 226–227
overview, 31–32, 112–113
sleep issues from, 139
using in Drained Brain program, 211
Pesticides
in fruits and vegetables, 62–63
GMO foods and, 83–84
Pets, connection to, 185–186
Pharmaceutical medicines
antibiotics, 87–89
exercise compared to, 105, 109
natural sleep remedies *versus*, 128–129, 130
 (*See also* Cognitive behavioral therapy for
 insomnia)
pranayama (breath control) compared to,
 159
probiotics *versus*, 92
sleep aids, 5
tapering off/adjusting dose of, 203
PharmaGABA dietary supplement, 92
Physical activity. *See* Exercise
Physical poses as antidote (EBCT step 2),
 115–120. *See also* Energy-based cognitive
 therapy
Physical problems. *See also* Heart health
gut bacteria and, 89
physical brain drain, 41–42
physical tension release, 153–155
sleep disorders, 130–131
stress and mind-body connection, 26–30
Pigeon pose (EBCT exercise), 118–119
Pingala (energy), 166
Pink Lemonade Kombucha, 301
Pitfall thought patterns. *See also* Energy-based
 cognitive therapy
identifying (EBCT step 1), 114–115
moderate insomnia and, 138–141
overview, 31–32, 112–113
using in Drained Brain program, 210–211
Pizza, 55
Polarized thought patterns. *See also* Energy-
 based cognitive therapy
identifying, 114–115

Lifestyle Tracking exercise, 228–229
overview, 32, 113
sleep issues from, 139
spinal twist for, 119–120
using in Drained Brain program, 211
"Pole caught" tuna, 78
Polyphenols, 96
Polyunsaturated fats, 84
Positive behaviors, 181–186
connection, 184–186
gratitude, 183–184
kindness, 181–182
Lifestyle Tracking exercises, 244–245
using in Drained Brain program, 213
Positive stress, 22
Positive thoughts, 121–122. *See also* Energy-
 based cognitive therapy
Posttraumatic growth, 21
Power yoga, 109
Prakti paksha bhavana, 121
Pranayama (breath control), 159–171
activating breath, 167–168
advanced sequences, 168–171
calming breath, 161–167
Lifestyle Tracking exercise, 239
overview, 159–161
using in Drained Brain program, 213
Prefrontal cortex, 30, 93
Prescription sleep aids, 5
Prioritizing techniques, 192–193
Probiotics, 87–96
adding to diet, 205–207
boosters for, 95–96
gut as "second brain," 90–92
gut bacteria and, 88–90
prebiotics in foods, 94–95
probiotic-rich foods, 92–94
problems of antibiotics, 87–88
Processed foods
blood sugar and, 50–52
gut bacteria affected by, 89
soy protein isolate, 82–84
Progressive muscle technique
Lifestyle Tracking exercise, 235–236
overview, 153–155
using in Drained Brain program, 213
Prosocial behavior, kindness as, 181–182
Proteins and fats
confusion about, 71–72
fats in modified Mediterranean diet, 84–86
modified Mediterranean diet for, 76–86 (*See
 also* Modified Mediterranean diet)
omega-3 and omega-6 balance in, 72–76
Psychiatric service animals, 186

About the Author

Dr. Mike Dow is a psychotherapist, best-selling author, and brain-health expert. Dr. Mike has hosted shows on TLC, E!, VH1, and Investigation Discovery. He is a recurring guest co-host on *The Doctors*, is one of *The Dr. Oz Show*'s core experts, and has made regular appearances on *Today, Good Morning America, The Talk, Rachael Ray, The Wendy Williams Show, Dr. Drew on Call, The Meredith Vieira Show, Ricki Lake, Anderson Live,* and *Bethenny*. He is also a contributor for the *Huffington Post*. Dr. Mike holds a master of science degree in marriage and family therapy and a doctorate in psychology. He is in private practice in Los Angeles. You can hear him weekly on Hay House Radio's *The Dr. Mike Show*.

Hay House Titles of Related Interest

YOU CAN HEAL YOUR LIFE, the movie,
starring Louise Hay & Friends
(available as a 1-DVD program, an expanded 2-DVD set,
and an online streaming video)
Learn more at www.hayhouse.com/louise-movie

THE SHIFT, the movie,
starring Dr. Wayne W. Dyer
(available as a 1-DVD program, an expanded 2-DVD set,
and an online streaming video)
Learn more at www.hayhouse.com/the-shift-movie

———

Breaking the Habit of Being Yourself:
How to Lose Your Mind and Create a New One,
by Dr. Joe Dispenza

Power Up Your Brain: The Neuroscience of Enlightenment,
by David Perlmutter, M.D., FACN, and Alberto Villoldo, Ph.D.

Fat for Fuel: A Revolutionary Diet to Combat Cancer, Boost Brain Power,
and Increase Your Energy, by Dr. Joseph Mercola

The MindBody Self: How Longevity Is Culturally Learned and the
Causes of Health Are Inherited, by Dr. Mario Martinez

All of the above are available at your local bookstore,
or may be ordered by contacting Hay House (see next page).

———

We hope you enjoyed this Hay House book. If you'd like to receive our online catalog featuring additional information on Hay House books and products, or if you'd like to find out more about the Hay Foundation, please contact:

Hay House, Inc., P.O. Box 5100, Carlsbad, CA 92018-5100
(760) 431-7695 or (800) 654-5126
(760) 431-6948 (fax) or (800) 650-5115 (fax)
www.hayhouse.com® • www.hayfoundation.org

———

Published and distributed in Australia by:
Hay House Australia Pty. Ltd., 18/36 Ralph St., Alexandria NSW 2015
Phone: 612-9669-4299 • *Fax:* 612-9669-4144 • www.hayhouse.com.au

Published and distributed in the United Kingdom by:
Hay House UK, Ltd., Astley House, 33 Notting Hill Gate, London W11 3JQ
Phone: 44-20-3675-2450 • *Fax:* 44-20-3675-2451 • www.hayhouse.co.uk

Published in India by: Hay House Publishers India,
Muskaan Complex, Plot No. 3, B-2, Vasant Kunj, New Delhi 110 070
Phone: 91-11-4176-1620 • *Fax:* 91-11-4176-1630 • www.hayhouse.co.in

Distributed in Canada by:
Raincoast Books, 2440 Viking Way, Richmond, B.C. V6V 1N2
Phone: 1-800-663-5714 • *Fax:* 1-800-565-3770 • www.raincoast.com

———

Access New Knowledge.
Anytime. Anywhere.

Learn and evolve at your own pace
with the world's leading experts.

www.hayhouseU.com

Free e-newsletters
from Hay House, the Ultimate
Resource for Inspiration

Be the first to know about Hay House's free downloads, special offers, giveaways, contests, and more!

 Get exclusive excerpts from our latest releases and videos from *Hay House Present Moments*.

 Our *Digital Products Newsletter* is the perfect way to stay up-to-date on our latest discounted eBooks, featured mobile apps, and Live Online and On Demand events.

 Learn with real benefits! *HayHouseU.com* is your source for the most innovative online courses from the world's leading personal growth experts. Be the first to know about new online courses and to receive exclusive discounts.

 Enjoy uplifting personal stories, how-to articles, and healing advice, along with videos and empowering quotes, within *Heal Your Life*.

 Have an inspirational story to tell and a passion for writing? Sharpen your writing skills with insider tips from *Your Writing Life*.

Sign Up Now!

Get inspired, educate yourself, get a complimentary gift, and share the wisdom!

Visit www.hayhouse.com/newsletters to sign up today!

 HAY HOUSE

 HAYHOUSE RADIO
radio for your soul®

 HAYHOUSE online learning

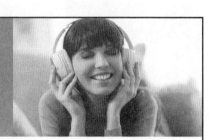

Hay House Podcasts
Bring Fresh, Free Inspiration Each Week!

Hay House Meditations Podcast

Features your favorite Hay House authors guiding you through mediations designed to help you relax and rejuvenate. Take their words into your soul and cruise through the week!

Dr. Wayne W. Dyer Podcast

Discover the timeless wisdom of Dr. Wayne W. Dyer, world-renowned spiritual teacher and affectionately known as "the father of motivation". Each week brings some of the best selections from the 10-year span of Dr. Dyer's talk show on HayHouseRadio.com.

Hay House World Summit Podcast

Over 1 million people from 217 countries and territories participate in the massive online event known as the Hay House World Summit. This podcast offers weekly mini-lessons from World Summits past as a taste of what you can hear during the annual event, which occurs each May.

Hay House Radio Podcast

Listen to some of the best moments from HayHouseRadio.com, featuring expert authors such as Dr. Christiane Northrup, Anthony William, Caroline Myss, James Van Praagh, and Doreen Virtue discussing topics such as health, self-healing, motivation, spirituality, positive psychology, and personal development.

Hay House Live Podcast

Enjoy a selection of insightful and inspiring lectures from Hay House Live, an exciting event series that features Hay House authors and leading experts in the fields of alternative health, nutrition, intuitive medicine, success, and more! Feel the electricity of our authors engaging with a live audience, and get motivated to live your best life possible!

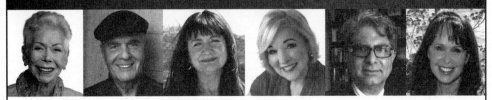